Gynecologic and Obstetric Pathology

Editor

CARLOS PARRA-HERRAN

SURGICAL PATHOLOGY CLINICS

www.surgpath.theclinics.com

Consulting Editor
JASON L. HORNICK

June 2022 • Volume 15 • Number 2

ELSEVIER

1600 John F. Kennedy Boulevard • Suite 1800 • Philadelphia, Pennsylvania, 19103-2899

http://www.theclinics.com

SURGICAL PATHOLOGY CLINICS Volume 15, Number 2
June 2022 ISSN 1875-9181, ISBN-13: 978-0-323-84987-6

Editor: Katerina Heidhausen
Developmental Editor: Diana Grace Ang

© **2022 Elsevier Inc. All rights reserved.**

Surgical Pathology Clinics (ISSN 1875-9181) is published quarterly by Elsevier Inc., 360 Park Avenue South, New York, NY 10010. Months of issue are March, June, September, and December. Business and Editorial Office: Elsevier Inc., 1600 John F. Kennedy Blvd., Ste. 1800, Philadelphia, PA 19103-2899. Accounting and Circulation Offices: Elsevier Inc., 3251 Riverport Lane, Maryland Heights, MO 63043. Periodicals postage paid at New York, NY and at additional mailing offices. Subscription prices are $237.00 per year (US individuals), $376.00 per year (US institutions), $100.00 per year (US students/residents), $283.00 per year (Canadian individuals), $395.00 per year (Canadian Institutions), $284.00 per year (foreign individuals), $395.00 per year (foreign institutions), and $120.00 per year (international students/residents), $100.00 per year (Canadian students/residents). Foreign air speed delivery is included in all *Clinics'* subscription prices. All prices are subject to change without notice. **POSTMASTER:** Send address changes to *Surgical Pathology Clinics*, Elsevier, 3251 Riverport Lane, Maryland Heights, MO 63043. **Customer Service: 1-800-654-2452 (US). From outside the United States, call 1-314-447-8871. Fax: 1-314-447-8029. E-mail:** JournalsCustomerServiceusa@elsevier.com **(for print support)** and JournalsOnlineSupport-usa@elsevier.com **(for online support).**

Reprints. For copies of 100 or more, of articles in this publication, please contact the Commercial Reprints Department, Elsevier Inc., 360 Park Avenue South, New York, NY 10010-1710. Tel. 212-633-3874; Fax: 212-633-3820; E-mail: reprints@elsevier.com.

Surgical Pathology Clinics of North America is covered in *MEDLINE/PubMed (Index Medicus).*

Contributors

CONSULTING EDITOR

JASON L. HORNICK, MD, PhD
Director of Surgical Pathology and
Immunohistochemistry, Brigham and Women's
Hospital, Professor of Pathology, Harvard
Medical School, Boston, Massachusetts, USA

EDITOR

CARLOS PARRA-HERRAN, MD
Pathologist, Department of Pathology,
Brigham and Women's Hospital, Associate
Professor, Harvard Medical School, Boston,
Massachusetts, USA

AUTHORS

JENNIFER A. BENNETT, MD
Associate Professor, Department of Pathology,
University of Chicago Medicine, Chicago,
Illinois, USA

NATALIA BUZA, MD
Professor, Department of Pathology, Yale
School of Medicine, New Haven, Connecticut,
USA

LEE-MAY CHEN, MD
Gynecologic Oncology Division,
Department of Obstetrics, Gynecology
and Reproductive Sciences, University of
California, San Francisco, San Francisco,
California, USA

SABRINA CROCE, MD, PhD
Biopathology Department, Anticancer Center,
Institut Bergonié, INSERM U 1218, Action Unit,
Bordeaux, France

W. PATRICK DEVINE, MD, PhD
Molecular Pathology Division, Pathology
Department, University of California,
San Francisco, San Francisco, California,
USA

RAJI GANESAN, FRCPath
Department of Cellular Pathology, Birmingham
Women's Hospital, Birmingham, United
Kingdom

LYNN N. HOANG, MD
Consultant Pathologist, Clinical Assistant
Professor, Vancouver General Hospital,
University of British Columbia, Vancouver,
British Columbia, Canada

PHILIP P.C. IP, MBChB, FRCPath
Clinical Associate Professor, Department of
Pathology, School of Clinical Medicine, The
University of Hong Kong, Queen Mary Hospital,
Hong Kong SAR

JUSTIN T. KELLEY, MD, MPH
Pathology House Officer IV, Department of
Pathology, University of Michigan, Ann Arbor,
Michigan, USA

**ELIZABETH C. KERTOWIDJOJO, MD, MPH,
PhD**
Assistant Professor, Department of Pathology,
University of Chicago Medicine, Chicago,
Illinois, USA

TAKAKO KIYOKAWA, MD, PhD
Professor, Department of Pathology, The Jikei
University School of Medicine, Tokyo, Japan

FRANÇOIS LE LOARER, MD, PhD
Biopathology Department, Anticancer Center,
Institut Bergonié, INSERM U 1218, Action Unit,
Bordeaux, France; University of Bordeaux,
Talence, France

JOSHUA J.X. LI, MBChB, FHKCPath
Honorary Clinical Assistant Professor,
Department of Anatomical and Cellular
Pathology, Prince of Wales Hospital, The
Chinese University of Hong Kong, Hong Kong
SAR

EMILY R. McMULLEN–TABRY, MD
Pathologist, Department of Pathology, Grand
Traverse Pathology, PLLC, Traverse City,
Michigan, USA

JELENA MIRKOVIC, MD, PhD
Staff Pathologist, Division of Laboratory
Medicine and Molecular Diagnostics, Anatomic
Pathology, Sunnybrook Health Sciences
Centre, Assistant Professor, Department of
Laboratory Medicine and Pathobiology,
University of Toronto, Toronto, Ontario, Canada

ZEHRA ORDULU, MD
Department of Pathology, Immunology and
Laboratory Medicine, Assistant Professor,
University of Florida, Gainesville, Florida, USA

CARLOS PARRA-HERRAN, MD
Pathologist, Department of Pathology,
Brigham and Women's Hospital, Associate
Professor, Harvard Medical School, Boston,
Massachusetts, USA

RAUL PERRET, MD
Biopathology Department, Anticancer Center,
Institut Bergonié, INSERM U 1218, Action Unit,
Bordeaux, France

JOSEPH T. RABBAN, MD, MPH
Professor, Director, Gynecological Pathology
Fellowship, Surgical Pathology Division,
Pathology Department, University of California,
San Francisco, San Francisco, California, USA

STEPHANIE L. SKALA, MD
Clinical Assistant Professor of Pathology and
Gynecologic Pathology Fellowship Director,
Department of Pathology, University of
Michigan, Ann Arbor, Michigan, USA

JONATHAN C. SLACK, MD
Department of Pathology, Boston Children's
Hospital, Boston, Massachusetts, USA

ROBERT A. SOSLOW, MD
Department of Pathology, Memorial Sloan
Kettering Cancer Center, New York, New York,
USA

SIMONA STOLNICU, MD, PhD
Department of Pathology, University of
Medicine, Pharmacy, Sciences and
Technology of Targu Mures, Targu Mures,
Romania

KAREN L. TALIA, MBBS(Hons), FRCPA
Department of Pathology, Royal Women's
Hospital, Australian Centre for the Prevention
of Cervical Cancer, Melbourne, Victoria,
Australia

KELLY X. WEI, BSc
Undergraduate Program, Faculty of Medicine,
University of British Columbia, Vancouver,
British Columbia, Canada

Contents

The Amsterdam Placental Workshop Group Consensus Statement on Sampling and Definitions of Placental Lesions has become widely accepted and is increasingly used as the universal language to describe the most common pathologic lesions found in the placenta. This review summarizes the most salient aspects of this seminal publication and the subsequent emerging literature based on Amsterdam definitions and criteria, with emphasis on publications relating to diagnosis, grading, and staging of placental pathologic conditions. We also provide an overview of the recent expert recommendations on the pathologic grading of placenta accreta spectrum, with insights on their clinical context. Finally, we discuss the emerging entity of SARS-CoV2 placentitis.

Pathologic diagnosis of gestational trophoblastic disease (GTD)—hydatidiform moles and gestational trophoblastic neoplasms—underwent a major shift in the past decade from morphology-based recognition to precise molecular genetic classification of entities, which also allows for prognostic stratification of molar gestations. This article highlights these recent advances and their integration into the routine pathology practice. The traditional gross and histomorphologic features of each entity are also reviewed with special focus on differential diagnoses and their clinical implications.

Clinical testing for homologous repair (HR) deficiency (HRD) in ovarian cancers has emerged as a means to tailor the use of poly(ADP-ribose)polymerase (PARP) inhibitor therapy to the patients most likely to respond. The currently available HRD tests evaluate tumor tissue for genomic evidence of impairment of the HR pathway of DNA damage repair, which, if present, renders the tumor vulnerable to PARP inhibitors in conjunction with platinum chemotherapy. Germline or somatic mutation of BRCA1/2 is a major contributor HRD. Thus, tubo-ovarian/peritoneal high-grade serous carcinoma (HGSC) is enriched by HRD. After highlighting the general concepts underlying HRD testing and PARP inhibitor therapy, this review discusses practical roles for pathologists to maximize the opportunities for eligible patients with ovarian cancer to benefit from HRD testing, chiefly by applying contemporary diagnostic criteria for ovarian cancer tumor typing and navigating through potential pitfalls of tumor types that may mimic HGSC but are unlikely to harbor HRD.

Contents

and molecular features are highlighted for perivascular epithelioid cell tumors, uterine tumors resembling ovarian sex cord tumors, BCOR/BCORL1-altered high-grade endometrial stromal sarcomas, and inflammatory myofibroblastic tumors. Novel developments in epithelioid and myxoid leiomyosarcomas are briefly discussed, and differential diagnoses with key diagnostic criteria are provided for morphologic mimickers.

This article provides an update of the recent developments in mesenchymal tumors of lower genital tract. We focus on the characterization of recurrent molecular events in certain genital stromal tumors, for instance angiomyofibroblastomas and superficial myofibroblastomas. Moreover, fusions involving Tyrosine-kinases receptors (NTRK, FRFR1, RET, COL1A1-PDGFB) have been demonstrated in an emerging group of mesenchymal tumors characterized by a fibrosarcoma-like morphology and a predilection for uterine cervix of premenopausal women. We also cover the topic of smooth muscle tumors of the lower genital tract, which can be now classified using the same diagnostic criteria than their uterine counterpart.

Squamous cell carcinoma is the most frequent epithelial malignant tumor of the cervix and among the most frequent neoplasm in women worldwide. Endocervical adenocarcinoma is the second most common malignancy. Both tumors and their precursors are currently classified based on human papillomavirus status, with prognostic and predictive value. Various prognostic biomarkers and alternative morphologic parameters have been recently described and could be used in the management of these patients. This pragmatical review highlights recent developments, emerging issues as well as controversial areas regarding the cause-based classification, diagnosis, staging, and prognostic parameters of epithelial malignant tumors of the cervix.

A number of changes have been introduced into the 5th Edition of the World Health Organization (WHO) Classification of squamous and glandular neoplasms of the vulva and vagina. This review highlights the major shifts in tumor classification, new entities that have been introduced, recommendations for p16 immunohistochemical testing, biomarker use, molecular findings and practical points for pathologists which will affect clinical care. It also touches upon several issues that still remain answered in these rare but undeniably important women's cancers.

Neuroendocrine neoplasia is relatively uncommon in the female genital tract (FGT) and occurs at any site, most often the ovary and cervix. A unified dichotomous nomenclature, introduced by the World Health Organization Classification of Tumors in all fifth edition volumes, divides neuroendocrine neoplasms (NENs) into well-differentiated neuroendocrine tumors (NETs) and poorly differentiated neuroendocrine carcinomas (NECs). The term carcinoid tumor is retained in the ovary and represents the commonest FGT NEN. NEC is most common in the cervix and is usually admixed with another human papillomavirus-associated epithelial neoplasm. Despite shared neuroendocrine differentiation, NET and NEC show diverse etiology, morphology, and clinical behavior.

As gender-affirming surgeries become more routine, it is increasingly important for pathologists to recognize the expected histologic changes seen in various tissues secondary to gender-affirming hormone therapy. For example, exogenous testosterone-related squamous atrophy or transitional cell metaplasia of the cervix may be confused for high-grade squamous intraepithelial lesion. In addition to distinguishing between benign and dysplastic/malignant features, pathologists should be mindful of the phrasing of their reports and aim to use objective, nongendered language.

SURGICAL PATHOLOGY CLINICS

SERIES OF RELATED INTEREST

Clinics in Laboratory Medicine
http://www.labmed.theclinics.com/
Medical Clinics
https://www.medical.theclinics.com/

THE CLINICS ARE AVAILABLE ONLINE!
Access your subscription at:
www.theclinics.com

Preface

Gynecologic and Obstetric Pathology: A Review of Emerging Concepts and Relevant Topics

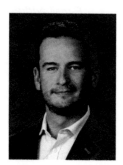

Carlos Parra-Herran, MD
Editor

Thank you for reading this new issue of the *Surgical Pathology Clinics* devoted to Gynecologic and Obstetric Pathology (and thank you for reading the always sidelined Preface section!). The authors and I framed this effort to include the latest published literature and the 2020 World Health Organization classification, and to concentrate on topics not covered in previous reviews. The end-result is a comprehensive, yet user-friendly and accessible review providing practical information and emerging concepts in gynecologic pathology, based on recent evidence and/or consensus-based information.

The issue starts with a review of key concepts in placental pathology in the framework of consensus terminology, and a review of the state-of-the-art in the diagnosis of gestational trophoblastic disease. I intentionally chose obstetric pathology topics, as they are not always included in gynecologic pathology reference materials, even though placental pathology represents a significant component of the specialty. I hope these reviews give you an up-to-date perspective and the information you need to handle (and even love!) placental pathology.

Subsequently, the issue follows a (more or less) traditional organ-based format. In the articles covering the upper genital tract, readers will find a tailored discussion on the value of BRCA and homologous recombination deficiency testing in patients with ovarian carcinoma, and a review of the most recently described features of ovarian sex-cord stromal neoplasia. We also include a review of lesions primarily involving (or arising from) the peritoneum, which are as challenging as they are important to the gynecologic pathologist.

Reviews on uterine pathology focus on the ever-changing challenges of high-grade endometrial carcinoma diagnosis, and a review of the most relevant features, pathologic and molecular, which determine the prognosis and management of patients with endometrial cancer. On the topic of mesenchymal neoplasia, two reviews address what is known about the most important entities in the uterus and lower genital tract, respectively.

Talking about lower genital tract, the evolving knowledge about the classification of cervical and vulvovaginal epithelial neoplasms is covered in detail in two dedicated reviews. As a separate article, we discuss the topic of neuroendocrine neoplasia of the gynecologic tract, now unified in terms of diagnosis and terminology as per the World Health Organization classification. The issue concludes with a review of the pathologic findings in specimens from patients undergoing gender-affirming surgery, which are increasingly encountered. This review underscores the role of the pathologist in the shift toward a more inclusive health care system in which gender identity is recognized and celebrated.

Surgical Pathology 15 (2022) xi–xii
https://doi.org/10.1016/j.path.2022.03.001
1875-9181/22/© 2022 Published by Elsevier Inc.

This issue is the product of collective work by a diverse group of experts, selected given their scholar contributions and commitment to academia. They represent eight countries and four continents. As a group they are reflective of the diversity and enormous talent of the gynecologic pathology community. I was humbled by their dedication toward this project and educated by their excellent contributions. Working with the authors and learning from them has been the most rewarding part of this experience. I hope that you, as the reader, find this *Surgical Pathology Clinics* issue equally rewarding.

Carlos Parra-Herran, MD
Department of Pathology
Brigham and Women's Hospital
Harvard Medical School
75 Francis Street
Boston, MA, 02115, USA

E-mail address:
cparra-herran@bwh.harvard.edu

Life After Amsterdam: Placental Pathology Consensus Recommendations and Beyond

Jonathan C. Slack, MD[a], Carlos Parra-Herran, MD[b],*

KEYWORDS

- Placenta • Amsterdam • Chorioamnionitis • Ascending infection • Villitis
- Maternal vascular malperfusion • Fetal vascular malperfusion • Placenta accreta

Key points

- Several placental lesions and disorders, as defined by the Amsterdam consensus statement, have been proven to be associated with maternal, obstetric, and neonatal outcomes.

- Emerging literature has underscored the value of staging and grading of placental lesions. The association with clinical outcomes is stronger with high-grade lesions; in turn, low-grade lesions have been shown in many settings to be frequent in placentas from uneventful pregnancies.

- From a pathology perspective, placenta accreta spectrum requires standardized reporting terminology for both gravid hysterectomy and in placentas with basal plate myometrial fibers.

ABSTRACT

The Amsterdam Placental Workshop Group Consensus Statement on Sampling and Definitions of Placental Lesions has become widely accepted and is increasingly used as the universal language to describe the most common pathologic lesions found in the placenta. This review summarizes the most salient aspects of this seminal publication and the subsequent emerging literature based on Amsterdam definitions and criteria, with emphasis on publications relating to diagnosis, grading, and staging of placental pathologic conditions. We also provide an overview of the recent expert recommendations on the pathologic grading of placenta accreta spectrum, with insights on their clinical context. Finally, we discuss the emerging entity of SARS-CoV2 placentitis.

OVERVIEW

Since its publication in 2016, the Amsterdam Placental Workshop Group Consensus Statement on Sampling and Definitions of Placental Lesions has become an essential resource for pathologists and obstetricians.[1] At press time, the article has been cited 215 times in PubMed and 799 times according to Google Scholar.[2,3] Major reference literature, including the American Registry of Pathology (formerly Armed Forces Institute of Pathology) AFIP Atlas of Placental Pathology, 5th series, have now introduced the recommendations outlined in the Amsterdam workshop.[4] Now, more than 5 years after their inception, several studies using the Amsterdam criteria have shown the clinical value of the recommendations and explored some of the many questions in the pathologic evaluation of placental lesions that remain unanswered. This review summarizes the Amsterdam criteria and the recent evidence underscoring their clinical applications. We also discuss current knowledge gaps that will hopefully be addressed in future investigations and consensus studies. The review goes beyond Amsterdam to discuss recent grading recommendations for patients with placenta accreta spectrum (PAS) and

[a] Department of Pathology, Boston Children's Hospital, 300 Longwood Avenue, Boston, MA 02115, USA;
[b] Department of Pathology, Brigham and Women's Hospital, 75 Francis Street, Boston, MA 02115, USA
* Corresponding author.
E-mail address: cparra-herran@bwh.harvard.edu

Surgical Pathology 15 (2022) 175–196
https://doi.org/10.1016/j.path.2022.02.001
1875-9181/22/© 2022 Elsevier Inc. All rights reserved.

present the current knowledge of the placental pathology related to severe acute respiratory syndrome coronavirus 2 (SARS-CoV-2) infection (COVID-19).

ASCENDING INTRAUTERINE INFECTION

Introduction: The Amsterdam recommendations for the histologic staging and grading of maternal and fetal inflammatory responses in ascending intrauterine infection is based on *the Society for Pediatric Pathology: Perinatal Section's* 2003 classification, wherein the fetal and maternal inflammatory responses are staged (1–3) and graded (1 or 2) separately.[5] The stage is predominantly determined by the anatomic compartment(s) involved by the acute inflammatory process, whereas the grade is determined by its severity. This was done to provide a clearly defined categorization with clinical relevance that would also provide a framework for future clinical research.[1,5] A summary of the definitions of ascending intrauterine infection stages and grades is provided in **Table 1**. Representative histologic examples are depicted in **Fig. 1**.

Emerging evidence: Recent studies have assessed the Amsterdam staging and grading criteria in normal deliveries without evidence of infection, explored the origin of the acute inflammatory infiltrate and dynamic interplay between fetal and maternal responses, and interrogated the significance of acute villitis.

Application of Amsterdam Criteria: Several studies have sought to evaluate the correlation between histologic chorioamnionitis, as defined by the Amsterdam criteria, and clinical chorioamnionitis. In their prospective study of 350 women and 380 newborns (including 145 preterm), Loverro and colleagues[6] found a significant correlation between cases of neonatal sepsis and placental inflammation. This supports the findings of an earlier study by Yamada and colleagues[7] who found that neonatal infection-related morbidity in a cohort of 245 preterm births was significantly associated with the histologic grading and staging system used in the Amsterdam consensus article. Moreover, Yamada and colleagues[7] demonstrated that adverse neonatal outcomes increased in a stepwise manner in concordance with the grade of the placental inflammation.

In a multiinstitution, retrospective cohort study, Romero and colleagues[8] sought to evaluate the incidence of placental lesions in 944 relatively young (mean age = 23 years) predominantly African American (81%) women with term deliveries (73.8% vaginal deliveries) who lacked significant chronic diseases and had no maternal or neonatal complications. They found that although acute inflammatory lesions were found in 42% of all placentas, 99% of these were low grade (G1 per Amsterdam) and were significantly more common in vaginal delivery (47.3%; 95% confidence interval [CI], 43.6% to 51.1%) than in Caesarean section (19.1%, 95% CI, 13.3%–26.1%; $P < .0001$). The relatively high incidence of acute inflammation in normal placentas in this study (42%) may be explained, at least in part, by their sampling methodology that exceeds the guidelines set forth by the Amsterdam Criteria (ie, up to 3 membrane rolls, 3 sections of umbilical cord, and up to 6 sections from the placental disc were routinely taken in each case). However, a prior study by Roberts and colleagues found histologic acute inflammation in a comparable proportion of low-risk gestations (34%). Most of these (78%)

Table 1
Staging and grading definitions for ascending intrauterine infection diagnosis

Staging and Grading of the Maternal and Fetal Responses in Ascending Intrauterine Infection	
Stage	**Grade**
Maternal Response	
1 Acute subchorionitis or chorionitis	1 Not severe as defined
2 Acute chorioamnionitis	2 Severe (confluent neutrophils or subchorionic microabcesses)
3 Necrotizing chorioamnionitis	
Fetal Response	
1 Chorionic vasculitis or umbilical phlebitis	1 Not severe as defined
2 Umbilical vein and one or more arteries	2 Severe (confluent intramural neutrophils with smooth muscle loss)
3 Necrotizing funisitis	

Modified from Khong TY et al "Sampling and Definitions of Placental Lesions: Amsterdam Placental Workshop Group Consensus Statement" (Arch Pathol Lab Med. 2016;140(7):698–713) with permission from Archives of Pathology & Laboratory Medicine. Copyright 2016. College of American Pathologists.

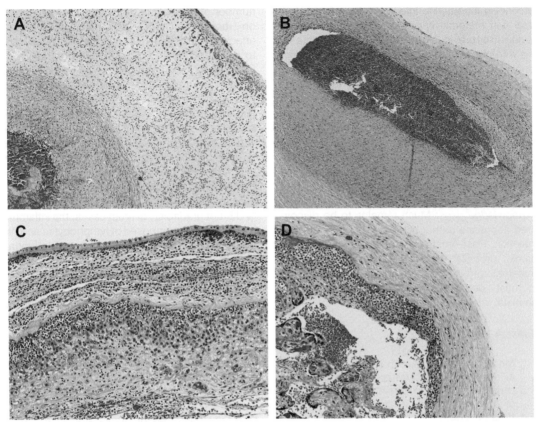

Fig. 1. Maternal and fetal responses to ascending intrauterine infection (same placenta in all 4 panels). (*A, B*) Fetal neutrophils migrate outward from an umbilical artery (*A*) or from a chorionic plate vessel (*B*) toward the infected amniotic fluid in this example of ascending intrauterine infection with necrotizing funisitis (Stage 3, grade 2 fetal inflammatory response). Maternal neutrophils migrate from decidual arteries to reach the chorion (namely chorionitis) and eventually the subamnniotic connective tissue of the placental membranes (namely chorioamnionitis) (*C*) similarly, they accumulate in the maternal intervillous space against the chorionic plate of the placental disk (namely subchorionitis) (*D*) toward the infected amniotic fluid. Figures C and D depict severe maternal inflammatory response (Stage 3, grade 2; focal area of viable amnion chosen in C for orientation).

were low grade, defined as grade 1, stage 1 or 2 maternal inflammation (whereas stage 3 or grade 2 at any stage was considered high-grade). Moreover, nearly all cases (96%) were shown to be negative for infection by concurrent microbiological testing (culture or molecular techniques).[9] These studies indicate that mild acute inflammation (defined by Roberts and colleagues[9] as grade 1, stage 1–2, fetal/maternal responses per the Amsterdam criteria) is a common finding in placentas from low-risk deliveries without complications, particularly vaginal births and is unlikely to represent an infectious process (at least one that is clinically significant). As such, the inclusion of mild/low grade inflammatory responses under the heading "ascending intrauterine infection," as is currently done in the Amsterdam criteria, may warrant reconsideration in future iterations of the guidelines.

Origin of inflammatory infiltrate: Historically considered of maternal origin, amniotic fluid

neutrophils have more recently been suggested to be of fetal origin as well.[10,11] In their 2017 study, Gomez-Lopez and colleagues[12] used DNA fingerprinting in amniotic fluid to show that the neutrophils can be entirely fetal, entirely maternal, or any admixture of both. Surprisingly, one of their cases, in which the patient received serial amniocentesis, showed progression from fetal to maternal neutrophil predominance as infection progressed.[12] Severe fetal inflammation was associated with premature birth, whereas severe maternal inflammation was associated with term or postterm delivery.[12]

Acute villitis: Acute villitis, defined by the presence of neutrophils in and around villous capillaries, is a rare entity that was not specifically addressed by the Amsterdam classification.[13] Narice and colleagues[13] reported a case of severe maternal sepsis caused by acute villitis with intravascular microorganisms associated with severe necrotizing ascending intrauterine infection (stage 3, grade 2 fetal and maternal inflammatory response). They reviewed all previously published cases of acute villitis with intravascular organisms and found the majority (15/17 cases; 88%) also had maternal chorioamnionitis, most were linked to common ascending organisms (*Escherichia coli* or Group B *Streptococcus*), and all cases resulted in fetal demise.[13] This suggests that acute villitis represents a rarely encountered, extreme, severe end of the spectrum of fetal response to ascending intrauterine infection and may warrant consideration into future revisions to the staging and grading of acute fetal inflammatory responses.

Knowledge gaps: Much remains to be discovered about the pathophysiology of amniotic fluid infection. Post-Amsterdam studies indicate a dynamic process wherein both the fetus and maternal immune systems are active participants in host defense mechanisms against intraamniotic infection.

Ascending Intrauterine Infection-Key Points

1. Mild acute inflammation (Grade 1, stage 1, as defined by the Amsterdam criteria) is a common finding in births without clinical or microbiological evidence of amniotic fluid infection.

2. Severe acute inflammation (Grade 2 or stage 3, as defined by Amsterdam criteria) is rare (<1%) in births without clinical or microbiological evidence of infection.

3. Amniotic fluid neutrophils may be of fetal, maternal, or mixed origin.

4. Severe fetal acute inflammation is associated with extremely preterm deliveries, whereas severe maternal inflammation is associated with term or late deliveries.

5. Acute villitis may represent the most extreme severe end of the histologic spectrum of fetal inflammatory response; it correlates strongly with maternal chorioamnionitis, presence of intravascular microorganisms, and fetal demise.

VILLITIS OF UNKNOWN ETIOLOGY AND RELATED LESIONS

Introduction: The Amsterdam consensus promotes the use of the term villitis of unknown etiology (VUE) over nonspecific chronic villitis and other such terms as it excludes, by definition, cases where a cause is identified.[1] VUE is divided into low and high-grade based on the greatest number of contiguous villi involved. Multiple foci on more than one slide, with inflammation affecting more than 10 contiguous villi, is required to diagnose high-grade VUE. High grade VUE is further subdivided into patchy (up to 30%) versus diffuse (more than 30% of all distal villi involved; **Fig. 2**A). Low grade VUE is defined as inflammation in less than 10 contiguous villi in 2 or more foci and is subdivided into focal (only one slide) versus multifocal (more than one slide involved). When avascular villi are found in a placenta with VUE the recommended terminology is "chronic villitis with associated avascular villi" (**Fig. 2**B). A solitary focus of chronic villitis can be reported as "VUE, not gradable." In most cases, the inflammatory infiltrate is composed of lymphocytes and histiocytes (**Fig. 2**C). The presence of abundant plasma cells does not exclude a diagnosis of VUE but should trigger a thorough workup to exclude an infectious origin (viral or spirochetes). Other inflammatory lesions linked to VUE include eosinophilic/T-cell chorionic vasculitis (ETCV), chronic deciduitis, chronic chorioamnionitis, and chronic histiocytic intervillositis [CHI].[1]

Emerging evidence: Recent studies have explored the relationship between obesity and chronic villitis, assessed the staging and grading criteria for VUE in "normal" deliveries, reviewed long-term outcomes of infants after VUE and the risk of recurrence in subsequent pregnancies, and further interrogated the pathogenesis of VUE.

Relationship to obesity: In a prospective study of 382 women from the Netherlands, Brouwers and colleagues[14] found a significant positive association between prepregnancy obesity and high-grade chronic villitis (odds ratio of 18.1), even in uncomplicated pregnancies. Their findings are concordant with prior epidemiologic data from Becroft and colleagues[15] that identified a positive correlation between chronic villitis and increased body mass index (BMI).

Chronic inflammatory lesions in normal pregnancies: The study by Romero and colleagues[8] found that 30% (282/944 pregnancies) had one or more chronic inflammatory placental lesions, including chronic deciduitis (19.3%), VUE (18.5%), high-grade VUE (1.2%), chronic chorioamnionitis (12.7%), CHI (0.4%), and ETCV (0.4%). Nulliparity was negatively associated with chronic inflammatory lesions (*P* < .001). They propose that in some cases, and if not associated with significant damage to the placental membranes, villous tree, or decidua basalis, maternal lymphocytes may indicate a maternal fetal cellular interaction rather than a pathologic process.[8]

Long-term significance of chronic villitis and risk of recurrence: In a prospective study of 261

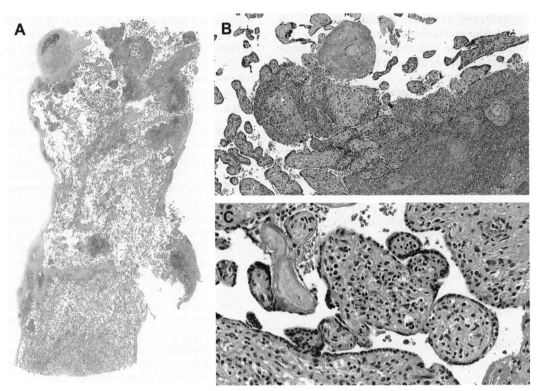

Fig. 2. VUE. (*A*) Diffuse high grade VUE spanning the full thickness of the placental disc with multiple large foci of agglutinated villi. (*B*) Avascular villi adjacent to high-grade VUE are commonly found and are thought to indicate "burnt out" villi. (*C*) Intravillous inflammation in VUE is typically composed of an admixture of histiocytes and lymphocytes.

deliveries from Japanese women, Yaguchi and colleagues[16] found that a history of VUE did not predict low body weight in the first 18 months of life. In a large study of 883 women with 2 placentas evaluated within a nearly 10-year study period, Freedman and colleagues[17] found that 54% women with chronic villitis in their first pregnancy developed chronic villitis in their subsequent pregnancy (2.59x corrected relative risk, 2.12–3.15 95% CI). This represents a substantially higher figure than the 10% to 15% range typically cited in review literature.[18]

Viral cause of VUE: Two major theories exist for the cause of VUE. The first, and most widely accepted theory, is that it represents a maternal inflammatory response directed against fetal alloantigens-analogous to what is seen in allograft rejection.[18,19] Evidence in favor of this hypothesis includes an increased incidence of VUE in egg donor pregnancies and in multigravid women, as well as a significant risk of recurrence in subsequent gestations (up to 50%).[15,18,20,21] In the second theory, chronic inflammatory infiltrates are thought to represent a maternal and/or fetal immune response to infection.[22,23] Evidence in favor of this mechanism includes

seasonal variation in incidence and the association of chronic villitis with many infectious agents (including Toxoplasma, Others [syphilis, varicella-zoster, parvovirus B19], Rubella, Cytomegalovirus and Herpes virus [TORCH] pathogens, COVID-19, and others).[18,24,25,26] In a recent retrospective case-control study, Ernst and colleagues[23] compared the prevalence of RNA and DNA viruses in placental tissues in a cohort of 20 placentas with high-grade VUE to an equally sized control group using viral metagenomic shotgun sequencing. They detected viruses in placental tissues approximately twice as frequently in high-grade VUEs (65% of cases) than in the control group (35% of cases). Moreover, they found a 5-fold higher prevalence of herpesviruses (50% of cases) in high-grade VUE than in the control group (10% of cases; *P* = .01). Papilloma and polyomaviruses were found in identical prevalence (25% of cases) in both groups. In addition, they used gene expression profiling to evaluate inflammatory profiles in each placenta and found inflammatory pathways associated with antiviral response to be upregulated in the VUE cases.[23] This study provides further evidence of a viral causative, specifically herpesviruses, in at least a subset of VUE.[23] As such, follow-up studies that interrogate the relationship between VUE and viral infection in larger numbers of patients and with broader numbers of viruses are needed.

Knowledge gaps: The pathophysiology of VUE remains poorly understood. Post-Amsterdam studies indicate a subset may be related to viral infection or maternal proinflammatory states such as obesity, but further exploration is needed because VUE—low-grade in particular—may be a normal finding and is common in uneventful low-risk gestations.

Villitis of Unknown Etiology-Key Points

1. Low-grade VUE, as defined by the Amsterdam criteria, is a common finding in low-risk and "normal" gestations.

2. High-grade VUE is rare, occurring in 1% of low-risk / "normal" gestations.

3. Obesity is associated with increased rates of high-grade VUE.

4. VUE is not associated with infant low body weight in the first 18 months of life.

5. RNA and DNA viruses, most notably herpesviruses, are more common in placentas with high-grade VUE than normal controls.

MATERNAL VASCULAR MALPERFUSION

Introduction: The term *maternal vascular malperfusion (MVM)* replaced formerly used names such as uteroplacental underperfusion and placental insufficiency. MVM encompasses a constellation of findings seen in the setting of abnormal blood supply to the feto-placental unit. The concept of "insufficiency" still applies: impaired spiral artery remodeling causes insufficient circulation to the placental bed leading to placental and fetal growth restriction and hypoxia.[27,28] However, it is recognized that incomplete remodeling can also cause turbulent and high-momentum blood ejection into the intervillous space, resulting in villous damage and ischemia-reperfusion injury.[29] A similar state of hyperperfusion of the placental bed has also been demonstrated in missed first trimester abortions, presumably secondary to oxidative damage to the trophoblast, which leads to defective implantation and placentation.[30]

Pathologic features of MVM are common. According to a recent report, the prevalence of MVM among placentas submitted for pathologic evaluation at the University Hospitals Cleveland Medical Center (2006–2015) was 14.2% at 37 to 42 weeks, 17.4% at 32 to 37 weeks, 22.7% at 23 to 32 weeks, and 4% for less than 23 weeks of gestation.[31] The pathologic lesions that are part of the MVM spectrum can be macroscopic or microscopic. The following paragraphs describe those recognized by the Amsterdam consensus (**Figs. 3** and **4**):

- *Placental growth restriction:* In the form of *low placental weight* (weight less than the tenth percentile for the stated gestational age[32]), and/or *thin umbilical cord* (cord diameter less than the tenth percentile for stated gestational age,[33] or < 8 mm at term).

- *Infarction:* Infarcts should be grossly described in terms of location (marginal vs central or paracentral), size (in cm, range if multiple) and the percentage of the placental parenchyma involved. Infarcts should be confirmed histologically; therefore, sampling should include at least the central infarcts. The presence of any infarct should be noted in the report; however, only infarcts before term and any non-marginal infarction involving greater than 5% of the parenchyma at term are considered significant and evidential of MVM.[1]

Histologically, early placental infarction is characterized by obliteration of the intervillous space, loss of villous stromal nuclear basophilia and smudgy syncytiotrophoblast. Late infarction shows additional loss of trophoblast nuclear integrity, ranging from pyknosis and karyorrhexis to full loss of basophilia resulting in "ghost" villi.

- *Retroplacental hemorrhage:* This lesion is defined as blood (fresh or coagulated) on the basal plate associated with compression of the parenchyma.[34] Grossly, this is seen as indentation or depression of the basal surface, which should always be described in terms of size (2 dimensions) and the percentage of basal plate surface area involved. Histologically, there is blood dissecting the decidua, and subjacent parenchyma shows obliteration of the intervillous space, intravillous hemorrhage and/or early ischemic changes in the villous trophoblast.

- *Accelerated villous maturation (AVM):* Defined as small or short hypermature villi, usually with an increased number of syncytial knots.[35] In a preterm placenta, assessment of this feature is straightforward, as any villi with morphology akin to a term placenta (small round villi with scant stroma and capillaries directly apposed to cytotrophoblast) indicates AVM. Conversely, in a term placenta, the assessment is more

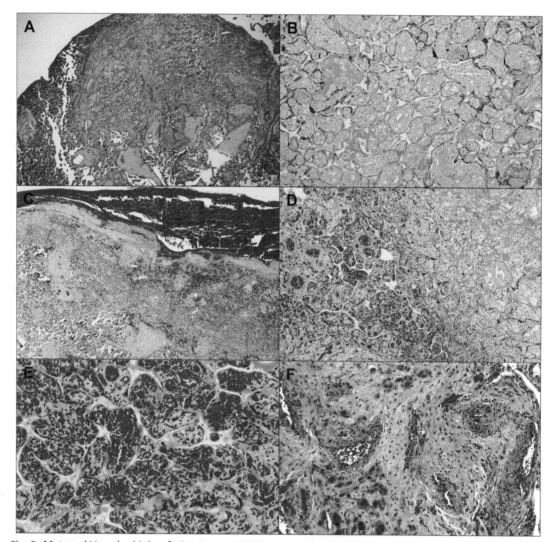

Fig. 3. Maternal Vascular Malperfusion. In our practice, we evoke this diagnosis in any placenta with low weight for gestational age and 2 or more of the diagnostic features listed in the Amsterdam consensus. These include grossly visible changes such as infarction and retroplacental hemorrhage. Placental infarction is seen as a well-defined zone of villi with collapse of the intervillous space (*A*). Consequently, villi become infarcted (*B*), with changes ranging from loss of stromal nuclear basophilia and smudgy syncytiotrophoblast appearance in early stages (*B*, periphery of image) to complete loss of trophoblast nuclear basophilia (ghost villi) in late stages (*B*, center of image). Retroplacental hemorrhage (*C*) often causes a depression or indentation on the basal surface with compression of the underlying parenchyma (*C*, right side). Compressed villi can be congested or pale (*D*) and often show intravillous hemorrhage (*E*). Decidual vasculopathy, appreciated in the decidua of the basal plate and membranes, is often seen as arteries with persistent musculoelastic layers (*F*).

subjective, although syncytial knots in more than a third of villi at term is generally accepted as AVM.[36]

- *Distal villous hypoplasia (DVH)*: Defined as regional paucity of villi, compared with the surrounding parenchyma, in the basal two-thirds of the placental thickness and representing 30% or more of a full-thickness slide. In addition, the villi in the hypoplastic area are

morphologically abnormal, showing reduced branching and being predominantly thin and slender rather than round. DVH is further graded as focal (1 slide only) or diffuse (2 or more full-thickness slides).[1]

- *Decidual arteriopathy*: The Amsterdam consensus applies this term to a variety of findings in the maternal vessels of the basal plate and/or extraplacental membranes.

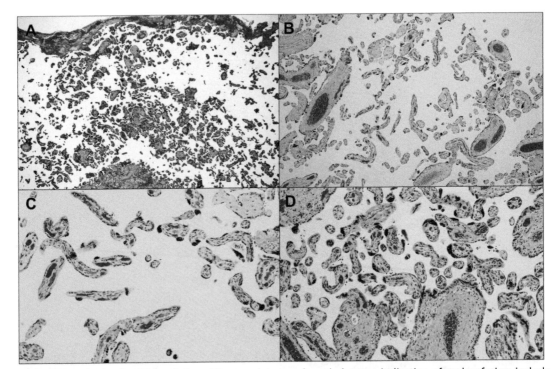

Fig. 4. Maternal Vascular Malperfusion. Microscopic parenchymal changes indicative of malperfusion include DVH and AVM. DVH should be appreciable at low-power magnification as areas of decreased villous density (villous paucity) in the basal two-thirds of the parenchyma (*A*). Villi in hypoplastic areas are small but with appreciable long and slender villous forms (*B*), which often display syncytial knots (*C*). AVM is diagnosed in the presence of "mature" terminal villi in any preterm placenta, or in any term placenta in which more than 33% of terminal villi contain syncytial knots (*D*).

These findings include the retention of musculoelastic elements in the arterial wall (with or without mural hypertrophy), arterial fibrinoid necrosis (with or without lipid-laden macrophages), chronic perivasculitis, arterial thrombosis, and persistent intramural endovascular trophoblast (into the third trimester).[1,37]

The Amsterdam consensus does not state how many of these findings are required to make a diagnosis of MVM. Some authors require the presence of AVM, with or without other findings.[31] Others recommend using the diagnosis of MVM when placental growth restriction (low placental weight) plus *at least* 2 histologic features are present.[38] Otherwise, listing the finding(s) separately in the report (without the heading of MVM) is sufficient.

Findings identified in some studies as suggestive of placental hypoxia, but not included as definitive evidence of MVM in the Amsterdam consensus, include excessive fibrinoid trophoblast islands,[39] chorion laeve pseudocysts,[40] and laminar decidual necrosis.[41,42] If present, these lesions should be noted in the report.

Emerging evidence: Recent studies have confirmed that MVM, as defined by the Amsterdam consensus, correlates with systemic hypertensive disorders. Bustamante Helfrich and colleagues[43] evaluated the association between selected maternal conditions and MVM in a cohort of 3074 patients. MVM was significantly more frequent in placentas from women with hypertensive disorders (chronic hypertension, eclampsia, preeclampsia, HELLP syndrome) than those without even after adjusting for demographics, substance use, diabetes, and BMI. Interestingly, no association was observed between MVM and diabetes or BMI categories including obesity.[43] Kulkarni and colleagues[44] also found a high frequency of MVM in patients with maternal hypertension (71.4%). Similarly, in their review of 755 placentas (>21 weeks gestation) from patients with hypertensive disorders, Stanek[45] found that patients with preeclampsia showed the highest rates of decidual arteriopathy (both hypertrophic and atherosis), infarction, and maternal floor multinucleate trophoblasts. Interestingly, patients with gestational hypertension and chronic hypertension had the highest perinatal mortality, but fewer hypoxic and thrombotic lesions.[45] Tateishi and colleagues[46] documented associations between pathologic lesions of MVM and pregnancy-induced hypertension (PIH) of early onset (<34 weeks) versus late-onset (≥34 weeks). Early onset PIH showed higher rates of acute arteriolar atherosis, DVH and AVM, compared with late-onset PIH, whereas the prevalence of infarction did not differ.[46]

MVM has also been found to be a potential marker or predictor of cardiovascular and metabolic risk. Catov and colleagues[47] found that MVM, in the setting of preterm delivery, is associated with a subsequent high-risk cardiometabolic profile. They examined the prevalence of placental findings, grouped as per Amsterdam criteria, in 115 women with preterm birth (with 210 patients with term birth as control) and found that patients with preterm birth and MVM had higher total cholesterol and systolic blood pressure at time of follow-up (4–12 years) compared with controls. Although Bustamante Helfrich and colleagues[43] found no association between MVM and obesity, Brouwers and colleagues[14] found a correlation between obesity and AVM, as well as obesity and high-grade chronic villitis (see previous section). In this study, placental weight was overall high and positively correlated with prepregnancy BMI, as well as with mean infant's birth weight.[14]

In addition to maternal morbidity, MVM as currently defined is also associated with adverse fetal and neonatal outcomes. A large study by Kulkarni and colleagues[44] included 1633 patients from India and Pakistan (814 with fetal death, 618 with preterm live birth and subsequent neonatal death, and 201 with term live birth). The study found higher prevalence of MVM (more commonly infarcts and DVH) in placentas from cases with fetal death (58%) and preterm neonatal death (31%) compared with those with term live births (15%), conferring on MVM relative risks of 3.88 (95% CI 2.7–5.59) for fetal death and 2.07 (95% CI 1.41–3.02) for neonatal death.[44] Similarly, Jaiman and colleagues[48] also documented a high frequency of MVM in placentas from patients with fetal death at greater than 20 weeks of gestation (76% vs 36% in controls). Interestingly, the authors document a high frequency of abnormal villous maturation in the setting of fetal death (44% vs 1% in controls), not only AVM but also delayed villous maturation and maturation arrest.

In a study by Oh and colleagues,[49] MVM was significantly associated with intraventricular hemorrhage in preterm neonates. Conversely, Parodi and colleagues[50] found an inverse correlation between MVM and intraventricular hemorrhage (the former being more frequent in cases with no hemorrhage), and no correlation with cerebellar hemorrhage.

The following paragraphs address important points related to some of the major lesions that comprise the MVM spectrum:

- *Placental weight*: To our knowledge, the most commonly used reference values for singleton and twin gestations are those published by Pinar and colleagues in 1996.[32] Reference values for triplet placentas have also been published.[51] Subsequent studies have provided more accurate reference values for second trimester gestations (weeks 23–27)[52] and twin gestations.[53] In addition, studies performed in selected populations such as Ireland[54] and northern Alberta[55] have shown that placental weights have increased compared with standard values, underscoring the need to update the reference or, ideally, identify population-specific reference values. To this end, dynamic reference value generation can provide better accuracy. For instance, the Hematogones.com Placental Weight Reference and Report Generator (https://hematogones.com/surg-path/placenta) shows real-time reference values obtained from entries of placental weight and gestational age placed anywhere in the world.[56] Interestingly, this resource is showing that current average placental weights are, overall, lower than those reported by Pinar and colleagues.[32] Admittedly, this shift may be due to selection bias (placentas submitted for pathologic examination and with weight available are more likely to be abnormal, depending on the local and regional indications for submission of placentas to pathology).

- *Infarction*: The so-called *rounded intraplacental hematoma/infarction hematoma* is defined as an infarct with prominent central hemorrhage. It is now recognized as a distinct type of infarction with a significantly higher incidence of stillbirth.[57,58] Rounded intraplacental hematoma can be mistakenly interpreted as an intervillous thrombus; however, it is distinguished from it by the presence of an encircling rim of infarcted villi spanning at least 4 to 5 villi in thickness.[31]

- *Retroplacental hemorrhage*: The presence of retroplacental hemorrhage on pathologic examination should not be interpreted automatically as an indication of *placental abruption*, which is a clinical diagnosis. However, histopathologic findings seem to correlate with the presence and timing of acute abruption as demonstrated by Chen and colleagues.[59] The study showed that basal plate indentation and/or villous compression, intravillous hemorrhage, trophoblastic ischemic changes, and infarction were significantly more frequent in patients clinically diagnosed with acute abruption compared to clinically normal placentas. Importantly, pathologic finding(s) were found in 58% of 177 patients with acute abruption, indicating that in a significant subset of patients (42%), abruption does not manifest in pathologic placental changes.[59] Related to this, Gonen and colleagues[60] showed that MVM is preferentially associated with abruption that occurs early (<34 weeks) during gestation.

- *AVM*: The interobserver reproducibility of AVM, as defined by the Amsterdam consensus, was found to be poor (Fleiss Kappa 0.16; CI, −0.03–0.34) in a recent study including 6 observers.[61] Agreement was poor even among the 4 observers who practice in settings with high volumes of placenta cases (3000–4000 per year; Fleiss Kappa 0.18; CI -0.21–0.56).[61] This underscores the need for better definitions of this lesion.
- *Distal villous hypoplasia*: The interobserver reproducibility of DVH was assessed by Mukherjee and colleagues.[62] The study included 4 international experts in placental pathology who evaluated a set of 30 placental images at 4× magnification obtaining moderate interobserver agreement (weighted Kappa 0.59, range: 0.42–0.70).[62] Although better than for AVM, this reported agreement also indicates that assessment of DVH can be difficult. Digital image analysis can potentially improve DVH diagnosis. The same study[62] showed correlation between DVH grade (determined by experts) and fractal dimension computation, which was estimated using the box counting method in transformed digital images.

Knowledge gaps: As a diagnostic term, MVM is applied inconsistently among practices, as it is unclear how many and which pathologic features are required for this diagnosis. In addition, standardized diagnostic criteria are needed for certain MVM lesions such as AVM, which suffers from poor interobserver reproducibility. Ancillary techniques, particularly image analysis, promise to improve the detection and quantification of pathologic changes characteristic of MVM. Finally, it is necessary to explore the biologic and clinical significance of lesions attributed to superficial or defective placental implantation, and their relationship with MVM.

> ## Maternal Vascular Malperfusion-Key Points
>
> 1. MVM is a constellation of macroscopic and microscopic findings.
>
> 2. MVM is associated with systemic maternal disorders, in particular hypertensive disorders (preeclampsia, pregnancy-induced hypertension, HELLP).
>
> 3. MVM is also associated with adverse fetal and neonatal outcomes, most importantly death.
>
> 4. Updated consensus is required to determine how many and which lesions are required (vs optional) for the diagnosis of MVM. Similarly, updating metrics such as placental weight normograms is imperative.
>
> 5. The interobserver reproducibility of AVM and DVH, as hallmarks of MVM, is poor. Improving definitions and developing a staging/grading system for MVM may address this issue and improve future research efforts to understand this condition.

FETAL VASCULAR MALPERFUSION

Introduction: Fetal vascular malperfusion (FVM) is an umbrella term for a constellation of lesions that are thought to result from impaired/obstructed fetal blood flow. This term was introduced by the Amsterdam group to standardize the terminology with that used for analogous lesions involving the maternal circulation (ie, MVM). Previous terms included fetal thrombotic vasculopathy,[63] hemorrhagic endovasculitis,[64] and others. Histologic findings of FVM include fetal vessel thrombosis, avascular villi, villous stromal karyorrhexis, stem vessel obliteration, vascular ectasia, and or vascular intramural fibrin deposition (**Fig. 5**). Two major patterns of FVM are recognized, both of which are subdivided further into low and high-grade. The first pattern, segmental, thought to represent irreversible thrombotic occlusion of a chorionic or stem villous vessels with subsequent involution of downstream villi, is characterized by larger amounts of contiguous avascular villi (>15 per slide). The second pattern, global, is thought to be secondary to partial or intermittent occlusion, and as such is characterized by haphazardly distributed small (usually <5 villi) clusters of avascular villi with less than 15

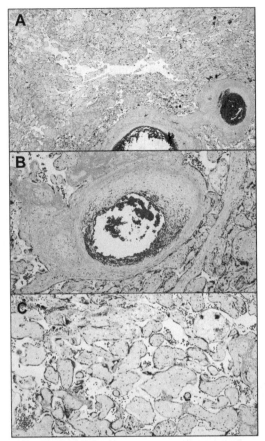

Fig. 5. Fetal Vascular Malperfusion. Histologically, occlusion of stem villous vessels (*A, bottom right*) is often associated with downstream changes in the vasculature of originating terminal villi (*A, top*). Occlusive fetal vascular thrombosis is seen as organizing thrombosis with accumulation of subendothelial loose fibro-myxoid tissue (intimal cushion) which often has entrapped blood elements (*B*). Villi distal to the occlusion show obliteration of the villous capillaries (avascular villi), and often show karyorrhexis of the stromal nuclei (*C*).

affected villi on average per slide. Most cases are thought to be caused by umbilical cord obstruction. Other, less common, causes include the following: maternal diabetes, fetal cardiac insufficiency, hyperviscosity syndromes, and inherited or acquired thrombophilias.[65]

Emerging evidence: Recent studies have evaluated the reproducibility of FVM diagnosis, the specificity of the Amsterdam criteria in a healthy normal control cohort and further explored the possibility that, in a limited number of specific settings, a subset of FVM may be genetically determined.

The interobserver reproducibility by Redline and colleagues[61] reported fair to poor agreement for FVM and avascular villi in different proportions. Agreement improved to fair–moderate when agreement was limited to 4 highly subspecialized pathologists.

Applicability of Amsterdam Criteria in normal deliveries: A single lesion of FVM can be identified in nearly 20% of normal deliveries, typically small foci of hyalinized avascular villi (6.6%), or nonocclusive intimal fibrin deposition in large fetal vessels (6.5%).[8] High burden lesions, which the authors defined as 2 or more lesions of FVM, were seen in only 0.7% of normal deliveries (7 of 944).[8] Although this deviates slightly from the proposed Amsterdam definition of high-grade FVM (average of >15 avascular villi per section or 2 or more chorionic plate/major vessel thrombi or multiple nonocclusive thrombi), their findings mirror that of prior studies which found high-grade FVM in less than 1% of normal placentas.[66,67] It may warrant mention that their low reported incidence of high-grade FVM is despite sampling methods that exceeded the Amsterdam recommendations of 3 sections of placental disc, as they examined up to 6 sections of placental disc in each case.

Hereditary cases of FVM: Although Ariel colleagues[68] found no association between fetal thrombophilia and fetal vascular lesions, investigators have continued exploring the possibility that a small subset of cases of FVM may have a hereditary cause. At least 2 unique scenarios have been identified in which this phenomenon may occur: hereditary coagulation disorders and recurrent pregnancy losses due to excessively long and hypercoiled umbilical cords.

Maternal hypercoagulability has long been recognized as a hereditary cause of MVM.[69,70] Likewise, it has been speculated that fetal/paternal hypercoagulability is related to FVM. In 2018, Nevalainen and colleagues[71] compared a study group consisting of 126 Finnish mothers, 58 matched fathers and 72 matched fetuses from gestations with one or more severe complications (severe preeclampsia, abruption, stillbirth, or intrauterine growth restriction) to a similarly sized normal control group (111 mothers, 91 matched fathers, and 50 fetuses). Unsurprisingly, they found that maternal thrombophilias were more than 5 times as common in women with severe pregnancy complications than in the control group (9.5% vs 1.8%). Somewhat unexpectedly, fetal and parental thrombophilias were noted at statistically similar rates in the study and control groups and suggest that they may not be associated with severe pregnancy complications. It warrants mention that smaller numbers of positive cases in fetuses (6 of 72 fetuses with thrombophilia vs 7 of 50 control fetuses) and fathers (4 of 58 fathers

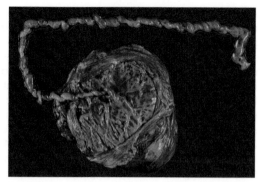

Fig. 6. Long and/or hypercoiled umbilical cords, such as this example, have been associated with a variety of adverse outcomes like stillbirth as in this case.

with thrombophilia vs 5 of 48 control fathers) may have influenced their results.[71] To this end, one study reported a nearly 6-fold increased risk of recurrent pregnancy loss with paternal thrombophilia (Factor V Leiden heterozygotes),[72] whereas another reported a tenfold increase in Factor V Leiden mutation in fetuses with placentas showing

more than 10% infarction (42% vs 3%–4%, $P < .0001$, odds ratio of 37, $n = 396$).[73]

Although excessively long and/or hypercoiled umbilical cords (**Fig. 6**) have generally been considered sporadic nongenetic events, rare instances of recurrent intrauterine fetal demise due to such phenomenon have been reported. The first series was reported by Bakotic and colleagues,[74] which described 3 consecutive second trimester intrauterine demises that were otherwise normal aside from dramatically elongated and/or hypercoiled umbilical cords. Since then, 3 additional case series have been reported with similar findings.[75–77] In total, 13 of 16 cumulative fetuses/neonates have been male.[74–77] No recurrent genetic/molecular alteration has identified. Hypercoiled umbilical cords have been subclassified into 4 main gross patterns by Ernst and colleagues[78] (**Fig. 7**), with segmented and linked patterns being most strongly associated with stillbirth. It may prove informative, when assessing future series of recurrent stillbirth due to excessively long and/or hypercoiled umbilical cords to determine if

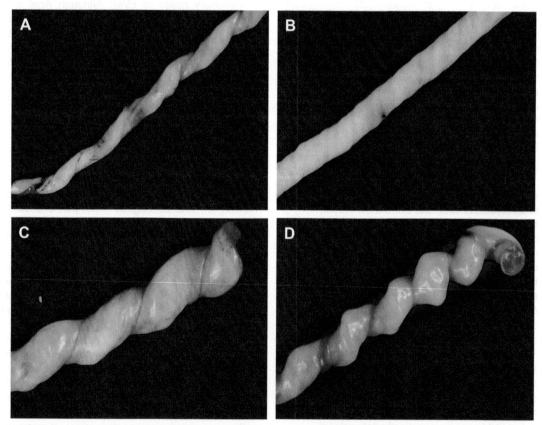

Fig. 7. Gross patterns of umbilical cord hypercoiling. (*A*) Undulating pattern shows irregular loose coils without significant indentation between coils. (*B*) Rope pattern is characterized by tight coils with a flat external surface. (*C*, *D*) Segmental and linked patterns show significant indentations between relatively tight coils with indentations less than 50% of cord diameter in segmental (*C*), but exceeding 50% of cord diameter in linked pattern (*D*).

these recurrent cases also share similar gross morphologies. These examples of recurrent long and hypercoiled umbilical cords within families may suggest a genetic contribution to umbilical cord length and coiling index.

In 2021, FVM was linked COL4A1 mutations, which may be transmitted in an autosomal dominant fashion. Three of 4 placentas in fetuses with COL4A1 mutations showed FVM (2 of which were high-grade).[79] In 2 of 4 cases, the COL4A1 mutations were inherited from the mother, whereas the remaining half were de novo. In 2 cases, where umbilical cord examination was possible, no gross or histologic cord abnormalities were noted.[78] In a single case, there was concurrent large vessel arteriopathy and microvascular thrombosis, which the authors believed suggested multiple tissue level pathogenic events from a single mutation—although they acknowledge a larger systematic evaluation of placentas in COL4A1 disease is needed.[79]

Knowledge gaps: Although many significant improvements have been made in recent years relating to the diagnosis of FVM, much remains to be explored in subsequent studies. Low-grade FVM is a relatively common finding in normal placentas,[8] suggesting that revisions to the current diagnostic cutoffs according to clinical risk and outcomes may be necessary. The studies to date regarding fetal and parental hypercoagulability syndromes being a hereditary cause of FVM have been contradictory. Systematic evaluations of larger numbers of patients are needed to further explore this possibility. Although a few small series[74–77] of intrafamilial recurrent long and hypercoiled umbilical cords that have resulted in intrauterine fetal demise have been reported, an underlying genetic (or other) cause has not been uncovered. Additional studies to expand our knowledge of the genetic, environmental, and other drivers of umbilical cord development are needed. COL4A1 mutations have recently been associated with FVM.[79] Additional investigation may help clarify the genetic pathways involved and uncover additional hereditary causes of FVM.

Fetal Vascular Malperfusion-Key Points

1. Diagnosis of FVM and avascular villi have a fair interobserver agreement.

2. Low-grade FVM, as defined by the Amsterdam criteria, is a relatively common finding in placentas from normal gestations.

3. High-grade FVM, as defined by the Amsterdam criteria, is exceedingly uncommon in placentas from normal gestations, being found in less than 1% of these.

4. Unlike maternal thrombophilia, which has been convincingly linked to MVM, it remains equivocal if fetal/paternal thrombophilia is associated with FVM.

5. Intrafamilial clustering of excessively long and hypercoiled cords leading to recurrent pregnancy loss suggests a genetic contribution to umbilical cord coiling.

6. Four patterns of umbilical cord hypercoiling have been described: undulating, rope, segmented, and linked. Of these, segmented and linked are thought to be the most significant.

7. COL4A1 mutations have recently been associated with FVM and may be a rare hereditary cause of this phenomenon.

PLACENTA ACCRETA SPECTRUM

Introduction: The term Placenta Accreta Spectrum (PAS) is recommended over other nomenclature such as placenta creta and morbidly adherent placenta.[80,81] The incidence of PAS has increased 10-fold in the past 50 years with an incidence of 3 per every 1000 pregnancies in the last decade.[82,83] Indeed, PAS is now the leading cause of peripartum hysterectomy, accounting for a majority (50%–65%) of cases.[83–85] This lesion is strongly associated with placenta previa, as well as factors predisposing to endometrial and uterine scarring, most importantly Caesarian sections but also uterine curettage and myomectomy, among others.[86–89] These predisposing factors alter the amount and functionality of the decidua, which in turn leads to excessive intermediate trophoblast proliferation, uterine scar dehiscence, and intrusion of the placental tissue into myometrial vessels.[89–91] Microscopically, the diagnosis of PAS requires: 1) chorionic villi adjacent to myometrial fibers, either directly in contact or with an intervening layer of fibrinoid and 2) absence of intervening decidua[91] (Fig. 8).

Emerging recommendations and evidence: Historically, there has been a multitude of names applied to this condition (accreta placentation, abnormal placental adherence, and morbidly adherent placenta, among others). However, in recent past, the term PAS has gained popularity, culminating in the diagnostic guidelines issued by the International Federation of Gynecology and Obstetrics (FIGO) in 2019, which endorse the PAS nomenclature and propose a comprehensive

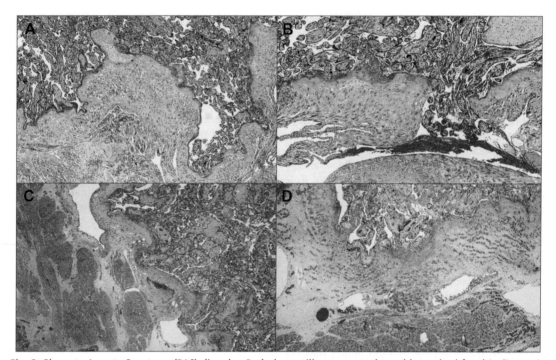

Fig. 8. Placenta Accreta Spectrum (PAS) disorder. Pathology still represents the gold standard for this diagnosis, which unfortunately can only be done definitively on a gravid hysterectomy specimen. The diagnosis requires the presence of placental tissue (chorionic villi) in direct contact with the myometrial wall. There is often a layer of fibrinoid material in between villi and myometrial fibers (*A*) or intrusion of villi into dilated myometrial vascular spaces (*B*). Extrauterine tissue involvement by PAS (*C*) can be demonstrated in cases in which such tissue is submitted, as in this case in which the placenta invades the outer urinary bladder muscle wall (*C*, muscular wall on left). Placental tissue invasion in PAS is associated with proliferation of mononuclear extravillous trophoblast, in this case also infiltrating bladder muscle fibers (*D*).

grading system.[81] This system has clinical criteria and corresponding histologic criteria for each grading category.[81] Thus, the grade can be obtained using clinical characteristics, with confirmation using pathologic evaluation of the gravid uterus if such specimen is available. The grading mirrors the traditional categorization of PAS into placenta accreta (placental tissue *adhered* to myometrium), increta (placental tissue *invades* myometrium), and percreta (placental tissue *perforates* uterine serosa).[81]

The new FIGO grading schema has been used to describe institutional cohorts of PAS. For instance, Aalipour and colleagues[92] retrospectively established the clinical FIGO grade in a cohort of 185 cases of PAS confirmed with histopathology. The cohort was distributed as follows: 41 (22%) with placenta accreta, 44 (24%) with placenta increta, and 100 (54%) with placenta percreta. The authors found significant correlation between FIGO clinical grading parameters and the histologic grading ($P < .001$). However, there was no association between FIGO clinical grading parameters and maternal complications (including

estimated blood loss, amount of blood products transfused, and postoperative complications). Similarly, an institutional series of PAS patients by Bluth and colleagues[93] included retrospective PAS grading following the FIGO guidelines. The cohort consisted of 46 patients with the following distribution: accreta in 26 patients (56%), increta in 18 (39%), and percreta in 2 (4%). Interestingly, only 25 patients had histopathologic analysis and of those only 17 (68%) had confirmation of PAS diagnosis and 11 (44%) had concordant clinical and histologic PAS grading.[93] Ishibashi and colleagues[94] recently studied PAS using FIGO grading criteria in a series of patients with placenta previa. They found that patients with placenta previa and PAS, either by clinical or clinical plus histologic criteria, had greater blood loss at delivery, and a greater rate of massive hemorrhage (>2500 mL) compared with patients with placenta previa but no PAS.[94]

Assessing gravid hysterectomy specimens for PAS has inherent limitations, such as disruption of the uterine wall due to dehiscence or surgical manipulation, as well as absence of anatomic landmarks to evaluate for extrauterine tissue invasion, which may preclude grading using clinical definitions established by FIGO. In 2020, a subcommittee of the Society for Pediatric Pathology published recommendations for the histopathologic diagnosis and grading of PAS.[80] The descriptive grading system in this publication somewhat parallels the clinical grading endorsed by FIGO. A comparison between systems is depicted in **Table 2**.

These PAS consensus recommendations by Hecht and colleagues[80] distinguish PAS from uterine scar dehiscence. The guideline describes dehiscence as a thinned portion of the anterior lower uterine segment wall associated with an extruding placental disk (clinically referred to as a "uterine window"). A gradual "wedge" shaped transition from scar to normal myometrium is characteristic of dehiscence; in contrast, PAS shows

Table 2
Placenta Accreta Spectrum grading according to the International Federation of Obstetrics and Gynecology (FIGO) and a recent consensus group from the Society for Pediatric Pathology

Placenta Accreta Spectrum Pathologic Grading			
Clinical Grading (FIGO[81])—Histologic Criteria		**Pathologic Grading (Hecht and Coworkers[80])—Criteria**	
Grade 1	Accreta - Histology shows extended areas of absent decidua between villous tissue and myometrium; placental villi attached directly to the superficial myometrium	Grade 1	Noninvasive: grossly adherent placenta. Myometrial cross sections show a smooth placental–myometrial interface and uniform myometrial thickness without thinning
Grade 2	Increta - Histology shows placental villi within the muscular fibers and sometimes in the lumen of the deep uterine vasculature	Grade 2	Superficial invasion: irregular placental–myometrial interface with preservation of at least 25% of the myometrial wall thickness relative to the uninvolved myometrium
Grade 3	3a: Percreta - Histology shows villous tissue within or breaching the uterine serosa	Grade 3	3a: Deep invasion: Irregular placental–myometrial interface with preservation of <25% of the myometrial wall thickness relative to the uninvolved myometrium. The serosa is intact.
	3b: Percreta - Histology shows villous tissue breaching the uterine serosa and invading the bladder wall tissue or urothelium		3d: Deep invasion with disruption of the serosa
	3c: Percreta - Histology shows villous tissue breaching the uterine serosa and invading pelvic tissues/organs (with or without invasion of the bladder)		3e: Placental invasion into adjacent organs (most commonly bladder) or extrauterine fibroadipose tissue, confirmed by microscopy

an irregular and abrupt interface between the area of invasion and the adjacent uninvolved wall.[80] Microscopically, these differences in transition are also observed; in addition, in dehiscence the wall underneath the placenta is entirely composed of scar tissue. Assessment of PAS in this setting should be done in areas away from any scar tissue.

Another important contribution of the consensus effort by Hecht and colleagues[80] is the reporting recommendations for the presence of basal plate myometrial fibers (BPMF) in placentas submitted for pathologic evaluation. This finding has been associated with PAS in subsequent gestations, particularly when there is no decidua associated with the adhered smooth muscle fibers.[95,96] The consensus panel recommends the diagnosis of BPMF, as well as a staging and additional information to be provided in every case (Table 3).

Knowledge gaps: Although the study by Aalipour and colleagues[92] showed significant concordance between clinical and histologic PAS grading as defined by FIGO, this is not seen in all cases as evidenced in other reports.[93] Moreover, the concordance rate between FIGO clinical grading and the novel pathologic grading proposed by Hecht and colleagues[80] needs to be evaluated. Most importantly, it remains to be determined whether the novel PAS grading system correlates with obstetric and/or neonatal outcomes.

Although helpful, the PAS pathologic grading proposed by Hecht and colleagues[80] can be potentially confusing, particularly in grade 3 cases. Grade 3A is defined as invasive placenta with preservation of less than 25% of the wall, in principle because in the setting of extensive wall involvement, it is often difficult to determine whether underlying scar or serosa have been breached (personal communication). Nonetheless, this definition brings confusion because it could also be interpreted as placenta increta with more than 75% uterine wall invasion (hence a FIGO grade 2). In fact, clinical PAS grade 3A as per FIGO better corresponds to pathologic PAS grade 3D as per Hecht and colleagues in which the defining feature is serosal involvement (see Table 2). In addition, pathologic PAS grade 3E under Hecht and colleagues is not further subdivided into categories that would mirror clinical grades 3B (bladder wall involvement) and 3C (invasion into other pelvic tissues) as such distinction is more often done intraoperatively rather than on pathologic examination. If these potential confounders hinder widespread adoption of the proposed classification, a revised nomenclature may be warranted.

The PAS consensus recommendations by Hecht and colleagues[80] emphasize the distinction between PAS and dehiscence. However, it can be difficult to reliably distinguish between the 2 on pathologic evaluation (Fig. 9). Moreover, some authors believe dehiscence is an integral component of the pathophysiology of PAS, not a phenomenon independent from it.[97] Further research is needed to clarify whether the distinction between uterine scar dehiscence and PAS can be made reproducibly, and whether such distinction is biologically and/or clinically relevant.

Finally, the clinical significance of stage 1 BPMF needs to be further elucidated. Literature indicates that stage 2 (BPMF without associated decidua) has an association with PAS in subsequent gestations. Although it seems that such correlation does not apply to stage 1 BPMF, its identification through routine staging of BPMF is for now encouraged until further evidence emerges.

PLACENTAL INFECTION BY SEVERE ACUTE RESPIRATORY SYNDROME CORONAVIRUS 2

Most studies describing the pathologic changes seen in placentas from patients with COVID-19 have concentrated on patients with infection during the third trimester. They report a spectrum of changes including inflammatory processes (chronic villitis, chronic deciduitis, ascending intrauterine infection), MVM (placental infarction, AVM, decidual arteriopathy) and FVM (fetal vascular thrombosis).[98–100] Although the incidence of such findings does not seem to be significantly different than in patients without SARS-CoV-2 infection,[98] evidence accumulated during the course of the COVID-19 global pandemic shows that this

Table 3
Diagnosis and reporting elements of basal plate myometrial fibers

BPMF—Reporting Parameters	
Parameter	**Definition**
Stage	Stage 1: With accompanying decidua Stage 2: Without decidua
Size (in mm)	Linear dimension along the basal plate of the largest focus
Number of foci	In all sections including basal plate

Data from Hecht JL., Baergen R., Ernst LM., et al. Classification and reporting guidelines for the pathology diagnosis of placenta accreta spectrum (PAS) disorders: recommendations from an expert panel. Mod Pathol 2020;33(12):2382–96. 10.1038/s41379-020-0569-1.

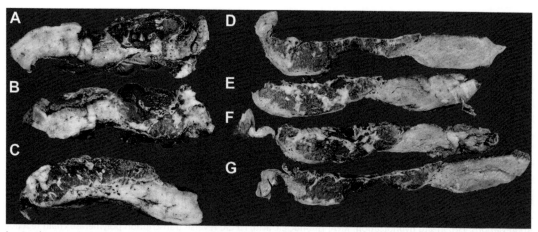

Fig. 9. Placenta Accreta Spectrum (PAS) disorder. Macroscopically, PAS with invasion into the myometrium (FIGO PAS grade 2 or greater) is often seen as placental parenchyma replacing the wall (*A, B,* anterior wall sections) with a rather sharp and vertical interface with the adjacent uninvolved wall (*A, B*). Sometimes, however, the invasion into the wall is more "gradual" and seems as progressive thinning of the myometrial wall (*C*). This appearance could be confused as uterine scar dehiscence; however, this section is from the posterior wall, in which no transmural scar is present (*A–C* correspond to the same gravid uterus). Placenta percreta (FIGO PAS grade 3) is often grossly visible as the serosal surface is disrupted and placental tissue is visible through the disruption (*D,* area or perforation is marked with orange ink). Note the very thin layer of residual myometrium in the wall adjacent to the perforation (*E–G; D–G* correspond to the same gravid uterus).

Placenta Accreta Spectrum Disorders-Key Points

1. PAS disorders are increasing in frequency and represent a significant cause of obstetric morbidity.

2. The 2019 FIGO definitions and grading for PAS outline clinical criteria for accreta, increta, and percreta categories, with corresponding histologic criteria.

3. An alternative pathologic grading system has been developed by a Society for Pediatric Pathology working group, aiming at improving applicability in gravid hysterectomy specimens.

4. Further consensus and investigation are needed to harmonize the current grading systems and establish their correlation with clinical characteristics and outcomes.

5. The presence of BPMF needs to be included in the pathology report, along with the corresponding stage (decidua present or not), size (in millimeters) and number of foci.

disease indeed carries an increased risk of obstetric and neonatal complications.[101,102] Preterm labor occurs in 15% to 43% of women with COVID-19 during the third trimester, compared with the national average of 10% preterm labor in prepandemic times.[101,102] Moreover, COVID-19 during pregnancy has been associated with elevated rates of intrauterine growth restriction (10%) and pregnancy loss (2%).[102]

Vertical transmission of SARS-CoV-2 to the placenta has been documented in some,[103–105] but not all studies.[106] Studies demonstrating SARS-CoV-2 positivity in placental tissue (by immunohistochemistry, in situ hybridization [ISH], and real time polymerase chain reaction [RT-PCR]) have described syncytiotrophoblast and cytotrophoblast damage as a major finding. For instance, Watkins and colleagues[103] described 7 placentas with *COVID-19 placentitis,* all with detection of SARS-CoV-2 by in situ hybridization, displaying villous trophoblast necrosis, histiocytic intervillositis, extensive perivillous fibrin deposition and intervillous space collapse.[105] While villous trophoblast seems most susceptible to SARS-CoV-2, a recent study by de Gioia and colleagues[107] has also identified endothelial cell infection. The extent of these findings seems to correlate with obstetric outcomes because diffuse and severe infection has been observed in the setting of intrauterine fetal demise.[105] The National Institutes of Health/Eunice Kennedy Shriver National Institute of Child Health and Human Development (NIH/NICHD) developed definitions of placental infection by SARS-CoV-2.[108] The expert panel recommended that placental infection by SARS-CoV-2 be classified as definitive, probable, possible, or unlikely based on the techniques

Table 4
Categories of placental infection by SARS-CoV-2

Categories of Placental Infection with SARS-CoV-2		
Category	Definition	Testing Method
Definite	Evidence of active replicating virus with location in the placental tissues	RNA ISH with probe for antisense strand or for double-strand RNA
Probable	Evidence of viral RNA or protein located in placental tissues	RNA ISH with probe for positive-sense strand, or immunohistochemistry for viral proteins
Possible	Evidence of viral RNA in placental homogenates or viral-like particles	rtPCR or quantification of viral RNA in placental homogenates; electron microscopy
Unlikely	No evidence of placental viral infection	Any methodology

Abbreviations: ISH, in situ hybridization; RNA, ribonucleic acid; rtPCR, reverse transcription polymerase chain reaction.
Adapted from Roberts DJ., Edlow AG., Romero RJ., et al. SPECIAL REPORT: A standardized definition of placental infection by severe acute respiratory syndrome coronavirus 2 (SARS-CoV-2), a consensus statement from the National Institutes of Health/Eunice Kennedy Shriver National Institute of Child Health and Human Development (NIH/NICHD) SARS-CoV-2 placental infection workshop. Am J Obstet Gynecol 2021:S0002-9378(21)00832-2. 10.1016/j.ajog.2021.07.029.

used for virus detection in the placental tissue (**Table 4**).[108] This standardized terminology, if applied strictly, will allow for a more uniform appraisal of future research, and help define the spectrum of placental changes under SARS-CoV-2 infection.

COVID-19 Placentitis-Key Points

1. COVID-19 is associated with obstetric complications including preterm labor, intrauterine growth restriction, and early pregnancy loss.

2. Placental infection by SARS-CoV-2 is characterized by villous trophoblast necrosis, histiocytic intervillositis, extensive perivillous fibrin deposition, and intervillous space collapse.

3. Testing methodologies for detection of SARS-CoV-2 in placental tissue have been developed and are instrumental in documenting placental infection by this pathogen.

SUMMARY

We provide an overview of the main entities discussed in the Amsterdam Placental Workshop Group Consensus Statement on Sampling and Definitions of Placental Lesions. The consensus has become widely accepted as the definitive reference pertaining to major aspects of placental pathologic conditions. Subsequent literature has supported many of the definitions and criteria outlined by the Amsterdam group and unveiled novel associations between placental lesions and clinical outcomes. Continued utilization of the pathologic definitions, staging and grading proposed by the Amsterdam consensus provides a common language for further investigations, hopefully uncovering evidence to refine criteria, improve reproducibility, and further integrate pathologic findings into clinical care. An updated consensus considering the emerging evidence discussed here (and the one that is yet to come) would also be highly beneficial. Equally important is the need to produce a similar level of consensus and recommendations on entities not covered by the first Amsterdam consensus.

CLINICS CARE POINTS

- Adoption and consistent use of Amsterdam terminology is strongly recommended because it provides a common language for the diagnosis and management of the most common placental lesions.

- Definitions and criteria for certain lesions need refinement in order to improve interobserver agreement and strengthen their clinical significance.

- Recommendations in the reporting of PAS disorders by the FIGO align clinical and pathologic definitions.

- COVID19 placentitis is a recently recognized complication of SARS-CoV-2 infection that requires histologic recognition and, ideally, confirmation by viral testing methods.

ACKNOWLEDGMENTS

The authors thank Dr. Marie-Anne Bründler, MD (Alberta Children's Hospital/University of Calgary, Calgary, AB, Canada) and Chris Horn, Pathology Scientist (Alberta Children's Hospital, Calgary, AB, Canada) for providing images for inclusion in **Figs. 6** and **7**. The authors further thank Dr. Marie-Anne Bründler for reviewing the article and providing insightful critiques, comments, and suggestions.

DISCLOSURE

The authors have no financial or other conflicts of interest to disclose.

REFERENCES

1. Khong TY, Mooney EE, Ariel I, et al. Sampling and definitions of placental lesions: amsterdam placental workshop group consensus statement. Arch Pathol Lab Med 2016;140(7):698–713.
2. PubMed - National Library of Medicine n.d. Available at: https://pubmed.ncbi.nlm.nih.gov/. Accessed December 9, 2021.
3. Google scholar n.d. Available at: https://scholar.google.com/. Accessed December 9, 2021.
4. AFIP Atlas of tumor pathology series 5 | Fascicle 6 atlas of placental pathology. Available at: Www.Arppress.Org https://www.arppress.org/product-p/5f06.htm. Accessed November 29, 2021.
5. Redline RW, Faye-Petersen O, Heller D, et al. Amniotic Infection syndrome: nosology and reproducibility of placental reaction patterns. Pediatr Dev Pathol 2003;6(5):435–48.
6. Loverro MT, Damiani GR, Di Naro E, et al. Analysis of relation between placental lesions and perinatal outcome according to Amsterdam criteria: a comparative study. Acta Biomed 2020;91(3):e2020061.
7. Yamada N, Sato Y, Moriguchi-Goto S, et al. Histological severity of fetal inflammation is useful in predicting neonatal outcome. Placenta 2015;36(12):1490–3.
8. Romero R, Kim YM, Pacora P, et al. The frequency and type of placental histologic lesions in term pregnancies with normal outcome. J Perinat Med 2018;46(6):613–30.
9. Roberts DJ, Celi AC, Riley LE, et al. Acute Histologic Chorioamnionitis at Term: Nearly Always Noninfectious. PLoS One 2012;7(3):e31819.
10. Blanc WA. Pathology of the placenta and cord in ascending and in haematogenous infection. Ciba Found Symp 1979;77:17–38.
11. Sampson JE, Theve RP, Blatman RN, et al. Fetal origin of amniotic fluid polymorphonuclear leukocytes. Am J Obstet Gynecol 1997;176(1 Pt 1):77–81.

12. Gomez-Lopez N, Romero R, Xu Y, et al. Are amniotic fluid neutrophils in women with intraamniotic infection and/or inflammation of fetal or maternal origin? Am J Obstet Gynecol 2017;217(6):693.e1–16.
13. Narice BF, Trzeszcz M, Cohen M, et al. Acute villitis and intravascular microorganisms in fetal vessels: a case report and literature review of an unusual histopathological finding. Pediatr Dev Pathol 2021;24(3):246–51.
14. Brouwers L, Franx A, Vogelvang TE, et al. Association of Maternal Prepregnancy Body Mass Index With Placental Histopathological Characteristics in Uncomplicated Term Pregnancies. Pediatr Dev Pathol 2019;22(1):45–52.
15. Becroft DM, Thompson JM, Mitchell EA. Placental villitis of unknown origin: epidemiologic associations. Am J Obstet Gynecol 2005;192(1):264–71.
16. Yaguchi C, Itoh H, Tsuchiya KJ, et al. Placental pathology predicts infantile physical development during first 18 months in Japanese population: Hamamatsu birth cohort for mothers and children (HBC Study). PLoS One 2018;13(4):e0194988.
17. Freedman AA, Miller GE, Ernst LM. Chronic villitis: refining the risk ratio of recurrence using a large placental pathology sample. Placenta 2021;112:135–40.
18. Redline RW. Villitis of unknown etiology: noninfectious chronic villitis in the placenta. Hum Pathol 2007;38(10):1439–46.
19. Redline RW, Patterson P. Villitis of Unknown Etiology Is Associated with Major Infiltration of Fetal Tissue by Maternal Inflammatory. Cells 1993;143(2):7.
20. Styer AK, Parker HJ, Roberts DJ, et al. Placental villitis of unclear etiology during ovum donor in vitro fertilization pregnancy. Am J Obstet Gynecol 2003;189(4):1184–6.
21. Redline RW. Classification of placental lesions. Am J Obstet Gynecol 2015;213(4, Supplement):S21–8.
22. Kim CJ, Romero R, Chaemsaithong P, et al. Chronic inflammation of the placenta: definition, classification, pathogenesis, and clinical significance. Am J Obstet Gynecol 2015;213(4, Supplement):S53–69.
23. Ernst LM, Bockoven C, Freedman A, et al. Chronic villitis of unknown etiology: Investigations into viral pathogenesis. Placenta 2021;107:24–30.
24. Freedman AA, Goldstein JA, Miller GE, et al. Seasonal variation of chronic villitis of unknown etiology. Pediatr Dev Pathol 2020;23(4):253–9.
25. Baergen RN, Heller DS. Placental pathology in Covid-19 positive mothers: preliminary findings. Pediatr Dev Pathol 2020;23(3):177–80.
26. Benirschke K, Coen R, Patterson B, et al. Villitis of known origin: varicella and toxoplasma. Placenta 1999;20(5):395–9.
27. Khong TY, De Wolf F, Robertson WB, et al. Inadequate maternal vascular response to placentation in pregnancies complicated by pre-eclampsia

and by small-for-gestational age infants. Br J Obstet Gynaecol 1986;93(10):1049–59.

28. Kovo M, Schreiber L, Bar J. Placental vascular pathology as a mechanism of disease in pregnancy complications. Thromb Res 2013;131(Suppl 1): S18–21.

29. Burton GJ, Woods AW, Jauniaux E, et al. Rheological and physiological consequences of conversion of the maternal spiral arteries for uteroplacental blood flow during human pregnancy. Placenta 2009;30(6):473–82.

30. Jauniaux E, Hempstock J, Greenwold N, et al. Trophoblastic oxidative stress in relation to temporal and regional differences in maternal placental blood flow in normal and abnormal early pregnancies. Am J Pathol 2003;162(1):115–25.

31. Redline RW, Ravishankar S, Bagby CM, et al. Four major patterns of placental injury: a stepwise guide for understanding and implementing the 2016 Amsterdam consensus. Mod Pathol 2021;34(6): 1074–92.

32. Pinar H, Sung CJ, Oyer CE, et al. Reference values for singleton and twin placental weights. Pediatr Pathol Lab Med 1996;16(6):901–7.

33. Proctor LK, Fitzgerald B, Whittle WL, et al. Umbilical cord diameter percentile curves and their correlation to birth weight and placental pathology. Placenta 2013;34(1):62–6.

34. Redline RW, Boyd T, Campbell V, et al. Maternal vascular underperfusion: nosology and reproducibility of placental reaction patterns. Pediatr Dev Pathol 2004;7(3):237–49.

35. Morgan TK, Tolosa JE, Mele L, et al. Placental villous hypermaturation is associated with idiopathic preterm birth. J Matern Fetal Neonatal Med 2013;26(7):647–53.

36. Loukeris K, Sela R, Baergen RN. Syncytial knots as a reflection of placental maturity: reference values for 20 to 40 weeks' gestational age. Pediatr Dev Pathol 2010;13(4):305–9.

37. Zhang P. Decidual vasculopathy in preeclampsia and spiral artery remodeling revisited: shallow invasion versus failure of involution. AJP Rep 2018;8(4): e241–6.

38. Crum CP, Nucci MR, Granter SR, et al. Diagnostic gynecologic and obstetric pathology. 3rd edition. Elsevier; 2017.

39. Stanek J. Utility of diagnosing various histological patterns of diffuse chronic hypoxic placental injury. Pediatr Dev Pathol 2012;15(1):13–23.

40. Stanek J, Weng E. Microscopic chorionic pseudocysts in placental membranes: a histologic lesion of in utero hypoxia. Pediatr Dev Pathol 2007; 10(3):192–8.

41. Stanek J, Al-Ahmadie HA. Laminar necrosis of placental membranes: a histologic sign of uteroplacental hypoxia. Pediatr Dev Pathol 2005;8(1):34–42.

42. Goldenberg RL, Faye-Petersen O, Andrews WW, et al. The alabama preterm birth study: diffuse decidual leukocytoclastic necrosis of the decidua basalis, a placental lesion associated with preeclampsia, indicated preterm birth and decreased fetal growth. J Matern Fetal Neonatal Med 2007; 20(5):391–5.

43. Bustamante Helfrich B, Chilukuri N, He H, et al. Maternal vascular malperfusion of the placental bed associated with hypertensive disorders in the Boston Birth Cohort. Placenta 2017;52:106–13.

44. Kulkarni VG, Sunilkumar KB, Nagaraj TS, et al. Maternal and fetal vascular lesions of malperfusion in the placentas associated with fetal and neonatal death: results of a prospective observational study. Am J Obstet Gynecol 2021;225(6):660.e1–12.

45. Stanek J. Placental pathology varies in hypertensive conditions of pregnancy. Virchows Arch 2018;472(3):415–23.

46. Tateishi A, Ohira S, Yamamoto Y, et al. Histopathological findings of pregnancy-induced hypertension: histopathology of early-onset type reflects two-stage disorder theory. Virchows Arch 2018;472(4):635–42.

47. Catov JM, Muldoon MF, Reis SE, et al. Preterm birth with placental evidence of malperfusion is associated with cardiovascular risk factors after pregnancy: a prospective cohort study. BJOG 2018; 125(8):1009–17.

48. Jaiman S, Romero R, Pacora P, et al. Disorders of placental villous maturation are present in one-third of cases with spontaneous preterm labor. J Perinat Med 2021;49(4):412–30.

49. Oh MA, Barak S, Mohamed M, et al. Placental pathology and intraventricular hemorrhage in preterm and small for gestational age infants. J Perinatol 2021;41(4):843–9.

50. Parodi A, De Angelis LC, Re M, et al. Placental pathology findings and the risk of intraventricular and cerebellar hemorrhage in preterm neonates. Front Neurol 2020;11:761.

51. Pinar H, Stephens M, Singer DB, et al. Triplet placentas: reference values for weights. Pediatr Dev Pathol 2002;5(5):495–8.

52. Hecht JL, Kliman HJ, Allred EN, et al. Reference weights for placentas delivered before the 28th week of gestation. Placenta 2007;28(10):987–90.

53. Gielen M, Lindsey PJ, Derom C, et al. Curves of placental weights of live-born twins. Twin Res Hum Genet 2006;9(5):664–72.

54. O'Brien O, Higgins MF, Mooney EE. Placental weights from normal deliveries in Ireland. Ir J Med Sci 2020;189(2):581–3.

55. Dy CL, Chari RS, Russell LJ. Updating reference values for placental weights in Northern Alberta. Am J Obstet Gynecol 2004;190(5):1458–60.

56. Krishnan C. Placenta weights reference and report generator. Hematogones n.d. Available at: https://

hematogones.com/surg-path/placenta. Accessed November 29, 2021.

57. Bendon RW. Nosology: infarction hematoma, a placental infarction encasing a hematoma. Hum Pathol 2012;43(5):761–3.

58. Neville G, Russell N, O'Donoghue K, et al. Rounded intraplacental hematoma - A high risk placental lesion as illustrated by a prospective study of 26 consecutive cases. Placenta 2019;81:18–24.

59. Chen AL, Goldfarb IT, Scourtas AO, et al. The histologic evolution of revealed, acute abruptions. Hum Pathol 2017;67:187–97.

60. Gonen N, Levy M, Kovo M, et al. Placental histopathology and pregnancy outcomes in "Early" vs. "Late" Placental Abruption. Reprod Sci 2021; 28(2):351–60.

61. Redline RW, Vik T, Heerema-McKenney A, et al. Interobserver reliability for identifying specific patterns of placental injury as defined by the amsterdam classification. Arch Pathol Lab Med 2021. https://doi.org/10.5858/arpa.2020-0753-OA.

62. Mukherjee A, Chan ADC, Keating S, et al. The placental distal villous hypoplasia pattern: interobserver agreement and automated fractal dimension as an objective metric. Pediatr Dev Pathol 2016;19(1):31–6.

63. Redline RW, Pappin A. Fetal thrombotic vasculopathy: the clinical significance of extensive avascular villi. Hum Pathol 1995;26(1):80–5.

64. Sander CH, Stevens NG. Hemorrhagic endovasculitis of the placenta: an indepth morphologic appraisal with initial clinical and epidemiologic observations. Pathol Annu 1984;19(Pt 1):37–79.

65. Redline RW, Ravishankar S. Fetal vascular malperfusion, an update. APMIS 2018;126(7):561–9.

66. Saleemuddin A, Tantbirojn P, Sirois K, et al. Obstetric and perinatal complications in placentas with fetal thrombotic vasculopathy. Pediatr Dev Pathol 2010;13(6):459–64.

67. Tantbirojn P, Saleemuddin A, Sirois K, et al. Gross abnormalities of the umbilical cord: related placental histology and clinical significance. Placenta 2009;30(12):1083–8.

68. Ariel I, Anteby E, Hamani Y, et al. Placental pathology in fetal thrombophilia. Hum Pathol 2004;35(6): 729–33.

69. Raspollini MR, Oliva E, Roberts DJ. Placental histopathologic features in patients with thrombophilic mutations. J Matern Fetal Neonatal Med 2007; 20(2):113–23.

70. Gogia N, Machin GA. Maternal thrombophilias are associated with specific placental lesions. Pediatr Dev Pathol 2008;11(6):424–9.

71. Nevalainen J, Ignatius J, Savolainen E-R, et al. Placenta-mediated pregnancy complications are not associated with fetal or paternal factor V Leiden mutation. Eur J Obstet Gynecol Reprod Biol 2018; 230:32–5.

72. Udry S, Aranda FM, Latino JO, et al. Paternal factor V Leiden and recurrent pregnancy loss: a new concept behind fetal genetics? J Thromb Haemost 2014;12(5):666–9.

73. Dizon-Townson DS, Meline L, Nelson LM, et al. Fetal carriers of the factor V Leiden mutation are prone to miscarriage and placental infarction. Am J Obstet Gynecol 1997;177(2):402–5.

74. Bakotic BW, Boyd T, Poppiti R, et al. Recurrent umbilical cord torsion leading to fetal death in 3 subsequent pregnancies: a case report and review of the literature. Arch Pathol Lab Med 2000;124(9): 1352–5.

75. Hoffman JD, Kleeman L, Kennelly K, et al. Three new families with recurrent male miscarriages and hypercoiled umbilical cord. Clin Dysmorphol 2015;24(3):128–31.

76. Beggan C, Mooney EE, Downey P, et al. A case of recurrent familial male miscarriages with hypercoiled umbilical cord: a possible X-linked association? Clin Dysmorphol 2014;23(1):26–8.

77. Slack JC, Boyd TK. Fetal vascular malperfusion due to long and hypercoiled umbilical cords resulting in recurrent second trimester pregnancy loss: a case series and literature review. Pediatr Dev Pathol 2021;24(1):12–8.

78. Ernst LM, Minturn L, Huang MH, et al. Gross patterns of umbilical cord coiling: correlations with placental histology and stillbirth. Placenta 2013; 34(7):583–8.

79. Shannon P, Hum C, Parks T, et al. Brain and placental pathology in Fetal COL4A1 related disease. Pediatr Dev Pathol 2021;24(3):175–86.

80. Hecht JL, Baergen R, Ernst LM, et al. Classification and reporting guidelines for the pathology diagnosis of placenta accreta spectrum (PAS) disorders: recommendations from an expert panel. Mod Pathol 2020;33(12):2382–96.

81. Jauniaux E, Ayres-de-Campos D, Langhoff-Roos J, et al. FIGO classification for the clinical diagnosis of placenta accreta spectrum disorders. Int J Gynaecol Obstet 2019;146(1):20–4.

82. Publications Committee, Society for Maternal-Fetal Medicine, Belfort MA. Placenta accreta. Am J Obstet Gynecol 2010;203(5):430–9.

83. Khong TY. The pathology of placenta accreta, a worldwide epidemic. J Clin Pathol 2008;61(12): 1243–6.

84. Bodelon C, Bernabe-Ortiz A, Schiff MA, et al. Factors associated with peripartum hysterectomy. Obstet Gynecol 2009;114(1):115–23.

85. Kastner ES, Figueroa R, Garry D, et al. Emergency peripartum hysterectomy: experience at a community teaching hospital. Obstet Gynecol 2002;99(6): 971–5.

86. Eshkoli T, Weintraub AY, Sergienko R, et al. Placenta accreta: risk factors, perinatal outcomes,

and consequences for subsequent births. Am J Obstet Gynecol 2013;208(3):219.e1-7.

87. Bowman ZS, Eller AG, Bardsley TR, et al. Risk Factors for placenta accreta: a large prospective cohort. Am J Perinatol 2013. https://doi.org/10.1055/s-0033-1361833.

88. Kamara M, Henderson JJ, Doherty DA, et al. The risk of placenta accreta following primary elective caesarean delivery: a case-control study. BJOG 2013;120(7):879–86.

89. Tantbirojn P, Crum CP, Parast MM. Pathophysiology of placenta creta: the role of decidua and extravillous trophoblast. Placenta 2008;29(7):639–45.

90. Khong TY, Robertson WB. Placenta creta and placenta praevia creta. Placenta 1987;8(4):399–409.

91. Parra-Herran C, Djordjevic B. Histopathology of placenta creta: chorionic villi intrusion into myometrial vascular spaces and extravillous trophoblast proliferation are frequent and specific findings with implications for diagnosis and pathogenesis. Int J Gynecol Pathol 2016;35(6):497–508.

92. Aalipour S, Salmanian B, Fox KA, et al. Placenta accreta spectrum: correlation between FIGO Clinical classification and histopathologic findings. Am J Perinatol 2021. https://doi.org/10.1055/s-0041-1728834.

93. Bluth A, Schindelhauer A, Nitzsche K, et al. Placenta accreta spectrum disorders-experience of management in a German tertiary perinatal centre. Arch Gynecol Obstet 2021;303(6):1451–60.

94. Ishibashi H, Miyamoto M, Iwahashi H, et al. Criteria for placenta accreta spectrum in the International Federation of Gynaecology and Obstetrics classification, and topographic invasion area are associated with massive hemorrhage in patients with placenta previa. Acta Obstet Gynecol Scand 2021;100(6):1019–25.

95. Linn RL, Miller ES, Lim G, et al. Adherent basal plate myometrial fibers in the delivered placenta as a risk factor for development of subsequent placenta accreta. Placenta 2015;36(12):1419–24.

96. Khong TY, Werger AC. Myometrial fibers in the placental basal plate can confirm but do not necessarily indicate clinical placenta accreta. Am J Clin Pathol 2001;116(5):703–8.

97. Einerson BD, Comstock J, Silver RM, et al. Placenta accreta spectrum disorder: uterine dehiscence, not placental invasion. Obstet Gynecol 2020;135(5):1104–11.

98. Levitan D, London V, McLaren RA, et al. Histologic and immunohistochemical evaluation of 65 placentas from women with polymerase chain reaction-proven severe acute respiratory syndrome Coronavirus 2 (SARS-CoV-2) infection. Arch Pathol Lab Med 2021;145(6):648–56.

99. Bertero L, Borella F, Botta G, et al. Placenta histopathology in SARS-CoV-2 infection: analysis of a consecutive series and comparison with control cohorts. Virchows Arch 2021;479(4):715–28.

100. Menter T, Mertz KD, Jiang S, et al. Placental Pathology Findings during and after SARS-CoV-2 Infection: Features of Villitis and Malperfusion. Pathobiology 2021;88(1):69–77.

101. Elshafeey F, Magdi R, Hindi N, et al. A systematic scoping review of COVID-19 during pregnancy and childbirth. Int J Gynaecol Obstet 2020;150(1):47–52.

102. Dashraath P, Wong JLJ, Lim MXK, et al. Coronavirus disease 2019 (COVID-19) pandemic and pregnancy. Am J Obstet Gynecol 2020;222(6):521–31.

103. Watkins JC, Torous VF, Roberts DJ. Defining severe acute respiratory syndrome Coronavirus 2 (SARS-CoV-2) placentitis: a report of 7 cases with confirmatory in situ hybridization, distinct histomorphologic features, and evidence of complement deposition. Arch Pathol Lab Med 2021;145(11):1341–9.

104. Hecht JL, Quade B, Deshpande V, et al. SARS-CoV-2 can infect the placenta and is not associated with specific placental histopathology: a series of 19 placentas from COVID-19-positive mothers. Mod Pathol 2020;33(11):2092–103.

105. Garrido-Pontnou M, Navarro A, Camacho J, et al. Diffuse trophoblast damage is the hallmark of SARS-CoV-2-associated fetal demise. Mod Pathol 2021;34(9):1704–9.

106. Edlow AG, Li JZ, Collier AY, et al. Assessment of maternal and neonatal SARS-CoV-2 viral load, transplacental antibody transfer, and placental pathology in pregnancies during the COVID-19 pandemic. JAMA Netw Open 2020;3(12):e2030455.

107. di Gioia C, Zullo F, Bruno Vecchio RC, et al. Stillbirth and fetal capillary infection by SARS-CoV-2. Am J Obstet Gynecol MFM 2022;4(1):100523.

108. Roberts DJ, Edlow AG, Romero RJ, et al. SPECIAL REPORT: a standardized definition of placental infection by severe acute respiratory syndrome coronavirus 2 (SARS-CoV-2), a consensus statement from the National Institutes of Health/Eunice Kennedy Shriver National Institute of Child Health and Human Development (NIH/NICHD) SARS-CoV-2 placental infection workshop. Am J Obstet Gynecol 2021;225(6):593.e1–9.

Gestational Trophoblastic Disease
Contemporary Diagnostic Approach

Natalia Buza, MD

KEYWORDS

- Hydatidiform mole • Complete mole • Partial mole • Genotyping • p57 immunohistochemistry
- Gestational choriocarcinoma • Epithelioid trophoblastic tumor • Placental site trophoblastic tumor

Key points

- Hydatidiform moles are fundamentally defined by their genetic composition
- Morphologic features are not reliable for recognition of partial hydatidiform mole
- Algorithmic diagnostic approach is recommended for molar gestations using p57 immunohistochemistry and short tandem repeat genotyping
- Gestational trophoblastic tumors need to be differentiated from reactive trophoblastic proliferations and from neoplasms of nongestational origin, due to the significant therapeutic and prognostic implications

ABSTRACT

Pathologic diagnosis of gestational trophoblastic disease (GTD)—hydatidiform moles and gestational trophoblastic neoplasms—underwent a major shift in the past decade from morphology-based recognition to precise molecular genetic classification of entities, which also allows for prognostic stratification of molar gestations. This article highlights these recent advances and their integration into the routine pathology practice. The traditional gross and histomorphologic features of each entity are also reviewed with special focus on differential diagnoses and their clinical implications.

placental site trophoblastic tumor (PSTT). These entities continue to pose a diagnostic challenge because of their rarity and often unusual clinical presentations. However, there have been significant advances in recent years in their diagnostic workup utilizing ancillary studies—immunohistochemistry and molecular genotyping—as part of various proposed diagnostic algorithms. This article provides a systematic practical overview of the traditional gross and microscopic pathologic features of different forms of GTDs, their differential diagnoses, and potential prognostic and therapeutic implications in the context of the 2020 WHO classification.

OVERVIEW

Diagnostic classification of gestational trophoblastic disease (GTD) includes complete and partial hydatidiform moles (PHM) and gestational trophoblastic tumors, that is, choriocarcinoma, epithelioid trophoblastic tumor (ETT), and

HYDATIDIFORM MOLES

Hydatidiform moles are non-neoplastic proliferations of the chorionic villous trophoblast with unique genetic composition and a risk for persistent GTD and gestational trophoblastic neoplasia (GTN). The two forms of molar gestations—complete and PHM—share some features on the clinical, histologic, and genetic levels: both are

---

Department of Pathology, Yale School of Medicine, 310 Cedar Street LH 108, PO Box 208023, New Haven, CT 06520-8023, USA
E-mail address: natalia.buza@yale.edu

Surgical Pathology 15 (2022) 197–218
https://doi.org/10.1016/j.path.2022.02.002
1875-9181/22/© 2022 Elsevier Inc. All rights reserved.

surgpath.theclinics.com

abnormal gestations incompatible with fetal survival, they have hydropic changes and villous trophoblastic hyperplasia, and demonstrate paternal dominance in their genomes. However, distinction and precise classification of the two entities is crucial because of the marked differences in their risk of subsequent aggressive clinical behavior. In addition, hydatidiform moles have several nonmolar morphologic mimics necessitating the use of modern ancillary diagnostic tools.

GENETIC BASIS OF HYDATIDIFORM MOLES

Complete hydatidiform moles (CHM) typically have a diploid paternal-only genome, resulting from one sperm fertilizing an empty oocyte with reduplication of its genome (monospermic, homozygous CHM) in 80% to 90% of cases, whereas the remaining 10% to 20% of CHM are dispermic, heterozygous, as a result of 2 sperms fertilizing an empty egg.[1,2] Rare cases of tetraploid CHMs containing 4 haploid paternal chromosome sets have also been reported.[3,4] In addition, a small subset of CHM—representing approximately 0.6% to 2.6% of all hydatidiform moles—are familial biparental complete moles (FBCHM) that contain both maternal and paternal genomes and result from mutations in maternal effect genes NALP7/NLRP7 on chromosome 19q13.4 or KHDC3L on chromosome 6q13 leading to disruption of genomic imprinting.[5–10]

   PHM are characterized by their diandric monogynic triploid genome, arising from 2 sperms fertilizing an egg (dispermic/heterozygous PHM) in at least 95% of cases, and less commonly from one sperm with reduplication of its genome (monospermic/homozygous PHM).[3,11] Triploidy is one of the most common chromosomal abnormalities, occurring in up to 3% of all gestations[12,13] and in 8% to 10% of spontaneous abortions.[14] Approximately one-third of them are digynic monoandric nonmolar triploid gestations, arising from meiotic nondisjunction of maternal chromosomes,[11,12] with the remaining being diandric monogynic triploid gestations (namely, partial moles). Tetraploid PHMs may rarely also occur and contain 3 haploid paternal chromosome sets in addition to 1 set of maternal chromosomes.[15–19]

GROSS FEATURES

Specimens from well-developed CHMs typically have a large tissue volume with grossly visible villous hydrops, sometimes reminiscent of a "bunch of grapes" (Fig. 1A, Box 1). However, villous hydrops is often not grossly apparent in very early CHMs evacuated in the first trimester.

Regardless of the gestational age, fetal parts are absent in CHM. The gross appearance of partial moles is usually unremarkable until well into the second trimester of gestation, when focal hydropic changes may be observed (Box 2, Fig. 1B). A fetus may be present in PHM and may show symmetric intrauterine growth restriction, syndactyly, spina bifida, and other malformations.[20–23]

MICROSCOPIC FEATURES

Well-developed CHM (typically presenting after 11–12 weeks of gestation) can be recognized by diffuse villous enlargement, marked villous hydrops with cistern formation, and circumferential trophoblastic hyperplasia (see Box 1, Fig. 2). Cytologic atypia of intermediate trophoblasts at the implantation site is often present and may be quite striking.[2] The villous contours are usually smooth and round, but surface invaginations with trophoblastic pseudoinclusions may occur. The villous stroma is devoid of any vessels and fetal red blood cells. Fetal tissues are also absent.

   Very early complete moles (evacuated early during the first trimester, typically 10 weeks of gestation or earlier) often lack the aforementioned morphologic features: the villi are polypoid, irregularly shaped, and the villous size is usually within the normal range for the gestational age. Trophoblastic pseudoinclusions are uncommon and the trophoblastic proliferation may be less conspicuous; however, concentric growth is often appreciated, instead of the distinct polarization seen in early normal gestations. Instead of the hydrops, the villous stroma in very early CHM appears hypercellular and myxoid with stellate fibroblasts and prominent karyorrhectic debris (see Fig. 2). Rarely primitive fetal vessels and even nucleated red blood cells have been reported in CHM evacuated at a very early gestational age.[24]

   The morphologic features of PHM include heterogeneity in villous size and shape at scanning magnification due to the presence of 2 villous populations—large, hydropic villi in the background of a small, fibrotic, or normal-appearing villi; irregular, scalloped villous contours with surface invaginations and round to oval trophoblastic pseudoinclusions; prominent syncytiotrophoblastic knuckles, and mild to moderate trophoblastic hyperplasia[25–27] (see Box 2, Fig. 3). Unlike in CHM, significant cytologic atypia is typically absent in partial moles. Cistern formation may be seen in nearly 60% of cases. Fetal vessels with nucleated red blood cells are usually present, and fetal tissues may also be identified microscopically.

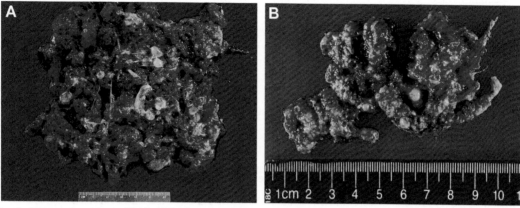

Fig. 1. Gross appearance of hydatidiform moles. (*A*) Well-developed complete hydatidiform mole with a large tissue volume and grossly visible villous hydrops. (*B*) Partial hydatidiform moles typically have a smaller volume of evacuation specimen (notice the scale difference between the 2 images) and may show focal hydropic changes.

DIFFERENTIAL DIAGNOSIS

Complete and partial moles can show overlapping morphologic features with each other and with various other nonmolar gestations. Nonmolar hydropic abortions may show significant villous hydrops, although typically they have smooth villous contours and lack trophoblastic hyperplasia (**Fig. 4**). Early nonmolar gestations and tubal ectopic pregnancies may have hypercellular and myxoid villous stroma similar to very early CHM. In addition, ectopic gestations may also be associated with significant, albeit noncircumferential, trophoblast proliferation. Chromosomal trisomy syndromes (especially trisomies 6, 7, 13, 15, 16, 18, 21, and 22) often demonstrate markedly irregular villous contours, trophoblastic pseudoinclusions, and variable degree of hydropic change, mimicking PHM[27–30] (see **Fig. 4**). Marked trophoblastic hyperplasia may also be seen in trisomies 7, 15, 21, and 22. Abnormal villous morphology reminiscent of PHM is often present in the second or third trimester of placental mesenchymal dysplasia (PMD), which encompasses a spectrum of entities, such as Beckwith-Wiedemann syndrome and androgenetic/biparental mosaic gestations.[31–33] In addition, nonmolar digynic monoandric triploid conceptions may also mimic PHM not only morphologically, but by karyotyping and ploidy analysis as well, as these tests would result in triploidy in both conditions, and the parental origin of the chromosomal content cannot be determined through these methods.[12,21] Interestingly, abnormal villous morphology has also been reported in nonmolar gestations conceived with egg donations, which may also complicate the interpretation of genotyping data (see details later).[34,35] Twin gestations with coexisting CHM and nonmolar fetus show two morphologically distinct villous populations, which may be intimately admixed with each other in curettings, simulating PHM.

The morphologic diagnosis of PHM is especially problematic because of the significant overlap with its mimics and the high rate of interobserver variability.[36] Systematic morphologic comparison of PHM, nonmolar hydropic abortions, and chromosomal trisomies suggests that presence of at least one of the following 3 features: cistern formation, 2 villous populations, and pseudoinclusions—in addition to a maximum villous size of $\geq$ 2.5 mm yields the highest sensitivity (61%) and specificity (84%) for the diagnosis of PHM in this setting.[27]

ANCILLARY STUDIES

P57 Immunohistochemistry

P57 protein is a cyclin-dependent kinase inhibitor, encoded by *CDKN1C* (*p57KIP2*) located on chromosome 11p15.5.[37] The gene is paternally imprinted, that is, expressed only by the maternal allele. Hence, normal p57 immunostaining pattern—strong nuclear staining in villous cytotrophoblasts, intermediate trophoblasts, and villous stromal cells—is seen in gestations containing maternal genetic material: nonmolar hydropic abortions, chromosomal trisomies, digynic triploidy, and PHM (**Fig. 5**). However, sporadic complete moles, including very early complete moles, are p57 negative in the aforementioned cell types (or show no more than focal expression in <10% of cells) due to lack of maternal genetic material.[37–41] In addition, p57 expression is also absent in familial biparental CHM due to disrupted

---

Box 1
Complete hydatidiform mole (CHM)—pathologic key features

Genotype
- Sporadic (Androgenetic) CHM
  - Homozygous (monospermic) 80% to 90%
  - Heterozygous (dispermic) 10% to 20%
- Familial Biparental CHM (0.6%–2.6%)
  - Mutations in *NALP7/NLRP7* or *KHDC3L*

Gross appearance
- Large specimen volume with villous hydrops (well-developed CHM)
- May not show gross abnormalities if evacuated at an early gestational age (very early CHM)

Histologic features
- Well developed CHM
  - Diffuse villous enlargement
  - Marked villous hydrops with cistern formation
  - Circumferential trophoblastic hyperplasia
  - Cytologic atypia of intermediate trophoblasts at the implantation site
  - Smooth and round villous contours, but surface invaginations with trophoblastic pseudoinclusions may also occur
  - Absence of fetal vessels and fetal red blood cells
- Very early CHM
  - No significant villous enlargement or hydrops
  - Polypoid, irregular villous shape
  - Hypercellular, myxoid villous stroma with prominent karyorrhexis
  - Rare primitive fetal vessels and fetal red blood cells

Immunohistochemistry
- Lack of p57 expression in villous cytotrophoblasts, intermediate trophoblasts and villous stromal cells

Differential diagnosis
- Partial hydatidiform mole
- Nonmolar hydropic abortion
- Uniparental disomy of chromosome 11
- Very early nonmolar gestations (mimicking very early CHM)
- Tubal ectopic gestations

Prognosis
- Persistent/invasive mole in 20% to 25%
- Gestational choriocarcinoma in 3% to 5%
- Risk of postmolar GTD/GTN is approximately 3-fold higher for heterozygous (dispermic) CHM compared with homozygous (monospermic) CHM

---

genomic imprinting affecting the expression of maternal alleles. Consequently, differential p57 expression can be used to distinguish between complete mole and its mimics; however, p57 cannot differentiate between PHM and other nonmolar gestations with abnormal villous morphology. Similarly, p57 cannot differentiate homozygous CHM from heterozygous CHM.

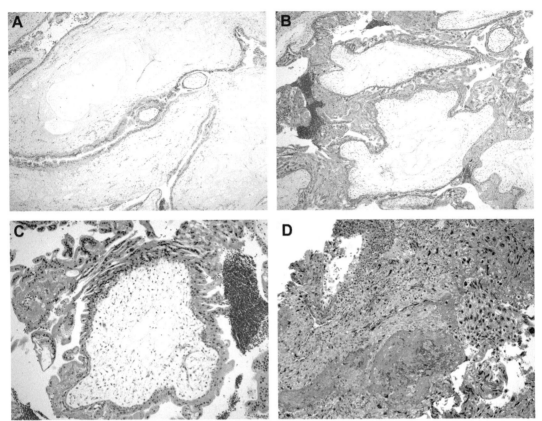

Fig. 2. Microscopic features of CHM. Well-developed CHM shows marked villous hydrops with cistern formation (A) and circumferential trophoblast hyperplasia (B). In very early CHM, the villi are smaller and have hypercellular, myxoid stroma with prominent karyorrhexis (C). Marked trophoblast atypia at the implantation site may also be present (D).

The interpretation of p57 immunohistochemistry is not without pitfalls and discordant/equivocal p57 staining patterns may occur, albeit infrequently. Rare cases of CHM may have normal p57 protein expression due to retained maternal chromosome 11,[42,43] and PHM may rarely be p57 negative as a result of loss of maternal chromosome 11.[32,44] Discordant p57 immunostaining patterns—p57-positive villous cytotrophoblast and p57-negative villous stromal cells, or vice versa—have also been described in rare androgenetic/biparental mosaic or chimeric gestations and PMD.[32,45,46] Furthermore, paternal uniparental disomy involving chromosome 11 (ie, both homologous chromosomes or part of the chromosome are inherited from the father and the maternal homologous chromosome is lost) is also associated with lack of p57 expression and abnormal morphologic features mimicking hydatidiform moles.[47] Twin gestations with a CHM and a non-molar fetus may show an admixture of p57-negative and p57-positive chorionic villi, which may complicate the diagnostic interpretation as well.[48]

The diagnostic utility of other immunohistochemical stains—including the proliferation marker Ki-67—has also been explored in this setting. CHMs generally have a higher proliferative index compared with PHM and nonmolar gestations; however, Ki-67 cannot reliably distinguish PHM from its nonmolar mimics, limiting its use in routine practice.[49]

Short Tandem Repeat Genotyping

The number of short tandem repeats (STR)—genetically stable, highly prevalent repetitive DNA sequences of 2 to 7 nucleotides—differs between individuals at each STR locus. Therefore, genetic analysis of these loci (STR genotyping) can be exploited to distinguish between individuals and is used for identity testing in forensics, paternity testing, and for tissue floater analysis in pathology laboratories.[50] Similarly, comparison of the allelic profiles between maternal decidua and chorionic villi using STR genotyping provides information about the parental genetic contribution to the villous tissue and the relative proportions of

---

Box 2
Partial hydatidiform mole—pathologic key features

Genotype
- Diandric triploidy
  - Heterozygous (dispermic) > 95%
  - Homozygous (monospermic) < 5%
- Triandric tetraploidy (~2%)

Gross appearance
- Unremarkable (first trimester)
- Focal placental hydrops (second trimester)
- Fetus may be present with developmental anomalies (eg, symmetric intrauterine growth restriction, syndactyly, spina bifida)

Histologic features
- Two villous populations (large hydropic and small fibrotic villi)
- Villous enlargement (≥2.5 mm)
- Villous hydrops with cistern formation
- Scalloped villous contours with surface invaginations and trophoblastic pseudoinclusions
- Prominent syncytiotrophoblastic knuckles
- Mild to moderate trophoblastic hyperplasia
- No significant cytologic atypia
- Fetal vessels with nucleated red blood cells are usually present

Immunohistochemistry
- Nuclear p57 expression is present in villous cytotrophoblasts, intermediate trophoblasts, and villous stromal cells

Differential diagnosis
- Complete hydatidiform mole
- Nonmolar hydropic abortion
- Chromosomal trisomies
- Digynic triploidy
- Placental mesenchymal dysplasia/Uniparental disomy of chromosome 11
- Twin gestation with CHM and normal fetus

Prognosis
- Persistent/invasive mole in 4% to 5%
- Gestational choriocarcinoma in less than 0.5%

---

maternal and paternal genetic material, allowing precise genetic classifications of molar gestations.[3,28,51,52]

A biallelic profile on STR genotyping analysis with balanced maternal and paternal contributions indicates a nonmolar gestation. CHMs show paternal-only alleles, either in a homozygous or heterozygous pattern (**Fig. 6**A), whereas PHM is characterized by the presence of 2 unique paternal alleles in addition to 1 maternal allele (dispermic or heterozygous PHM) or 1 paternal allele in duplicate quantity and 1 maternal allele at every STR locus (monospermic or homozygous PHM) (**Fig. 6**B). Unlike morphology and immunohistochemistry, genotyping can reliably distinguish PHM from its mimics: the presence of 1 paternal and 2 maternal alleles is diagnostic of nonmolar digynic monoandric triploidy, whereas chromosomal trisomies

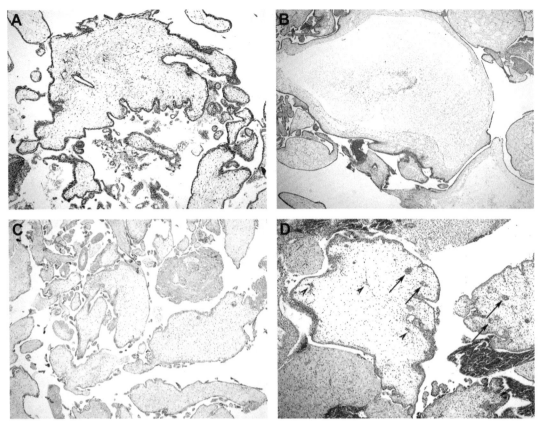

Fig. 3. Microscopic features of PHM include 2 populations of villi (*A*), cistern formation (*B*), trophoblast hyperplasia with syncytiotrophoblastic knuckles (*C*), and irregular, scalloped villous contours with trophoblastic pseudoinclusions (*D, arrows*). Fetal blood vessels with nucleated red blood cells are often present (*D, arrowheads*).

have a biparental genetic contribution, which are balanced at most STR loci, except those involved in trisomy, which can be recognized as a single allelic gain on genotyping.[27]

Rare pitfalls of genotyping include familial biparental complete moles and egg donor pregnancy. In contrast to sporadic CHM, familial biparental complete moles have a diploid biparental genome, which may be misinterpreted as a nonmolar gestation on genotyping. Gestations conceived with egg donation do not contain alleles from the recipient mother, mimicking a diandric complete mole on genotyping.[34,35] Both of the aforementioned scenarios require careful correlation between the genotyping results, morphologic findings, and p57 immunostaining patterns to make the correct diagnosis.

DIAGNOSTIC ALGORITHM

Various algorithmic approaches have been recently proposed for hydatidiform moles to integrate p57 immunohistochemistry and STR genotyping.[2,41,51–53] All algorithms begin with morphologic evaluation as the critical first step in triaging specimens for ancillary studies (**Fig. 7**). One algorithm advocates for p57 immunohistochemistry in all cases with histomorphologic suspicion for hydatidiform mole (either complete or partial), followed by genotyping only if normal p57 expression is observed. Another approach recommends primary genotyping analysis of all morphologically suspicious gestations and performing p57 only in rare cases with discrepancy between the morphology and genotyping results. The third approach combines the first 2 algorithms, pursuing p57 immunohistochemistry only for cases suspicious of CHM, and genotyping only without p57 if the morphology suggests PHM.

Although all 3 recommended algorithms incorporate genotyping, this technique is currently not uniformly available to all practices. If genotyping is unavailable, gestations with retained p57 expression and morphologic suspicion for PHM may be signed out descriptively acknowledging the differential diagnosis and the possibility of a partial mole. Review of the patient's routine prenatal work-up or karyotyping results (if available) may

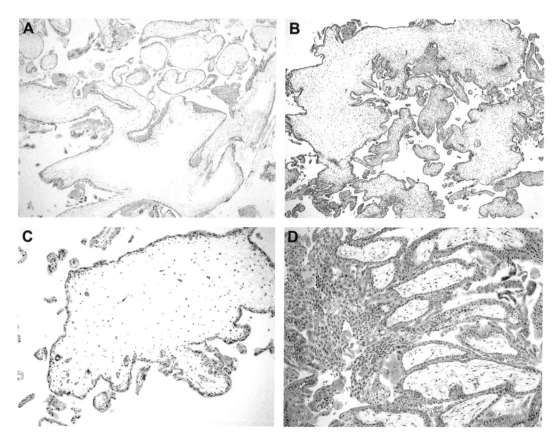

Fig. 4. Morphologic mimics of hydatidiform moles include nonmolar hydropic abortions (*A*), chromosomal trisomies (*B*, trisomy 13), digynic monoandric triploidy (*C*), and early nonmolar gestations (*D*, 5 + 3/7 weeks gestational age).

reveal results helpful in the differential diagnosis, such as a chromosomal trisomy. If karyotyping or other form of ploidy analysis (eg, FISH) demonstrates triploidy, the descriptive differential diagnosis should include PHM and nonmolar digynic triploidy. It needs to be acknowledged that this approach cannot provide a definitive diagnostic exclusion of PHM, and the patient will likely be subjected to serial hCG monitoring and contraception for up to 6 months as part of the postmolar surveillance program.[54] **Box 3** includes suggestions for diagnostic write-up depending on the local practice and the availability of ancillary testing modalities.

PROGNOSIS

Hydatidiform moles are associated with increased risk of persistent GTD and GTN. The level of risk is directly linked to the diagnosis and genotype of these entities, thus accurate diagnostic classification—preferably at the genetic level—is paramount for clinical prognostic assessment. Persistent GTD is primarily a clinical term, defined by plateauing or rising serum beta-hCG levels during postmolar surveillance. Histologic confirmation is usually not necessary to establish the diagnosis, although persistent molar villi, invasive mole, or choriocarcinoma may be seen if endometrial curettage or hysterectomy is performed.

CHM has a risk of progression into persistent/invasive mole in 20% to 25%, and into gestational choriocarcinoma in 3% to 5% of cases.[2,55] Recent studies also highlighted the prognostic importance of the precise genotype among complete moles: heterozygous (dispermic) CHMs have a significantly higher frequency (approximately 3-fold) of postmolar GTD compared with homozygous (monospermic) ones.[56–62] The risk of persistent/invasive mole and choriocarcinoma following a partial mole is lower, 4% to 5%, and less than 0.5%, respectively.[2,55]

GESTATIONAL TROPHOBLASTIC TUMORS

Gestational trophoblastic tumors may arise from villous intermediate—and cytotrophoblast—choriocarcinoma; intermediate trophoblast at the

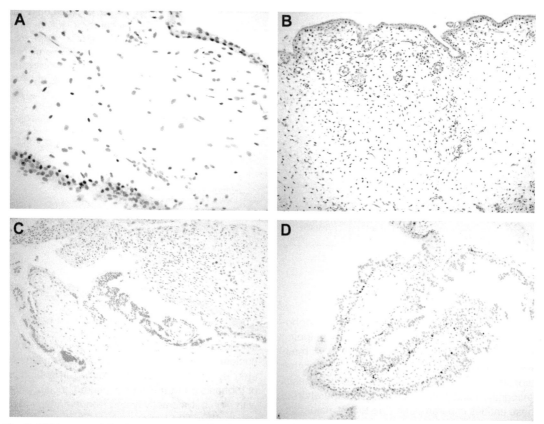

Fig. 5. P57 immunostain demonstrates retained nuclear expression in villous cytotrophoblast and stromal cells in nonmolar abortions (*A*) and in partial moles (*B*), whereas p57 is negative in the same cell types in complete moles (*C*). (Note the presence of internal positive control in decidua in the upper right portion of image.) Discordant p57 pattern (*D*) may be observed in some complete moles due to androgenetic/biparental mosaicism or relaxation of genomic imprinting.

Fig. 6. Short tandem repeat genotyping of hydatidiform moles. (*A*) Dispermic (heterozygous) complete mole shows 2 unique paternal alleles and absence of maternal alleles at several loci (**). (*B*) Dispermic (heterozygous) partial mole with 2 paternal alleles (***) or 1 paternal allele in duplicate quantity (*) in addition to 1 maternal allele at several loci.

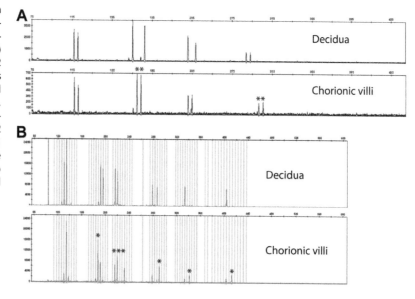

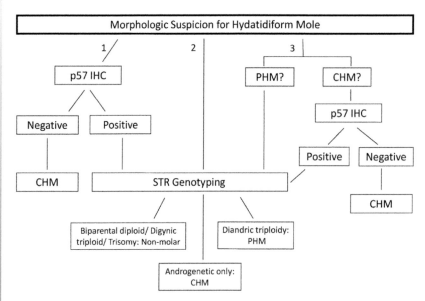

Fig. 7. Prposed diagnostic algorithms for hydatidiform moles. CHM, complete hydatidiform mole; IHC, immunohistochemistry; PHM, partial hydatidiform mole; STR, short tandem repeat.

chorion laeve—ETT; or implantation site trophoblast—PSTT. They often have overlapping morphologic features with each other, with reactive trophoblastic proliferations, and with other neoplasms of nongestational pathogenesis. Recognition and precise diagnostic separation of these entities is paramount, due to the major clinical differences in their therapeutic approaches and prognostic implications.

GESTATIONAL CHORIOCARCINOMA

CLINICAL AND GROSS FEATURES

Gestational choriocarcinoma usually presents during the reproductive years (mean age: 30 years), following a CHM, term pregnancy, or nonmolar abortion.[63–65] The average time interval between choriocarcinoma and the antecedent gestation is 1 to 3 months after a term pregnancy and 13 months after a complete mole, but rarely it may be over 20 years.[66] Most patients present with vaginal bleeding, although the first presentation may also be extrauterine hemorrhage from distant metastases (ie, lung, brain, liver, kidney, or gastrointestinal tract).[67] The serum beta-hCG level is typically very high, exceeding 10,000 mIU/mL[68] (**Box 4**).

On gross examination, the tumor forms a bulky, extensively hemorrhagic, and necrotic mass lesion within the uterus or in the fallopian tube or ovary if it is arising from an ectopic pregnancy.[69,70] Intraplacental choriocarcinoma may rarely be identified as a small hemorrhagic lesion within a term placenta.[71–73]

MICROSCOPIC FEATURES

Choriocarcinoma is composed of sheets of mononuclear trophoblastic cells rimmed by multinucleated syncytiotrophoblasts growing in a biphasic or triphasic pattern. There is marked nuclear atypia with high mitotic activity and frequent atypical mitoses. Abundant tumor necrosis and hemorrhage are also characteristic (**Fig. 8**).

Although the traditional histopathological definition of choriocarcinoma requires absence of chorionic villi, rare cases of CHM may be associated with exuberant biphasic trophoblastic proliferation with marked cytologic atypia and have been termed "emerging" or "in situ" choriocarcinoma.[74,75] In addition, intraplacental choriocarcinoma is expected to have chorionic villi in the vicinity of the tumor, and sometimes entrapped within the lesion. This is an evolving entity with no definitive cut-off for size or other distinct morphologic parameters at the time of this review.

IMMUNOHISTOCHEMISTRY

Choriocarcinoma is typically positive for cytokeratins, GATA3, inhibin, and hCG, and shows variable staining with hPL, p63, and p40.[76–79] Expression of SALL4—a frequently used germ cell marker—has also been reported in gestational choriocarcinomas.[80,81]

DIFFERENTIAL DIAGNOSIS

Gestational choriocarcinoma needs to be distinguished from other gestational trophoblastic tumors—ETT and PSTT—and from nongestational

---

Box 3
Recommended diagnostic write-up for molar and nonmolar aneuploid gestations

Complete Hydatidiform Mole

Final Diagnosis: Complete Hydatidiform Mole. See note.

Note (option 1): By immunohistochemistry, there is loss of p57 expression in cytotrophoblast and villous stroma (with adequate positive control staining). These results support the above diagnosis.

Note (option 2): By immunohistochemistry, there is loss of p57 expression in cytotrophoblast and villous stroma (with adequate positive control staining). Short tandem repeat genotyping shows [homozygous/heterozygous] diandric diploidy. These results are confirmatory of the above diagnosis.

Partial Hydatidiform Mole (confirmed or suspected)

Final Diagnosis: Partial Hydatidiform Mole. See note.

Note (option 1): By immunohistochemistry, there is retained p57 expression in cytotrophoblast and villous stroma (with adequate internal controls). Short tandem repeat genotyping shows [homozygous/heterozygous] diandric monogynic triploidy. These results are confirmatory of the above diagnosis.

Final Diagnosis: Mildly hydropic chorionic villi with abnormal villous morphology. See note.

Note (option 1): By immunohistochemistry, there is retained p57 expression in cytotrophoblast and villous stroma (with adequate internal controls). The differential diagnosis includes partial hydatidiform mole versus nonmolar gestation. Short tandem repeat genotyping is recommended if clinically indicated.

Note (option 2): By immunohistochemistry, there is retained p57 expression in cytotrophoblast and villous stroma (with adequate internal controls). Ploidy analysis by [karyotype/in situ hybridization/microarray] reveals triploidy. The differential diagnosis includes partial hydatidiform mole versus nonmolar triploidy (monoandric digynic). Short tandem repeat genotyping is recommended for definitive diagnosis.

Nonmolar Aneuploidy

Final Diagnosis: Mildly hydropic chorionic villi with abnormal villous morphology consistent with nonmolar aneuploidy. See note.

Note (option 1): By immunohistochemistry, there is retained p57 expression in cytotrophoblast and villous stroma (with adequate internal controls). [Short tandem repeat genotyping/karyotype/in situ hybridization/microarray] testing shows a biparental diploid chromosomal content with [trisomy/monosomy] of chromosome [13/18/21/X, other]. These results are confirmatory of the above diagnosis.

---

tumors of germ cell or somatic origin exhibiting trophoblastic differentiation.

ETT and PSTT are gestational neoplasms of intermediate trophoblastic origin with unique clinicopathologic features. Both tumors typically arise from a prior term gestation and present with amenorrhea or abnormal vaginal bleeding often years after the index pregnancy. The serum beta-hCG level may be elevated, but it is much lower compared with the levels seen in choriocarcinoma (**Table 1**). Histologically, the degree of nuclear atypia and the amount of necrosis and hemorrhage are less pronounced than those of choriocarcinoma. In addition, differences in the tumor immunoprofiles can also be used to facilitate the diagnostic distinction (**Table 2**).

The differential diagnosis of gestational choriocarcinoma also includes nongestational choriocarcinoma of germ cell origin and somatic carcinomas with trophoblastic differentiation, which have marked differences in their clinical management and prognosis. The morphology and immunophenotype of both types of choriocarcinoma are essentially identical. However, nongestational choriocarcinoma may be a part of a mixed germ cell tumor containing other nonchoriocarcinomatous components and somatic carcinomas with trophoblastic differentiation usually also contain a distinct somatic carcinoma component (eg, adenocarcinoma), although it may be focal and may be missed in a small biopsy. Nongestational pathogenesis can be determined

---

Box 4
Gestational choriocarcinoma—pathologic key features

Clinical presentation

- Usually presents during the reproductive years (mean 30 years) with vaginal bleeding
- May follow a CHM, term pregnancy, or nonmolar abortion
- Interval is 1 to 3 months after a term pregnancy and 13 months after CHM
- Very high serum beta-hCG levels (>10,000 mIU/mL)

Gross appearance

- Bulky mass lesion with extensive hemorrhage and necrosis

Microscopic features

- Sheets of mononuclear trophoblasts rimmed by syncytiotrophoblasts in a biphasic or triphasic pattern
- Marked nuclear atypia
- High mitotic activity with frequent atypical mitoses
- Abundant necrosis and hemorrhage

Immunohistochemistry

- Positive for cytokeratins, GATA3, inhibin, hCG, and SALL4
- Variable staining with hPL, p63, and p40

Differential diagnosis

- Epithelioid trophoblastic tumor (ETT)
- Placental site trophoblastic tumor (PSTT)
- Nongestational choriocarcinoma of germ cell origin
- Somatic carcinoma with trophoblastic differentiation

Prognosis

- Highly chemosensitive
- Overall survival rate 90% to 100%

---

based on the clinicopathologic features in some cases: choriocarcinoma in a prepubertal patient is germ cell derived, whereas older age, postmenopausal status, and lower serum beta-hCG levels are in favor of somatic origin. Uterine location and a recent gestational event (especially CHM) are essentially consistent with gestational origin. In equivocal cases, STR genotyping should be considered to provide definitive determination of gestational versus nongestational etiology by identifying the presence or absence of unique paternal alleles in the tumor compared with the patient's normal tissues.[70,78,82]

PROGNOSIS

The WHO scoring system and FIGO staging is used for the evaluation of the risk level of GTN based on various clinical factors.[83] Gestational choriocarcinoma is highly chemosensitive and responds well to single-agent or combination chemotherapy, with overall survival rates approaching 100% for low risk (FIGO stages I-III: score <7), and approximately 90% for high-risk disease (FIGO stages II-III WHO score >=7, and FIGO stage IV).[63]

EPITHELIOID TROPHOBLASTIC TUMOR

CLINICAL AND GROSS FEATURES

ETT—a gestational trophoblastic neoplasm arising from chorion laeve intermediate trophoblast—typically occurs in patients aged between 15 and 48 years most commonly following a full-term pregnancy and less often after a spontaneous abortion or a hydatidiform mole.[84] The average latency period between the antecedent gestation and ETT is 6 years (range: 1–25 years) (see Table 1). Patients may present with abnormal vaginal bleeding and the serum beta-hCG may be mildly elevated (Box 5). Macroscopically the tumor forms a discrete nodule or mass, often involving the lower uterine segment or cervix, ranging between

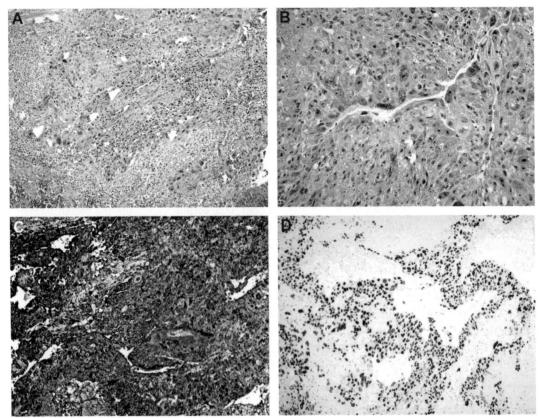

Fig. 8. Gestational choriocarcinoma is characterized by a biphasic or triphasic growth of markedly atypical trophoblastic cells with abundant hemorrhage and necrosis (*A, B*). The tumor cells are diffusely positive for hCG (*C*) and GATA3 (*D*) immunostains.

0.5 and 5 cm with white-tan to brown cut surfaces and foci of hemorrhage and necrosis.[84–86] Ulceration and fistula formation may also be present.

MICROSCOPIC FEATURES

ETT is composed of well-circumscribed, expansile proliferation of nests, cords, and sheets of relatively uniform medium-sized trophoblastic cells (**Fig. 9**). The tumor cells have round nuclei with small nucleoli, eosinophilic to clear cytoplasm, and distinct cell membranes. Eosinophilic hyaline-like material may be present and geographic necrosis and focal calcification are common.[87] The mitotic activity ranges from 0 to 47/10 high power field (HPF; average 2/10 HPF). The tumor may colonize the cervical mucosal surface mimicking a high-grade squamous intraepithelial lesion.

IMMUNOHISTOCHEMISTRY

ETTs are generally positive for cytokeratins, inhibin, GATA3, p63, and p40 immunostains (see **Table 2**). hPL and hCG are only focally expressed,

SALL4 is negative, and the Ki-67 labeling index is between 10% and 25% in most cases.[81,88–90]

DIFFERENTIAL DIAGNOSIS

In addition to other gestational trophoblastic tumors, choriocarcinoma and PSTT (see **Tables 1** and **2**), the differential diagnosis of ETT also includes other chorionic-type intermediate trophoblastic proliferations: placental site nodule (PSN) and atypical placental site nodule (APSN). Unlike ETT, PSN is small, typically measuring less than 0.5 cm, and most commonly it is an incidental finding in endometrial or endocervical curettings.[91] The cellularity is variable, and zonation with a hyalinized center is often present. Mild nuclear atypia and nuclear pseudoinclusions may be seen, but mitotic figures are rare or absent. The immunoprofile of PSN is similar to ETT, except the Ki-67 proliferation index is lower (<5%), and cyclin E is negative in contrast to the strong expression in ETT.[92] Lesions with intermediate microscopic features between ETT and PSN—size between 5 and 10 mm, increased cellularity, moderate nuclear atypia, presence of mitotic figures and Ki-67

Table 1
Clinicopathologic characteristics of gestational trophoblastic tumors

	CC	ETT	PSTT
Clinical presentation	Vaginal bleeding, persistent GTD	Vaginal bleeding	Vaginal bleeding
Time interval from antecedent pregnancy	Mean: 2 mo (term pregnancy) and 13 mo (CHM)	1–25 y (mean: 6 y)	2 weeks-17 years (median: 12–18 mo)
Pretreatment hCG (mIU/mL)	>10,000	<3000	<1000
Gross findings	Destructive, hemorrhagic mass	Expansile, circumscribed mass	Infiltrative mass
Location	Uterine corpus	Cervix, LUS, corpus	Uterine corpus
Cell of origin	Villous IT, cytotrophoblast, syncytiotrophoblast	Chorion laeve IT (chorionic IT at fetal membranes)	Implantation site IT
Growth pattern	Infiltrative	Expansile, pushing border	Infiltrative
Necrosis	Extensive	Extensive, geographic	Focal
Nuclear atypia	Marked	Mild to moderate	Moderate to marked
Multinucleated cells	Common (syncytiotrophoblast)	Rare	Common (implantation site IT)
Vasculature	No intrinsic vessels	No vessel wall invasion	Tumor cells invade and replace vessel walls

Abbreviations: CC, choriocarcinoma; CHM, complete hydatidiform mole; ETT, epithelioid trophoblastic tumor; GTD, gestational trophoblastic disease; IT, intermediate trophoblast; LUS, lower uterine segment; PSTT, placental site trophoblastic tumor.

proliferation index between 5% and 10%—have been termed APSN and have been postulated to be a precursor to ETT.[84,87,88,93]

The nuclear atypia, nested arrangement of tumor cells, hyalinized eosinophilic material, and frequent involvement of cervix and lower uterine segment in ETT may also mimic a cervical squamous cell carcinoma (SCC). The immunohistochemical profiles show a considerable overlap between the 2 entities: both are positive for cytokeratins, p63, and p40.[88] GATA3, which is typically positive in all trophoblastic tumors, also stains

Table 2
Immunohistochemistry in the differential diagnosis of gestational trophoblastic tumors

	CC	ETT	PSTT	SCC
Cytokeratins (AE1/AE3, CAM5.2)	+	+	+	+
P63	+/−	+	-	+
P40	+/−	+	-	+
GATA3	+	+	+	+/−
Inhibin	+	+	+	-
hPL	+ (IT)	+ (focal)	+ (diffuse)	-
hCG	+ (diffuse)	+ (focal)	+ (focal)	-
P16	-	-	-	+ (strong, diffuse)
SALL4	+	-	-	-
Ki-67	>90%	>10%	10%–30%	Variable

Abbreviations: CC, choriocarcinoma; ETT, epithelioid trophoblastic tumor; PSTT, placental site trophoblastic tumor; SCC, squamous cell carcinoma; IT, intermediate trophoblast.

Box 5
Epithelioid trophoblastic tumor—pathologic key features

Clinical presentation

- Presents between 15 and 48 years of age usually with abnormal vaginal bleeding
- Most often follows a full-term pregnancy
- Average interval from antecedent gestation is 6 years
- Serum beta-hCG level may be mildly elevated

Gross appearance

- Well-circumscribed 0.5 to 5 cm mass
- Often involves the lower uterine segment or cervix
- White-tan to brown cut surface with foci of hemorrhage and necrosis

Microscopic features

- Expansile nests, cords, and sheets of relatively uniform trophoblastic cells
- Eosinophilic to clear cytoplasm
- Average mitotic activity is 2/10 HPF (range: 0–47/10 HPF)
- Eosinophilic hyaline-like material and geographic necrosis

Immunohistochemistry

- Positive cytokeratins, inhibin, GATA3, p63, and p40
- Focal hPL and hCG
- Negative SALL4
- Ki-67 index 10% to 25%

Differential diagnosis

- Gestational choriocarcinoma
- Placental site trophoblastic tumor (PSTT)
- Squamous cell carcinoma
- Placental site nodule/Atypical placental site nodule

Prognosis

- Distant metastases in 25% of patients
- Approximately 10% of patients may die of the disease
- Primary treatment is surgical, chemotherapy/immunotherapy is reserved for recurrent or metastatic tumors

---

approximately one-third of cervical SCC.[94] P16, on the other hand, is usually strongly positive in cervical SCC and negative in ETT.[92] Genotyping offers a definitive separation of ETT from somatic carcinomas, including cervical SCC, by demonstrating the presence of unique paternal alleles in the tumor.[95]

PROGNOSIS

ETT is a malignant neoplasm with potential for spreading to adjacent extrauterine structures (ie, bladder, ureter, and vagina) and local recurrence. Distant metastases have been reported in 25% of

patients, and approximately 10% of patients die of the disease. The primary treatment is surgical–total hysterectomy with pelvic lymph node dissection, and chemotherapy is usually reserved for recurrent or metastatic tumors.[84,85] Immunotherapy has also been recently found to be a promising treatment option for ETT and PSTT.[96,97]

PLACENTAL SITE TROPHOBLASTIC TUMOR

CLINICAL AND GROSS FEATURES

PSTT is a neoplastic proliferation of implantation site intermediate trophoblast, typically presenting

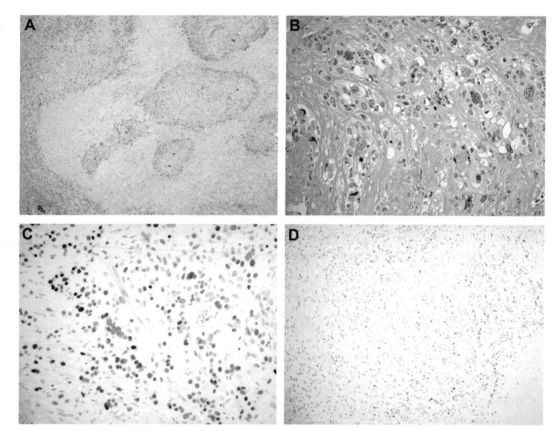

Fig. 9. Epithelioid trophoblastic tumor forms expansile nests with eosinophilic hyalin-like material and geographic necrosis (*A*). Nuclear atypia and abundant eosinophilic to clear cytoplasm are also characteristic (*B*). The tumor cells are diffusely positive for p63 immunostain (*C*) and show an increased Ki-67 proliferation index (*D*).

during the reproductive years with vaginal bleeding, amenorrhea, or abdominal pain several months after the antecedent pregnancy (median latency period: 12–18 months, range: 2 weeks–17 years)[98] (**Box 6**, see **Table 1**). The serum beta-hCG level may be mildly elevated and imaging studies show a uterine mass lesion. Grossly the tumor size ranges between 1 and 10 cm (mean: 5 cm) with fleshy, light tan-yellow cut surfaces and infiltrative borders, often with foci of hemorrhage and necrosis.[99,100] Deep myometrial involvement is present in 50% of patients and transmural invasion with perforation may also occur.

MICROSCOPIC FEATURES

The tumor cells in PSTT are large, predominantly mononuclear intermediate trophoblasts that form variably sized cords and sheets. Multinucleated tumor cells are also present and are usually irregularly distributed throughout the tumor. The tumor has a characteristic infiltrative growth pattern, separating the myometrial smooth muscle fibers

and replacing vessel walls while maintaining the overall vascular architecture (**Fig. 10**). There is moderate to marked nuclear atypia with hyperchromasia, nuclear pseudoinclusions, and conspicuous nucleoli. The cytoplasm is abundant, and may appear amphophilic, eosinophilic, or less often clear. The mitotic activity ranges between 0 and 22/10 HPF, falling between 2 and 4 mitoses/10 HPF in most tumors.[87]

IMMUNOHISTOCHEMISTRY

The tumor cells in PSTT diffusely express cytokeratins, inhibin, GATA3, and hPL, whereas hCG expression is only focal (see **Table 2**). Glypican-3 expression has also been reported in PSTT; however, SALL4, p63, and p40 immunostains are negative.[81,101–103] The Ki-67 proliferation index is usually 10% to 30%.

DIFFERENTIAL DIAGNOSIS

The differential diagnosis of PSTT includes other gestational trophoblastic tumors—ETT and

Box 6
Placental site trophoblastic tumor—pathologic key features

Clinical presentation

- Presents during the reproductive years
- Symptoms include vaginal bleeding, amenorrhea, or abdominal pain
- Median latency period is 12 to 18 months after the antecedent pregnancy
- Serum beta-hCG level may be mildly elevated

Gross appearance

- Infiltrative mass lesion
- Tumor size between 1 and 10 cm (mean: 5 cm)
- Fleshy, light tan-yellow cut surface
- Focal hemorrhage and necrosis

Microscopic features

- Infiltrative growth pattern
- Cords and sheets of large mononuclear intermediate trophoblasts
- Multinucleated trophoblasts in an irregular distribution
- Replacement of vessel walls
- Moderate to marked nuclear atypia with hyperchromasia
- Abundant amphophilic or eosinophilic cytoplasm
- Average mitotic activity 2-4/10 HPF (range: 0–22/10 HPF)

Immunohistochemistry

- Positive cytokeratins, inhibin, GATA3, hPL, and glypican-3
- Focal hCG expression
- Negative SALL4, p63, and p40
- Ki-67 index 10% to 30%

Differential diagnosis

- Gestational choriocarcinoma
- Epithelioid trophoblastic tumor (ETT)
- Exaggerated placental site

Prognosis

- Capacity for locally aggressive behavior, recurrence, and rarely for distant metastases
- Recurrence rate is 25% to 30%
- Primary treatment is surgical, chemotherapy/immunotherapy is used in advanced stage or recurrent tumors

choriocarcinoma—and reactive proliferation of implantation site intermediate trophoblasts, exaggerated placental site (EPS). ETT is usually well-circumscribed, often involving the cervix or lower uterine segment, whereas PSTT forms an infiltrative mass lesion in the uterine corpus. Similarly, the microscopic growth pattern of ETT is expansile in contrast with the infiltrative growth of PSTT. In addition, the tumor cells invade and replace vessel walls in PSTT, recapitulating a normal implantation site, whereas vascular wall invasion is absent in ETT. Compared with choriocarcinoma, the biphasic cellular appearance is absent and the degree of nuclear pleomorphism and mitotic activity, and the extent of necrosis is typically much less in PSTT. The immunohistochemical differences among gestational trophoblastic tumors are listed in **Table 2**.

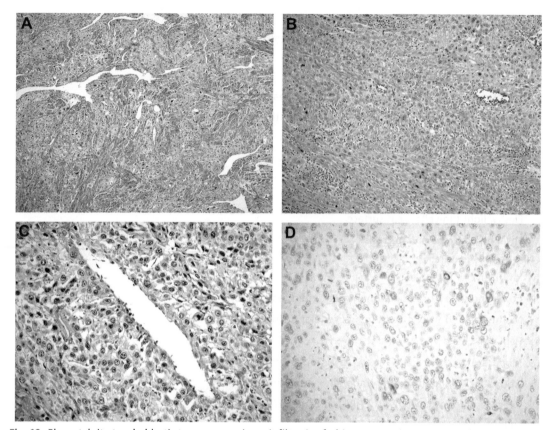

Fig. 10. Placental site trophoblastic tumor grows in an infiltrative fashion, separating myometrial smooth muscle fibers (*A*, *B*). The tumor cells form cords and sheets and replace existing vessel walls (*C*). hPL immunostain is weakly positive (*D*).

Unlike PSTT, EPS does not form a mass lesion and is invariably associated with a concurrent pregnancy. Additional helpful diagnostic clues in favor of EPS over PSTT include even distribution of the multinucleated cells (in contrast to irregular distribution in PSTT), presence of chorionic villi, and lack of necrosis and mitotic activity. Immuno-histochemistry is usually less useful in this setting, although the Ki-67 proliferation index is lower (<2%) in EPS, whereas it exceeds 10% in PSTT.[104]

PROGNOSIS

PSTT has a capacity for locally aggressive behavior, recurrence, and rarely for distant metas-tases, involving the lung or liver.[105,106] The recur-rence rate is reportedly between 25% and 30%, and half of patients with recurrence eventually die of the disease. The most important prognostic factor is FIGO stage, although prolonged interval (over 2 years) since the antecedent gestation, pa-tient age over 35 years, a prior term pregnancy, high mitotic activity, and large tumor size and ne-crosis have also been shown to correlate with

poor outcome. Most patients are successfully treated with surgery alone; however, advanced stage or recurrent tumors require chemotherapy. In addition, immunotherapy has also emerged as a novel treatment option for these tumors.[96,97]

CLINICS CARE POINTS

- Hydatidiform moles are fundamentally defined by their genetic composition

- Complete moles carry a 20% to 25% risk for persistent/invasive mole and 3% to 5% risk for gestational choriocarcinoma

- Risk of postmolar GTD/GTN is approximately 3-fold for heterozygous CHM compared with homozygous CHM

- Risk of persistent/invasive mole after a partial mole is 4% to 5%, gestational choriocarci-noma develops after less than 0.5% of PHM cases

- Morphologic features are not reliable for diagnostic separation of PHM from its mimics (particularly nonmolar aneuploid gestations)

- An algorithmic diagnostic approach is recommended for molar gestations. The highest degree of accuracy is obtained by using p57 immunohistochemistry and STR genotyping. Karyotype, in situ hybridization, and other forms of ploidy analysis offer inferior performance but can be helpful in narrowing the differential diagnosis depending on the local resources

- Gestational trophoblastic tumors need to be differentiated from reactive trophoblastic proliferations and from neoplasms of nongestational origin, due to the significant therapeutic and prognostic implications

- Gestational choriocarcinoma may have an unusual presentation—long time interval after pregnancy, distant metastases—and requires a high index of suspicion for prompt and accurate diagnosis and treatment

DISCLOSURE

The author has nothing to disclose.

REFERENCES

1. Kajii T, Ohama K. Androgenetic origin of hydatidiform mole. Nature 1977;268(5621):633–4.
2. Hui P, Buza N, Murphy KM, et al. Hydatidiform moles: genetic basis and precision diagnosis. Annu Rev Pathol 2017;12:449–85.
3. Bifulco C, Johnson C, Hao L, et al. Genotypic analysis of hydatidiform mole: an accurate and practical method of diagnosis. Am J Surg Pathol 2008; 32(3):445–51.
4. Fukunaga M, Endo Y, Ushigome S. Clinicopathologic study of tetraploid hydropic villous tissues. Arch Pathol Lab Med 1996;120(6):569–72.
5. Murdoch S, Djuric U, Mazhar B, et al. Mutations in NALP7 cause recurrent hydatidiform moles and reproductive wastage in humans. Nat Genet 2006;38(3):300–2.
6. Qian J, Deveault C, Bagga R, et al. Women heterozygous for NALP7/NLRP7 mutations are at risk for reproductive wastage: report of two novel mutations. Hum Mutat 2007;28(7):741.
7. Parry DA, Logan CV, Hayward BE, et al. Mutations causing familial biparental hydatidiform mole implicate c6orf221 as a possible regulator of genomic imprinting in the human oocyte. Am J Hum Genet 2011;89(3):451–8.
8. Moglabey YB, Kircheisen R, Seoud M, et al. Genetic mapping of a maternal locus responsible for familial hydatidiform moles. Hum Mol Genet 1999; 8(4):667–71.
9. Akoury E, Zhang L, Ao A, et al. NLRP7 and KHDC3L, the two maternal-effect proteins responsible for recurrent hydatidiform moles, co-localize to the oocyte cytoskeleton. Hum Reprod 2015; 30(1):159–69.
10. Rezaei M, Nguyen NM, Foroughinia L, et al. Two novel mutations in the KHDC3L gene in Asian patients with recurrent hydatidiform mole. Hum Genome Var 2016;3:16027.
11. Lawler SD, Fisher RA, Pickthall VJ, et al. Genetic studies on hydatidiform moles. I. The origin of partial moles. Cancer Genet Cytogenet 1982;5(4): 309–20.
12. Zaragoza MV, Surti U, Redline RW, et al. Parental origin and phenotype of triploidy in spontaneous abortions: predominance of diandry and association with the partial hydatidiform mole. Am J Hum Genet 2000;66(6):1807–20.
13. McFadden DE, Robinson WP. Phenotype of triploid embryos. J Med Genet 2006;43(7):609–12.
14. Szulman AE, Philippe E, Boue JG, et al. Human triploidy: association with partial hydatidiform moles and nonmolar conceptuses. Hum Pathol 1981;12(11):1016–21.
15. Surti U, Szulman AE, Wagner K, et al. Tetraploid partial hydatidiform moles: two cases with a triple paternal contribution and a 92,XXXY karyotype. Hum Genet 1986;72(1):15–21.
16. Sheppard DM, Fisher RA, Lawler SD, et al. Tetraploid conceptus with three paternal contributions. Hum Genet 1982;62(4):371–4.
17. Murphy KM, Descipio C, Wagenfuehr J, et al. Tetraploid partial hydatidiform mole: a case report and review of the literature. Int J Gynecol Pathol 2012; 31(1):73–9.
18. Bynum J, Batista D, Xian R, et al. Tetraploid partial hydatidiform moles: molecular genotyping and determination of parental contributions. J Mol Diagn 2020;22(1):90–100.
19. Xing D, Adams E, Huang J, et al. Refined diagnosis of hydatidiform moles with p57 immunohistochemistry and molecular genotyping: updated analysis of a prospective series of 2217 cases. Mod Pathol 2021;34(5):961–82.
20. Szulman AE, Surti U. The syndromes of hydatidiform mole. I. Cytogenetic and morphologic correlations. Am J Obstet Gynecol 1978;131(6): 665–71.
21. Genest DR. Partial hydatidiform mole: clinicopathological features, differential diagnosis, ploidy and molecular studies, and gold standards for diagnosis. Int J Gynecol Pathol 2001;20(4):315–22.
22. Doshi N, Surti U, Szulman AE. Morphologic anomalies in triploid liveborn fetuses. Hum Pathol 1983; 14(8):716–23.

23. Daniel A, Wu Z, Bennetts B, et al. Karyotype, phenotype and parental origin in 19 cases of triploidy. Prenat Diagn 2001;21(12):1034–48.

24. Fisher RA, Paradinas FJ, Soteriou BA, et al. Diploid hydatidiform moles with fetal red blood cells in molar villi. 2–Genetics. J Pathol 1997;181(2):189–95.

25. Fukunaga M. Histopathologic study of partial hydatidiform moles and DNA triploid placentas. Pathol Int 1994;44(7):528–34.

26. Sebire NJ, Fisher RA, Rees HC. Histopathological diagnosis of partial and complete hydatidiform mole in the first trimester of pregnancy. Pediatr Dev Pathol 2003;6(1):69–77.

27. Buza N, Hui P. Partial hydatidiform mole: histologic parameters in correlation with DNA genotyping. Int J Gynecol Pathol 2013;32(3):307–15.

28. Lipata F, Parkash V, Talmor M, et al. Precise DNA genotyping diagnosis of hydatidiform mole. Obstet Gynecol 2010;115(4):784–94.

29. Wilson Y, Bharat C, Crook ML, et al. Histological comparison of partial hydatidiform mole and trisomy gestation specimens. Pathology 2016;48(6):550–4.

30. Colgan TJ, Chang MC, Nanji S, et al. DNA genotyping of suspected partial hydatidiform moles detects clinically significant aneuploidy. Int J Gynecol Pathol 2017;36(3):217–21.

31. Kaiser-Rogers KA, McFadden DE, Livasy CA, et al. Androgenetic/biparental mosaicism causes placental mesenchymal dysplasia. J Med Genet 2006;43(2):187–92.

32. Xing D, Miller K, Beierl K, et al. Loss of p57 expression in conceptions other than complete hydatidiform mole: a case series with emphasis on the etiology, genetics, and clinical significance. Am J Surg Pathol 2022;46(1):18–32.

33. Buza N, Hui P. Gestational trophoblastic disease: histopathological diagnosis in the molecular era. Diagn Histopathol 2010;16(11):526–37.

34. Buza N, Hui P. Egg donor pregnancy: a potential pitfall in DNA genotyping diagnosis of hydatidiform moles. Int J Gynecol Pathol 2014;33(5):507–10.

35. Joseph NM, Pineda C, Rabban JT. DNA genotyping of nonmolar donor egg pregnancies with abnormal villous morphology: allele zygosity patterns prevent misinterpretation as complete hydatidiform mole. Int J Gynecol Pathol 2018;37(2):191–7.

36. Fukunaga M, Katabuchi H, Nagasaka T, et al. Interobserver and intraobserver variability in the diagnosis of hydatidiform mole. Am J Surg Pathol 2005;29(7):942–7.

37. Chilosi M, Piazzola E, Lestani M, et al. Differential expression of p57kip2, a maternally imprinted cdk inhibitor, in normal human placenta and gestational trophoblastic disease. Lab Invest 1998;78(3):269–76.

38. Fukunaga M. Immunohistochemical characterization of p57(KIP2) expression in early hydatidiform moles. Hum Pathol 2002;33(12):1188–92.

39. Merchant SH, Amin MB, Viswanatha DS, et al. p57KIP2 immunohistochemistry in early molar pregnancies: emphasis on its complementary role in the differential diagnosis of hydropic abortuses. Hum Pathol 2005;36(2):180–6.

40. McConnell TG, Murphy KM, Hafez M, et al. Diagnosis and subclassification of hydatidiform moles using p57 immunohistochemistry and molecular genotyping: validation and prospective analysis in routine and consultation practice settings with development of an algorithmic approach. Am J Surg Pathol 2009;33(6):805–17.

41. Buza N, Hui P. Immunohistochemistry and other ancillary techniques in the diagnosis of gestational trophoblastic diseases. Semin Diagn Pathol 2014;31(3):223–32.

42. Fisher RA, Nucci MR, Thaker HM, et al. Complete hydatidiform mole retaining a chromosome 11 of maternal origin: molecular genetic analysis of a case. Mod Pathol 2004;17(9):1155–60.

43. McConnell TG, Norris-Kirby A, Hagenkord JM, et al. Complete hydatidiform mole with retained maternal chromosomes 6 and 11. Am J Surg Pathol 2009;33(9):1409–15.

44. DeScipio C, Haley L, Beierl K, et al. Diandric triploid hydatidiform mole with loss of maternal chromosome 11. Am J Surg Pathol 2011;35(10):1586–91.

45. Lewis GH, DeScipio C, Murphy KM, et al. Characterization of androgenetic/biparental mosaic/chimeric conceptions, including those with a molar component: morphology, p57 immnohistochemistry, molecular genotyping, and risk of persistent gestational trophoblastic disease. Int J Gynecol Pathol 2013;32(2):199–214.

46. Hoffner L, Dunn J, Esposito N, et al. P57KIP2 immunostaining and molecular cytogenetics: combined approach aids in diagnosis of morphologically challenging cases with molar phenotype and in detecting androgenetic cell lines in mosaic/chimeric conceptions. Hum Pathol 2008;39(1):63–72.

47. Buza N, McGregor SM, Barroilhet L, et al. Paternal uniparental isodisomy of tyrosine hydroxylase locus at chromosome 11p15.4: spectrum of phenotypical presentations simulating hydatidiform moles. Mod Pathol 2019;32(8):1180–8.

48. Genest DR, Dorfman DM, Castrillon DH. Ploidy and imprinting in hydatidiform moles. Complementary use of flow cytometry and immunohistochemistry of the imprinted gene product p57KIP2 to assist molar classification. J Reprod Med 2002;47(5):342–6.

49. Alwaqfi R, Chang MC, Colgan TJ. Does Ki-67 have a role in the diagnosis of placental molar disease? Int J Gynecol Pathol 2020;39(1):1–7.

50. Much M, Buza N, Hui P. Tissue identity testing of cancer by short tandem repeat polymorphism: pitfalls of interpretation in the presence of microsatellite instability. Hum Pathol 2014;45(3):549–55.

51. Ronnett BM, DeScipio C, Murphy KM. Hydatidiform moles: ancillary techniques to refine diagnosis. Int J Gynecol Pathol 2011;30(2):101–16.

52. Buza N, Hui P. Genotyping diagnosis of gestational trophoblastic disease: frontiers in precision medicine. Mod Pathol 2021;34(9):1658–72.

53. Banet N, Descipio C, Murphy KM, et al. Characteristics of hydatidiform moles: analysis of a prospective series with p57 immunohistochemistry and molecular genotyping. Mod Pathol 2014;27(2):238–54.

54. Horowitz NS, Eskander RN, Adelman MR, et al. Epidemiology, diagnosis, and treatment of gestational trophoblastic disease: a society of gynecologic oncology evidenced-based review and recommendation. Gynecol Oncol 2021;163(3):605–13.

55. Seckl MJ, Sebire NJ, Berkowitz RS. Gestational trophoblastic disease. Lancet 2010;376(9742):717–29.

56. Baasanjav B, Usui H, Kihara M, et al. The risk of post-molar gestational trophoblastic neoplasia is higher in heterozygous than in homozygous complete hydatidiform moles. Hum Reprod 2010;25(5):1183–91.

57. Khawajkie Y, Mechtouf N, Nguyen NMP, et al. Comprehensive analysis of 204 sporadic hydatidiform moles: revisiting risk factors and their correlations with the molar genotypes. Mod Pathol 2020;33(5):880–92.

58. Usui H, Qu J, Sato A, et al. Gestational trophoblastic neoplasia from genetically confirmed hydatidiform moles: prospective observational cohort study. Int J Gynecol Cancer 2018;28(9):1772–80.

59. Wake N, Seki T, Fujita H, et al. Malignant potential of homozygous and heterozygous complete moles. Cancer Res 1984;44(3):1226–30.

60. Wake N, Fujino T, Hoshi S, et al. The propensity to malignancy of dispermic heterozygous moles. Placenta 1987;8(3):319–26.

61. Lawler SD, Fisher RA, Dent J. A prospective genetic study of complete and partial hydatidiform moles. Am J Obstet Gynecol 1991;164(5 Pt 1):1270–7.

62. Zheng XZ, Qin XY, Chen SW, et al. Heterozygous/dispermic complete mole confers a significantly higher risk for post-molar gestational trophoblastic disease. Mod Pathol 2020;33(10):1979–88.

63. Lurain JR. Gestational trophoblastic disease II: classification and management of gestational trophoblastic neoplasia. Am J Obstet Gynecol 2011;204(1):11–8.

64. Hui P. Gestational trophoblastic disease : diagnostic and molecular genetic pathology. New York: Springer; 2012.

65. Soper JT. Gestational trophoblastic disease. Obstet Gynecol 2006;108(1):176–87.

66. O'Neill CJ, Houghton F, Clarke J, et al. Uterine gestational choriocarcinoma developing after a long latent period in a postmenopausal woman: the value of DNA polymorphism studies. Int J Surg Pathol 2008;16(2):226–9.

67. Horn LC, Bilek K. Clinicopathologic analysis of gestational trophoblastic disease–report of 158 cases. Gen Diagn Pathol 1997;143(2–3):173–8.

68. Smith HO, Kohorn E, Cole LA. Choriocarcinoma and gestational trophoblastic disease. Obstet Gynecol Clin North Am 2005;32(4):661–84.

69. Ober WB, Maier RC. Gestational choriocarcinoma of the fallopian tube. Diagn Gynecol Obstet 1981;3(3):213–31.

70. Savage J, Adams E, Veras E, et al. Choriocarcinoma in women: analysis of a case series with genotyping. Am J Surg Pathol 2017;41(12):1593–606.

71. Liu J, Guo L. Intraplacental choriocarcinoma in a term placenta with both maternal and infantile metastases: a case report and review of the literature. Gynecol Oncol 2006;103(3):1147–51.

72. Ganapathi KA, Paczos T, George MD, et al. Incidental finding of placental choriocarcinoma after an uncomplicated term pregnancy: a case report with review of the literature. Int J Gynecol Pathol 2010;29(5):476–8.

73. Fox H, Laurini RN. Intraplacental choriocarcinoma: a report of two cases. J Clin Pathol 1988;41(10):1085–8.

74. Fukunaga M, Nomura K, Ushigome S. Choriocarcinoma in situ at a first trimester. Report of two cases indicating an origin of trophoblast of a stem villus. Virchows Arch 1996;429(2–3):185–8.

75. Fukunaga M, Ushigome S, Ishikawa E. Choriocarcinoma in situ: a case at an early gestational stage. Histopathology 1995;27(5):473–6.

76. Banet N, Gown AM, Shih Ie M, et al. GATA-3 expression in trophoblastic tissues: an immunohistochemical study of 445 cases, including diagnostic utility. Am J Surg Pathol 2015;39(1):101–8.

77. Shih IM, Kurman RJ. Immunohistochemical localization of inhibin-alpha in the placenta and gestational trophoblastic lesions. Int J Gynecol Pathol 1999;18(2):144–50.

78. Buza N, Baine I, Hui P. Precision genotyping diagnosis of lung tumors with trophoblastic morphology in young women. Mod Pathol 2019;32(9):1271–80.

79. Mao TL, Kurman RJ, Huang CC, et al. Immunohistochemistry of choriocarcinoma: an aid in differential diagnosis and in elucidating pathogenesis. Am J Surg Pathol 2007;31(11):1726–32.

80. Miettinen M, Wang Z, McCue PA, et al. SALL4 expression in germ cell and non-germ cell tumors: a systematic immunohistochemical study of 3215 cases. Am J Surg Pathol 2014;38(3):410–20.

81. Stichelbout M, Devisme L, Franquet-Ansart H, et al. SALL4 expression in gestational trophoblastic tumors: a useful tool to distinguish choriocarcinoma from placental site trophoblastic tumor and epithelioid trophoblastic tumor. Hum Pathol 2016;54: 121–6.

82. Buza N, Rutherford T, Hui P. Genotyping diagnosis of nongestational choriocarcinoma involving fallopian tube and broad ligament: a case study. Int J Gynecol Pathol 2014;33(1):58–63.

83. Ngan HYS, Seckl MJ, Berkowitz RS, et al. Update on the diagnosis and management of gestational trophoblastic disease. Int J Gynaecol Obstet 2018;143(Suppl 2):79–85.

84. Shih IM, Kurman RJ. Epithelioid trophoblastic tumor: a neoplasm distinct from choriocarcinoma and placental site trophoblastic tumor simulating carcinoma. Am J Surg Pathol 1998;22(11): 1393–403.

85. Fadare O, Parkash V, Carcangiu ML, et al. Epithelioid trophoblastic tumor: clinicopathological features with an emphasis on uterine cervical involvement. Mod Pathol 2006;19(1):75–82.

86. Allison KH, Love JE, Garcia RL. Epithelioid trophoblastic tumor: review of a rare neoplasm of the chorionic-type intermediate trophoblast. Arch Pathol Lab Med 2006;130(12):1875–7.

87. Shih IM, Kurman RJ. The pathology of intermediate trophoblastic tumors and tumor-like lesions. Int J Gynecol Pathol 2001;20(1):31–47.

88. Shih Ie M. Trophogram, an immunohistochemistry-based algorithmic approach, in the differential diagnosis of trophoblastic tumors and tumorlike lesions. Ann Diagn Pathol 2007;11(3):228–34.

89. Shih IM, Kurman RJ. p63 expression is useful in the distinction of epithelioid trophoblastic and placental site trophoblastic tumors by profiling trophoblastic subpopulations. Am J Surg Pathol 2004;28(9):1177–83.

90. Mirkovic J, Elias K, Drapkin R, et al. GATA3 expression in gestational trophoblastic tissues and tumours. Histopathology 2015;67(5):636–44.

91. Young RH, Kurman RJ, Scully RE. Placental site nodules and plaques. A clinicopathologic analysis of 20 cases. Am J Surg Pathol 1990;14(11):1001–9.

92. Mao TL, Seidman JD, Kurman RJ, et al. Cyclin E and p16 immunoreactivity in epithelioid trophoblastic tumor–an aid in differential diagnosis. Am J Surg Pathol 2006;30(9):1105–10.

93. Kaur B, Short D, Fisher RA, et al. Atypical placental site nodule (APSN) and association with malignant gestational trophoblastic disease; a clinicopathologic study of 21 cases. Int J Gynecol Pathol 2015;34(2):152–8.

94. Chang A, Amin A, Gabrielson E, et al. Utility of GATA3 immunohistochemistry in differentiating urothelial carcinoma from prostate adenocarcinoma and squamous cell carcinomas of the uterine cervix, anus, and lung. Am J Surg Pathol 2012; 36(10):1472–6.

95. Xu ML, Yang B, Carcangiu ML, et al. Epithelioid trophoblastic tumor: comparative genomic hybridization and diagnostic DNA genotyping. Mod Pathol 2009;22(2):232–8.

96. Veras E, Kurman RJ, Wang TL, et al. PD-L1 expression in human placentas and gestational trophoblastic diseases. Int J Gynecol Pathol 2017;36(2): 146–53.

97. Bolze PA, Patrier S, Massardier J, et al. PD-L1 expression in premalignant and malignant trophoblasts from gestational trophoblastic diseases is ubiquitous and independent of clinical outcomes. Int J Gynecol Cancer 2017;27(3):554–61.

98. Horowitz NS, Goldstein DP, Berkowitz RS. Placental site trophoblastic tumors and epithelioid trophoblastic tumors: Biology, natural history, and treatment modalities. Gynecol Oncol 2017;144(1):208–14.

99. Young RH, Scully RE. Placental-site trophoblastic tumor: current status. Clin Obstet Gynecol 1984; 27(1):248–58.

100. Baergen RN, Rutgers JL, Young RH, et al. Placental site trophoblastic tumor: a study of 55 cases and review of the literature emphasizing factors of prognostic significance. Gynecol Oncol 2006;100(3):511–20.

101. Ou-Yang RJ, Hui P, Yang XJ, et al. Expression of glypican 3 in placental site trophoblastic tumor. Diagn Pathol 2010;5:64.

102. McCarthy WA, Paquette C, Gundogan F, et al. Comparison of p63 and p40 immunohistochemical stains to distinguish epithelioid trophoblastic tumor from other trophoblastic lesions. Int J Gynecol Pathol 2018;37(4):401–4.

103. Buza N, Hui P. Immunohistochemistry in gynecologic pathology: an example-based practical update. Arch Pathol Lab Med 2017;141(8):1052–71.

104. Ichikawa N, Zhai YL, Shiozawa T, et al. Immunohistochemical analysis of cell cycle regulatory gene products in normal trophoblast and placental site trophoblastic tumor. Int J Gynecol Pathol 1998; 17(3):235–40.

105. Papadopoulos AJ, Foskett M, Seckl MJ, et al. Twenty-five years' clinical experience with placental site trophoblastic tumors. J Reprod Med 2002;47(6):460–4.

106. Hassadia A, Gillespie A, Tidy J, et al. Placental site trophoblastic tumour: clinical features and management. Gynecol Oncol 2005;99(3):603–7.

Homologous Recombination Deficiency and Ovarian Cancer Treatment Decisions

Practical Implications for Pathologists for Tumor Typing and Reporting

Joseph T. Rabban, MD, MPH[a],*, Lee-May Chen, MD[b],
W. Patrick Devine, MD, PhD[c]

KEYWORDS

- Ovarian cancer • High-grade serous carcinoma • PARP inhibitor • DNA repair
- Homologous recombination deficiency

Key points

- Patients with ovarian cancer may benefit from adding poly(ADP-ribose)polymerase inhibitor therapy to platinum chemotherapy if the tumor exhibits homologous repair (HR) deficiency (HRD).
- Clinical tests for HRD evaluate tumor tissue for genomic evidence of impairment of the HR pathway of DNA damage repair, of which germline or somatic mutation of *BRCA1/2* is a major contributor.
- High-grade serous carcinoma (HGSC) is the ovarian tumor type most enriched for HRD.
- Accurate diagnosis of HGSC and distinction from its morphologic mimics are key ways that pathologists may contribute toward optimal management decisions for patient care.
- The pathologist should make every effort to correctly identify and report HGSC at the time of index diagnostic biopsy or excision; using less specific descriptive terms such as "carcinoma of gynecologic origin" or "Mullerian carcinoma" and deferring specific tumor typing to the main surgical debulking specimen may not be in the best interest for management decisions.

ABSTRACT

Clinical testing for homologous repair (HR) deficiency (HRD) in ovarian cancers has emerged as a means to tailor the use of poly(ADP-ribose)polymerase (PARP) inhibitor therapy to the patients most likely to respond. The currently available HRD tests evaluate tumor tissue for genomic evidence of impairment of the HR pathway of DNA damage repair, which, if present, renders the tumor vulnerable to PARP inhibitors in conjunction with platinum chemotherapy. Germline or somatic mutation of *BRCA1/2* is a major contributor HRD. Thus, tubo-ovarian/peritoneal

Funding sources: none.
[a] Surgical Pathology Division, Pathology Department, University of California San Francisco, 1825 4th Street, M-2359, San Francisco, CA 94158, USA; [b] Gynecologic Oncology Division, Department of Obstetrics, Gynecology and Reproductive Sciences, University of California San Francisco, San Francisco, CA, USA; [c] Molecular Pathology Division, Pathology Department, University of California San Francisco, San Francisco, CA, USA
* Corresponding author.
E-mail address: joseph.rabban@ucsf.edu

surgpath.theclinics.com

high-grade serous carcinoma (HGSC) is enriched by HRD. After highlighting the general concepts underlying HRD testing and PARP inhibitor therapy, this review discusses practical roles for pathologists to maximize the opportunities for eligible patients with ovarian cancer to benefit from HRD testing, chiefly by applying contemporary diagnostic criteria for ovarian cancer tumor typing and navigating through potential pitfalls of tumor types that may mimic HGSC but are unlikely to harbor HRD.

OVERVIEW

Current treatment of pelvic carcinoma, specifically primary tubo-ovarian/peritoneal high-grade serous carcinoma (HGSC), is centered on agents that induce lethal damage to tumor cell DNA (platinum chemotherapy) and, more recently, on agents that cripple tumor cell attempts at repairing DNA damage (poly(ADP-ribose)polymerase [PARP] inhibitors), resulting in a form of so-called synthetic lethality in tumors that harbor genetic alterations that impair DNA damage repair pathways.[1–4] Predicting the sensitivity to platinum chemotherapy and to PARP inhibitors is central to tailoring management plans for individual patients that maximize patient benefits and minimize therapy-related morbidity.[4–7] Because these 2 major treatment strategies center on DNA damage and repair, it is not unexpected that biomarkers related to repair of DNA damage may predict treatment response. Indeed, the mutational status of BRCA1/2 genes, which are integral to the process that repairs double-strand DNA breaks (so-called homologous recombination repair [HRR]), generally predicts response to platinum therapy and to PARP inhibitors in pelvic HGSC.[2,4,8] However, BRCA mutational status is not a perfect predictor because mechanisms other than BRCA mutation can disrupt HRR.[9,10] Collectively, any alteration that leads to a defect in DNA repair via homologous recombination (HR), not just BRCA1/2 mutation, is referred to as HR deficiency (HRD).[11,12] Tumor testing for HRD has recently emerged as an approach to predict PARP inhibitor sensitivity and to guide management decisions.[4,9] The relationship between HRD and PARP inhibitor sensitivity is not simple for several reasons: (1) It is possible for tumor cells to harbor HRD at one time point and then subsequently acquire additional alterations that functionally reverse HRD by restoring HRR. (2) Tumor heterogeneity with respect to defects in HRR represents another challenge for HRD testing. (3) Currently available clinical HRD tests detect the downstream

consequences of HRD (a so-called genomic "scar," described in detail later) that may have occurred at some point in the past.[4,9,11] Even if HRR is functionally restored, the tumor retains this scar and thus would still seem to be responsive to PARP inhibitors with current testing modalities. These are some of the many explanations for imperfect correlation between current HRD tests and PARP inhibitor sensitivity. Tests that detect the real-time functionality of HRR are underdevelopment but not clinically available.[13] This review will summarize the background for understanding HRR and HRD, the clinical evidence for HRD testing as a predictor of PARP inhibitor sensitivity, and the different types of available HRD tests and their limitations. Although HRD testing is currently performed largely in a few select commercial laboratories, pathologists should be aware of the general concepts underling HRD testing as well as the testing and treatment implications of tumor histotype assignment in the evaluation of ovarian cancer. With this in mind, the article will also highlight practical issues and challenges in distinguishing HGSC from its morphologic mimics in the ovary.

NORMAL REPAIR OF DOUBLE-STRAND BREAKS IN DNA

DNA damage can accumulate from endogenous sources (ie, byproducts of normal daily cellular metabolism) and from exogenous sources (eg, radiation, viruses, mutagenic chemicals, and chemotherapy such as platinum therapy). Healthy cells avoid the deleterious effects of DNA damage through several molecular pathways generically referred to as the DNA damage response.[14–16] In mammalian cells, the repair of double-strand breaks (DSBs) in DNA is largely accomplished via one of 2 pathways: nonhomologous end joining (NHEJ) and HR. Left unrepaired, DNA damage, particularly DSBs, may lead to cell death or to carcinogenesis through the acquisition of inactivating mutations in tumor suppressors. Among the various types of DNA damage and DNA repair mechanisms, the most relevant to the discussion of ovarian cancer treatment are DSBs and their repair by the HRR pathway (including the BRCA1/2 genes). The term HRR refers to the fact that the repair process relies on a homologous copy of DNA to repair the DSB, and it is generally a conservative process, meaning no DNA sequence is lost or gained.[11,12] Although the actual biochemical details of the repair process are beyond the scope of this review, the main points include that the recognition and repair process is a multistep sequence that involves many proteins, beginning with the binding of the MRE11–Rad50–Nbs1 protein complex (also known as the MRN complex), continuing with nascent single strand invasion and displacement, and resolution resulting in conservative repair of the DNA DSB. The PARP enzymes (PARP1 and PARP2) and the ataxia telangiectasia mutated protein play key roles in the initial recognition of DSBs and facilitate chromatin decondensation, chromatin remodeling, and DNA end recognition.[17] The structure of the exposed DNA ends largely influences the choice between NHEJ and HRR as a pathway to repair the DSB, with activation of PARP (predominantly PARP1) at single-strand DNA gaps.

IMPAIRED HOMOLOGOUS RECOMBINATION REPAIR

Functional loss of HRR is defined as HRD (**Fig. 1**).[9] Germline or somatic mutation of BRCA1 or BRCA2 is a major cause of HRD, leading to an accumulation of DNA damage, particularly double-strand DNA breaks, and predisposing cells to oncogenesis, mostly notably breast cancer and pelvic HGSC. In addition to BRCA1/2 mutation, other causes of HRD include BRCA1 or RAD51C silencing by DNA methylation, alterations in microRNAs or transcription factors that regulate HRR genes, and alterations in chromatin regulation involved in repair. Tumor cells with HRD are able to survive because other mechanisms of repair of DSBs, such as NHEJ, and repair of single-strand breaks remain intact, although these are nonconservative repair mechanisms and can lead to a variety of secondary alterations including insertions, deletions, mutations, copy number alterations, and structural chromosomal abnormalities. These accumulated abnormalities induce a mutational signature or so-called genomic scar that can be detected by various molecular tests.[11]

EXPLOITING HRD TO TREAT PELVIC HIGH-GRADE SEROUS CARCINOMA: SYNTHETIC LETHALITY

Two strategies to exploit HRD in the treatment of patients with pelvic HGSC are currently in use. First, platinum-based chemotherapy works by inducing DSBs and, ultimately, cross-links in DNA, which are cytotoxic.[1,2] This can be effective in tumor cells with HRD because the tumor cell's impaired ability to repair such damage can lead to an overwhelming number of double-stranded breaks and ultimately tumor cell death. Second,

because HR-deficient tumor cells are dependent on alternate DNA repair pathways, particularly those using the PARP enzymes, PARP inhibitors eliminate one of the major remaining DNA repair tools on which tumor cells with HRD are dependent. In 2005, 2 groups described this dependency between PARP inhibition and BRCA1 and BRCA2 mutation,[18,19] a concept that had been described nearly a century earlier by geneticists in the study of Drosophila genetics and termed synthetic lethality.[1,20,21] The demonstration that BRCA-mutant cells were ~1000 times more sensitive than BRCA-wild type cells paved the way for clinical trials of synthetic lethality using PARP inhibitors in HRD tumors.[19]

TESTING PELVIC HIGH-GRADE SEROUS CARCINOMA FOR HRD

In concept, testing for the presence of HRD should identify patients whose pelvic HGSC is potentially responsive to platinum chemotherapy and PARP inhibition.[2,5,7,12,22] In reality, HRD testing is currently a complex array of available testing platforms, each of which measures different molecular end points of HRD.[9] This makes it challenging to compare clinical trials of PARP inhibitors using different HRD tests. Two approaches to assessing HRD exist: (1) germline and/or somatic testing for a pathogenic or likely pathogenic mutation in BRCA1/2 and (2) clinical HRD testing that identifies the so-called genomic scar in tumor cells, which results from the deficit in HRR and subsequent reliance on alternate DNA repair pathways.[14]

Currently, germline BRCA1/2 testing is typically performed as part of a multigene panel that includes other ovarian cancer-related genes BRIP1, RAD51C, RAD51D, and PALB2 and, in some panels, additional cancer-related genes beyond those associated with breast and ovarian cancer. Most testing is performed in commercial laboratories (eg, Myriad, Ambry, Invitae) or academic institutions/cancer centers (eg, University of Washington's BROCA Cancer Risk Panel, University of California San Francisco's Hereditary Cancer Panel). Up to 25% of ovarian cancers may harbor a germline mutation in one of the ovarian cancer risk genes.[2,23–26] BRCA1 accounts for approximately half of this cohort; BRCA2 accounts for about one-quarter; other genes, including BRIP1, RAD51C, RAD51D, and PALB2, account for the remainder. Testing of tumor tissue to identify somatic mutation or rearrangement of BRCA1/2 is available in commercial laboratories (Myriad MyChoice test, FoundationOne test) and some academic institutions/cancer centers. Up to 15% of ovarian cancers may harbor a somatic mutation in one of the genes involved in HRR.[2,26] A limitation of mutation testing to predict response to platinum chemotherapy and PARP inhibition is that, depending on which tumor specimen in the patient's course of disease is tested, reversion mutations in BRCA1/2 may partially restore HRR to a degree that results in resistance.[27] Another limitation is that not all pathogenic mutations in BRCA1/2 may equally affect HRR, and therefore, sensitivity/resistance may depend on the specific mutation.[28] Finally, certain genetic alterations (eg, deep intronic variants or epigenetic silencing) may not be easily detectable by routine sequencing panels and consequently result in a false-negative result.[26] Thus, BRCA1/2 mutation testing alone does not perfectly serve as a predictor of response to platinum chemotherapy or PARP inhibition.

Clinical HRD tests evaluate for a genomic scar that results from downstream effects of HRD, including mutations and structural abnormalities[9] (Fig. 1). Three major patterns of genomic scar are evaluated and quantified in current HRD tests (Box 1): (1) loss of heterozygosity (LOH),[29] (2) large-scale state transitions (LST),[30] and (3) telomeric allelic imbalances (TAI).[31] LOH and telomeric imbalance is typically detected by sequencing a panel of single-nucleotide polymorphisms (SNPs) in the tumor, whereas LST are evaluated by assays that look at copy number

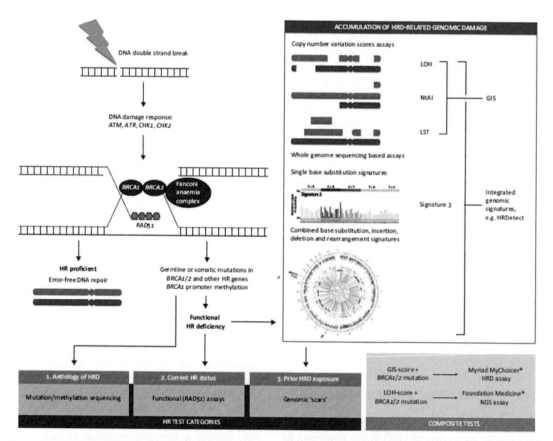

Fig. 1. Methods for detecting homologous recombination repair deficiency (HRD). HR, homologous recombination. Individual assays (HRDetect, LOH, NtAI [number of subchromosomal regions with allelic imbalance extending to the telomere], LST and genomic instability scores [GISs]) are described in the article. The 2 commercially available assays that combine BRCA mutation and GISs are described in the green box. Figure and legend reprinted with permission from the publisher. (From Miller RE, Leary A, Scott CL, Serra V, Lord CJ, Bowtell D, Chang DK, Garsed DW, Jonkers J, Ledermann JA, Nik-Zainal S, Ray-Coquard I, Shah SP, Matias-Guiu X, Swisher EM, Yates LR. ESMO recommendations on predictive biomarker testing for homologous recombination deficiency and PARP inhibitor benefit in ovarian cancer. Ann Oncol. 2020 Dec;31(12):1606-1622. https://doi.org/10.1016/j.annonc.2020.08.2102. Epub 2020 Sep 28. PMID: 33004253).

Box 1
Main alterations (so-called genomic scars) resulting from homologous recombination deficiency that are detected by current testing platforms

a. Loss of heterozygosity (LOH)

b. Large-scale state transitions (LST)

c. Telomeric allelic imbalances (TAI)

---

alterations across the tumor genome. Although defined differently, these 3 patterns of genomic scar are correlated with each other and with BRCA1/2 mutation.[29–32] The Myriad myChoice test, a Food and Drug Administration (FDA) approved companion diagnostic test, quantifies LOH, LST, and TAI to generate a "Genomic Instability Score." The threshold score defining HRD was based on a reference cohort of breast and ovarian cancers with biallelic loss of function of BRCA1/2. The FoundationFocus BRCA LOH, also an FDA approved companion diagnostic test, uses only LOH to define HRD by sequencing SNPs in the tumor and calculating the percentage of genomic regions showing LOH. The threshold score for defining HRD was based on ovarian cancer outcomes independent of BRCA1/2 status.[9]

A major limitation of defining HRD based on a genomic scar is that it does not necessarily reflect the real-time functionality of HRR if reversion mutations in HRR genes sufficiently restore functionality to HRR.[9] Such tumors will test positive for HRD but exhibit resistance to platinum chemotherapy and/or PARP inhibition. Similarly, tumor heterogeneity with respect to HRR functionality may also result in an HRD test score that does not correlate with the actual response to therapy. Real-time functional HRD tests are underdevelopment but not clinically available.[13] These include tests of RAD51 foci formation using immunohistochemistry (IHC) or immunofluorescence and tests of replication fork stability using immunofluorescence. Additional limitations to current clinical HRD tests are that direct comparisons of the different test platforms remain to be performed and consensus on cut-off scores for HRD tests remains to be established. Despite these issues, clinical HRD tests have been successfully used in phase III clinical trials to identify patients who respond to PARP inhibition, and as discussed above, some have been approved as companion diagnostic tests. Thus, further refinements in these tests will potentially maximize their ability to predict PARP inhibitor sensitivity.[9]

HOMOLOGOUS REPAIR DEFICIENCY TESTS AND FDA-APPROVED PARP INHIBITORS

To date, 3 PARP inhibitors are approved for patients with ovarian cancer by the United States FDA under varying clinical indications and varying requirements for demonstrating HRD: olaparib, niraparib, and rucaparib. The key clinical trials leading to FDA approval evaluated patients with pelvic HGSC (ARIEL2,[33] VELIA,[34] QUADRA,[35] NOVA,[36] and Study 19[37] trials) or patients with either pelvic HGSC or ovarian high-grade endometrioid carcinoma (SOLO-1,[38] SOLO-2,[39] PAOLA-1,[40] PRIMA,[41] ARIEL3,[42,43] Study 10[44] trials). Details of the clinical trial designs and results are beyond the scope of this review, but in general, these phase II and III trials each demonstrated benefit in progression-free survival among those who received PARP inhibitor therapy.[9] In general, in these studies, BRCA1/2 mutational status and/or HRD test status predicted response to PARP inhibitor therapy. As discussed earlier, these correlations are imperfect but are robust enough to have merited FDA approval. In the United States, the current National Comprehensive Cancer Network guidelines for ovarian cancer management now incorporate the use of PARP inhibitors and the use of BRCA testing and HRD testing in decision-making algorithms.[3]

Olaparib is approved for newly diagnosed ovarian cancer as maintenance therapy in platinum-sensitive patients with a germline or somatic BRCA1/2 mutation detected with an FDA approved companion diagnostic test (FoundationOne test; Myriad BRCAnalysis test), based on the SOLO-1 trial. In newly diagnosed platinum-sensitive patients with ovarian cancer receiving bevacizumab as part of first-line treatment, it is also approved as maintenance therapy in combination with bevacizumab in the setting of HRD using the Myriad myChoice test and/or BRCA1/2 mutation, based on the PAOLA-1 trial. For recurrent ovarian cancer, olaparib is approved as maintenance therapy in platinum-sensitive cancers independent of HRD testing and BRCA1/2 mutation status, based on the Study 19 trial. It is also approved for recurrent ovarian cancer after 3 or more lines of chemotherapy in patients with germline *BRCA1/2* mutation, based on the SOLO-2 trial.

Niraparib is approved for newly diagnosed ovarian cancer (PRIMA trial) and for recurrent ovarian cancer (NOVA trial) as maintenance therapy in platinum sensitive patients independent of HRD testing and *BRCA1/2* mutation status. For recurrent ovarian cancer after 3 or more lines of chemotherapy, niraparib is approved in the setting of HRD using the Myriad myChoice test and/or *BRCA1/2* mutation, based on the QUADRA study.

Rucaparib is approved for recurrent ovarian cancer independent of HRD testing and *BRCA1/2* mutation status, based on ARIEL2 trial and Study 10 trial. For recurrence after 2 or more lines of chemotherapy, rucaparib is approved for patients with a germline *BRCA1/2* mutation or somatic *BRCA1/2* mutation detected with FoundationFocus BRCA test, based on ARIEL3 trial.

ROLE OF THE PATHOLOGIST IN HRD TESTING OF OVARIAN CANCER

The key clinical trials demonstrating the efficacy of PARP inhibitors are based on patients with pelvic HGSC or based on patients with either pelvic HGSC or ovarian high-grade endometrioid carcinoma. Although the rationale for including pelvic HGSC stems from its association with *BRCA1/2* and related cancer risk genes, there is not a similar significant association with endometrioid carcinoma, although such tumors were included anyway in some of the clinical trials of PARP inhibition. These tumor type inclusion criteria raise a treatment-related mandate for pathologists to be as specific as possible in assigning a tumor type to ovarian cancer. Although most advanced stage ovarian cancers are HGSC, a minority consists of tumor types unrelated to HRD, including low-grade serous carcinoma (LGSC) and clear cell carcinoma, among other types.[45] Thus, the primary practical role for pathologists in the clinical management decisions for patients with ovarian cancer with potential HRD is to ensure accurate diagnosis of pelvic HGSC versus other tumor types. The recently published fifth edition of the *World Health Organization Classification of Female Genital Tumors* is internationally recognized as the reference standard for essential diagnostic criteria and classification terminology for ovarian cancer tumor types.[46] Molecularly validated IHC strategies for tumor typing are well described.[47,48] As with any laboratory test, optimal antibody titration, appropriate test controls, and standardized interpretative criteria and reporting are central to IHC for tumor typing.[49] The goals, challenges, and limitations of the pathologist's role in this setting can be divided into 4 major areas.

INDEX SPECIMEN ESTABLISHING THE DIAGNOSIS OF OVARIAN CANCER

Biopsy specimens that serve as the index diagnosis of advanced stage pelvic cancer merit particular attention to assigning the tumor type because patients with pelvic HGSC may be eligible for neoadjuvant chemotherapy, whereas other types are generally managed by primary cytoreduction followed by adjuvant therapy.[3,50] These index specimens often are small biopsies or fine needle aspirations of distant disease or cytologic preparations of malignant ascites or pleural fluid. Because some patients with HGSC may achieve a complete response to neoadjuvant chemotherapy and have no detectable cancer at subsequent interval surgery, the index specimen may be the sole opportunity to provide classification of the tumor type and primary origin. For this reason, the strategy of establishing general evidence for a primary gynecologic origin of the tumor in the index biopsy specimen but deferring specific tumor typing to the main surgical debulking specimen may not be in the best interest of the patient. For example, index biopsy diagnoses such as "adenocarcinoma of gynecologic origin" or "carcinoma consistent with ovarian origin" do not convey the granularity of tumor type details needed by the clinician to evaluate appropriateness of neoadjuvant chemotherapy or PARP inhibitor therapy.[3]

Ideally, clinicians arranging a biopsy of clinically suspected advanced stage ovarian cancer should consider a sampling procedure that maximizes the opportunity for potential immunohistochemical work up for tumor type, balanced alongside considering other relevant clinical characteristics that may define the best option for tumor sampling for the individual patient. This view is also endorsed by the Society of Gynecologic Oncology and American Society of Clinical Oncology's clinical practice guidelines for neoadjuvant chemotherapy for newly diagnosed ovarian cancer, which recommends using core biopsy technique to obtain adequate tissue for IHC for assessing tumor typing and origin.[50] Although not specifically mentioned in those guidelines, a cell block from a fine needle aspiration or malignant fluid specimen (eg, ascites, pleural effusion), if clinically appropriate to perform in the individual patient setting and if

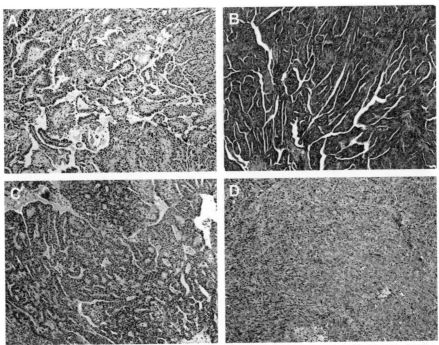

Fig. 2. Classic architectural patterns of HGSC include papillary growth consisting of branching (*A*) or resulting in slit-like clefted spaces (*B*), tubuloglandular growth (*C*), and solid growth (*D*).

performed with the goal of obtaining adequate tissue for IHC, can be a suitable alternative to a core biopsy.[51] Presuming sufficient tumor tissue is available in the index biopsy specimen and/or fluid, reasonable efforts should be made by pathologists to apply morphologic and, if appropriate, immunohistochemical criteria to arrive at a specific tumor type using the WHO classification system.[46]

DIAGNOSTIC DISTINCTION OF PELVIC HIGH-GRADE SEROUS CARCINOMA FROM ITS MORPHOLOGIC MIMICS

Tumor typing is typically straightforward in specimens with adequate tissue; however, there a few potential challenges and pitfalls that merit review. Classic morphologic features of pelvic HGSC include a constellation of complex papillary, solid, tubuloglandular, transitional cell-like, and/or cribriform architecture accompanied by severe nuclear pleomorphism and brisk mitotic activity, often with atypical mitotic figures (**Figs. 2** and **3**). However, not all cases exhibit classic morphology, and this may lead to challenges in distinguishing HGSC from a variety of other carcinomas. The diagnostic challenges may be compounded further if the index specimen is a small biopsy, fine needle aspiration, or cytologic preparation of malignant fluid. The immunophenotype of the major ovarian

cancer histologic types is for the most part distinct and improves classification in most cases. To this end, aberrant p53 immunohistochemical expression is a hallmark of pelvic HGSC (**Fig. 4**), as is WT1 staining, which is observed in most cases.[46] The following discussion summarizes the most important differential diagnoses and the tools helpful in their work-up (**Boxes 2** and **3**):

Distinction of Pelvic High-Grade Serous Carcinoma from Advanced Stage Primary Endometrial Serous Carcinoma

Currently, the role for PARP inhibitors is focused on primary pelvic HGSC. Thus, distinction from primary endometrial serous carcinoma is important. This distinction can be problematic based on the pathologic findings alone because both share similar morphology and aberrant p53 immunoexpression.[46] Clinically, however, primary endometrial serous carcinoma is not strongly associated with *BRCA1/2* mutation and tends to arise in a much older patient population than pelvic HGSC. Ideally, pathologists evaluating an index biopsy specimen of advanced stage gynecologic cancer should be provided relevant clinical context by the clinician, such as radiological distribution of disease (ie, presence of an endometrial mass) and *BRCA1/2* germline mutation status, if available. The presence of serous tubal

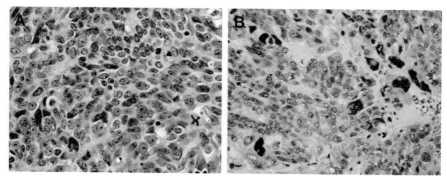

Fig. 3. Classic features of tumor cells of HGSC are high nucleus to cytoplasm ratio, moderate-to-severe nuclear pleomorphism, macronucleoli, high mitotic index, and atypical mitotic figures (*A*). Occasional scattered individual tumor cells with bizarre, anaplastic features can be seen in some HGSC and are in turn uncommon in other ovarian tumor histotypes (*B*).

intraepithelial carcinoma (STIC) in a patient with endometrial involvement by serous carcinoma does not, on its own, resolve the issue of tumor origin.[52] Approximately 20% of patients with endometrial serous carcinoma have a fallopian tube involved by STIC. WT1 IHC can be helpful because diffuse strong staining is a hallmark of pelvic HGSC, whereas most primary endometrial serous carcinoma are negative or exhibit limited staining. Comparison of WT1 staining between the endometrial and pelvic tumors may be useful because concordant results favor a single source of tumor. Acknowledging that objective criteria are currently lacking, the endometrial cancer

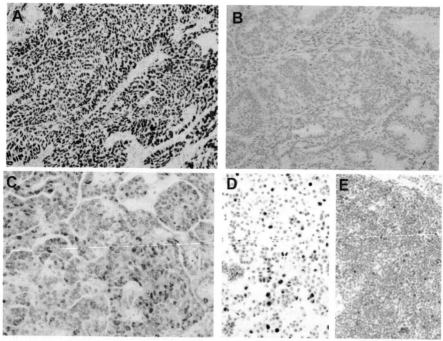

Fig. 4. Depending on the type of *TP53* mutation in HGSC, 3 p53 immunoexpression patterns may occur: overexpression pattern (uniform strong nuclear staining in ≥80% tumor nuclei) (*A*), null pattern (complete absence of any nuclear staining in any tumor cells, with appropriate wild-type staining in the background nontumor cells) (*B*), or, rarely, cytoplasmic staining (diffuse weak-to-moderate cytoplasmic staining of tumor cells with or without variable nuclear staining) (*C*). Wild-type p53 staining in tumors lacking *TP53* mutation is defined as an admixture of tumor nuclei with weak, moderate, or no nuclear staining (*D*). Normal tonsil or lymph node serves as a wild-type p53 stain control in which 10% to 20% of lymphoid cells should exhibit weak-to-moderate nuclear staining, whereas most nuclei show no staining (*E*).

Box 2
Aberrant patterns of p53 immunoexpression in tumors with *TP53* mutation

a. Overexpression pattern (uniformly strong nuclear staining in at least 80% of tumor cells)

b. Null pattern (complete absence of nuclear staining in tumor cells)

c. Cytoplasmic pattern (diffuse cytoplasmic staining of tumor cells with or without variable nuclear staining)

---

reporting guidelines from the International Society of Gynecologic Pathologists propose that most cases of concurrent endometrial and pelvic serous carcinoma originate from the endometrium and spread to extrauterine sites via transtubal dissemination; rare cases of the converse may represent transtubal dissemination from pelvic origin to the endometrium.[52]

Distinction of Pelvic High-Grade Serous Carcinoma from Pelvic Low-Grade Serous Carcinoma

Papillary and bud-like tumor growth can be present in both HGSC and LGSC, creating a potential diagnostic dilemma, especially in small biopsy specimens (**Fig. 5**). In addition, both tumor types are also WT1 positive. In this setting, the key morphologic criteria are nuclear atypia and mitotic index. HGSC is characterized by severe nuclear atypia and mitotic index of 12 mitoses or greater per 10 high power fields, whereas LGSC does not exhibit that degree of atypia or mitotic activity and tends to be more uniform and monotonous in appearance. Aberrant p53 immunohistochemical expression, often accompanied by positive (diffuse, strong staining) p16 immunoexpression, distinguishes HGSC from LGSC, the latter of which exhibits wild-type p53 immunoexpression and negative p16. Unlike pelvic HGSC, ovarian LGSC is not associated with *BRCA1/2* mutation. In resection specimens, the presence of STIC generally favors ovarian HGSC, whereas the presence of a background of serous borderline tumor often accompanies LGSC.[46]

Distinction of Pelvic High-Grade Serous Carcinoma from Ovarian High-Grade Endometrioid Carcinoma

Classical (also described as "confirmatory") features of ovarian endometrioid carcinoma include endometrioid gland formation, squamous differentiation, endometrioid borderline, or adenofibromatous architecture and the presence of ovarian endometriosis. However, they may not always be present in high-grade (FIGO grade 3) tumors.[46] This may result in a specimen exhibiting a poorly differentiated appearance that may overlap with that of HGSC and other poorly differentiated carcinomas, especially so in small biopsies of advanced sites of tumor. Rare ovarian endometrioid carcinomas may exhibit patterns resembling the transitional cell-like morphology seen in a subset of pelvic HGSC. Conversely, some pelvic HGSC may exhibit pseudoendometrioid/pseudocribriform growth mimicking that of lower grade endometrioid carcinoma (**Fig. 6**). *TP53* mutation is present in a subset of ovarian endometrioid carcinomas, which are often, but not always, higher grade and stage.[53,54] This further compounds the potential for diagnostic difficulty because such cases will exhibit aberrant p53 immunophenotype, as is expected in HGSC. WT1 is the most informative stain for this differential diagnosis.[47] Strong diffuse staining is a hallmark of pelvic HGSC.

Box 3
Common mimics of pelvic HGSC that should be considered in the differential diagnosis

a. Primary pelvic HGSC vs advanced staged endometrial serous carcinoma

b. Pelvic HGSC vs pelvic LGSC

c. Pelvic HGSC vs ovarian endometrioid carcinoma

d. Pelvic HGSC vs ovarian clear cell carcinoma

e. Pelvic HGSC versus ovarian metastasis from a nongynecological primary origin

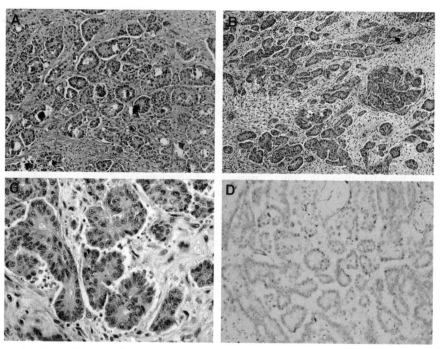

Fig. 5. HGSC may occasionally exhibit areas of uniform bud-like growth without severe nuclear pleomorphism or high mitotic index (*A*) that may be misinterpreted as LGSC (*B*) at scanning magnification. However, this is not a diffuse finding, and areas with high-grade cytomorphology can be appreciated. Conversely, LGSC exhibits only minimal nuclear atypia and minimal mitotic activity (*C*), as well as p53 wild type immunoexpression (*D*).

WT1 is negative in most endometrioid carcinoma, with rare exceptions. Immunohistochemical loss of PTEN, ARID1A, and/or mismatch repair proteins occurs in a subset of endometrioid carcinoma but not in HGSC. However, these alterations do not have high enough diagnostic sensitivity to identify all cases of endometrioid carcinoma, and therefore, intact staining results are noninformative in this setting. Tumor sequencing, if available, can also potentially provide insight regarding tumor type because there are additional genetic alterations of endometrioid differentiation for which there are no immunohistochemical markers; details are beyond the scope of this review.[26,55]

Distinction of Pelvic High-Grade Serous Carcinoma from Ovarian Clear Cell Carcinoma

Classic features of ovarian clear cell carcinoma include a constellation of architectural patterns (papillary, tubulocystic, tubuloglandular, solid, and/or hobnail growth), clear cytoplasm, specialized features (hyalinized stroma, hyaline globules, open tumor rings), and ovarian endometriosis.[46] In some cases, particularly small biopsies of advanced stage tumor, a solid pattern may predominate without any of the other classic findings. This may mimic solid pattern pelvic HGSC, which can exhibit variable degrees of clear cytoplasm,

particularly following neoadjuvant chemotherapy, further exacerbating the diagnostic dilemma (**Fig. 7**). As with the differential diagnosis with endometrioid carcinoma, WT1 is the most informative IHC as it is negative in clear cell carcinoma.[47] Napsin-A is positive in most clear cell carcinoma and, with rare exception, is negative in pelvic HGSC. ARID1A expression is completely absent in many clear cell carcinomas, but this is not a perfectly sensitive marker, and so the presence of staining is noninformative. Although most ovarian clear cell carcinomas show wild-type p53 staining, a rare subset may show aberrant p53 staining and so that result, on its own in isolation of other immunostain results, is noninformative in the differential diagnosis with pelvic HGSC.[56,57] In contrast, wild-type p53 staining would not be expected in pelvic HGSC, except in exceedingly rare instances.[58] As with endometrioid carcinoma, tumor sequencing, if available, may be of potential value to distinguish clear cell carcinoma from pelvic HGSC.[26]

Distinction of Residual Neoadjuvant-Treated Pelvic High-Grade Serous Carcinoma from Other Tumor Types

Chemotherapy can sometimes alter the morphologic appearance of residual pelvic HGSC. This

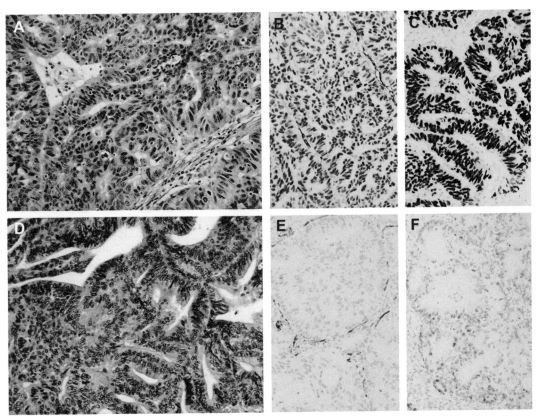

Fig. 6. HGSC with glandular architecture (*A*) may mimic lower grade endometrioid carcinoma but is WT1 positive (*B*) and p53 aberrant (*C*), whereas lower grade endometrioid carcinoma (*D*) is WT1 negative (*E*) and p53 wild type (*F*).

may potentially cause diagnostic difficulties with respect to tumor typing in an interval-debulking specimen following the initial management by neoadjuvant chemotherapy.[59,60] The classic brisk mitotic activity of HGSC may be significantly reduced following neoadjuvant treatment. This could lead to an appearance mimicking LGSC or lower grade endometrioid carcinoma, particularly in highly responsive tumors that leave minimal residual tumor in the debulking specimen. Conversely, residual neoadjuvant-treated HGSC may exhibit notable cytoplasmic clearing and vacuoles that mimic clear cell carcinoma. Thus, attention to these potential pitfalls is merited when evaluating residual ovarian cancer following neoadjuvant treatment. This variety of morphologic confounders also highlights the importance of establishing a histologic type in the pretreatment index diagnostic biopsy, whenever possible. It also underscores the value of reviewing the index biopsy to compare the tumor morphology with the posttreatment specimen, which can show morphologic similarities. Chemotherapy does not seem to interfere with the results of IHC and therefore can be used for tumor typing in this setting.[61]

Distinction of Pelvic High-Grade Serous Carcinoma from Metastatic Breast Cancer

The possibility of metastatic breast cancer involving the peritoneal cavity and/or gynecologic organs merits consideration particularly in patients known to have breast cancer or known to have *BRCA1/2* germline mutation. The possibility applies even in the absence of a primary breast cancer because distant metastasis could be the index presentation. Poorly differentiated breast cancer may exhibit architectural and cytologic features that resemble HGSC and some may also exhibit aberrant p53 immunoexpression. Thus, immunohistochemical staining can be valuable, particularly in small biopsies. The combination of positive PAX8 and WT1 but negative GATA3 is expected in HGSC, whereas the converse is expected in breast cancer.[62] CK7

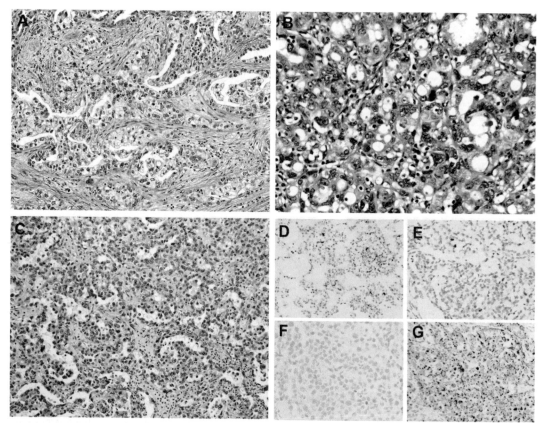

Fig. 7. HGSC may occasionally contain clear cytoplasm or vacuoles (*A*), particularly following neoadjuvant chemotherapy (*B*), mimicking ovarian clear cell carcinoma (*C*), which, unlike HGSC, is WT1 negative (*D*), typically p53 wild type (*E*), ER negative (*F*), and Napsin A positive (*G*).

and estrogen receptor (ER) are noninformative because both entities are typically positive for both markers.

Proper Use and Interpretation of p53 Immunohistochemistry

As discussed earlier, p53 IHC, a surrogate to *TP53* mutational analysis, serves a critical role in establishing a correct diagnosis of pelvic HGSC. Two issues are essential to the proper use of p53 IHC in this setting: optimal titration of the antibody and application of the criteria for aberrant versus wild-type staining (see **Fig. 4**). Both issues are discussed in detail in recently published practice guidelines from the International Society of Gynecologic Pathologists.[63] In summary, appropriate tissue controls are needed. The ideal wild-type tissue control is tonsil. Variable nuclear staining is expected in 20% of germinal center B cells, in occasional lymphocytes in the mantle zone, and in scattered keratinocytes of the lower third of squamous epithelium. Nonneoplastic cells in the tumor, such as fibroblasts, lymphocytes, and endothelium also exhibit a wild-type pattern of scattered weak-to-moderate nuclear staining. The ideal positive tissue control is a pelvic HGSC with the p53 overexpression pattern. Three patterns of aberrant expression correlate with the presence of a *TP53* mutation: (1) overexpression pattern, defined as uniformly strong staining of 80% or more of tumor nuclei, (2) null pattern, defined as complete absence of any nuclear staining, and (3) cytoplasmic pattern, defined as cytoplasmic staining in most tumor cells, with or without variable amounts of nuclear staining. The cytoplasmic pattern of aberrant p53 IHC, although rare, merits special attention because it is only a recent observation and prone to misinterpretation as a wild-type p53 IHC result or as an equivocal finding.[64–66] Concurrent use of p16 IHC can be helpful, particularly to serve as confirmation in cases with the p53 null pattern.[67] It is important to recognize, however, that p16 is not always positive in cases with aberrant p53 staining.

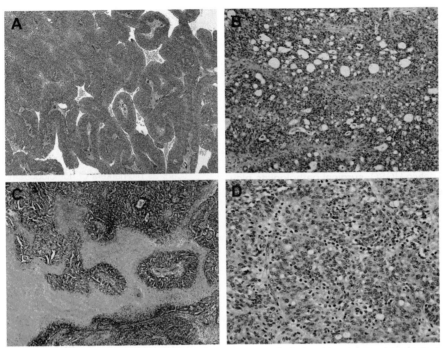

Fig. 8. HGSC in patients with a germline *BRCA1* or *BRCA2* mutation are associated with certain morphologic features such as transitional cell carcinoma-like growth (*A*), pseudoendometrioid growth (*B*), extensive tumor necrosis (*C*), and/or tumor infiltrating lymphocytes (*D*); however, these are neither sensitive nor specific enough to serve on their own in deciding whether PARP inhibitor therapy is indicated.

SELECTION OF MOST RECENT TUMOR FOR HRD TESTING

When a pathologist is asked to select a block of a patient's HGSC specimen, the ideal specimen is the most recent one available or, when there is only a primary or interval debulking specimen, the site of the most advanced disease (for instance, choosing tumor in the omentum over tumor in the fallopian tube or ovary). Although this does not guarantee that the HRD test is an accurate real-time functional reflection of HRR status, it mitigates against discrepancies that may occur by selecting a sample from an earlier presentation of the tumor before any reversion of HRR functionality may have occurred.[9] An equally important set of considerations are the tumor specimen requirements for HRD testing. Both of the currently available clinical HRD tests require a 25 mm^2 tissue block that ideally contains 30% or more tumor cellularity compared with normal tissue.[68,69] These requirements may be problematic in patients whose tumors partially respond to neoadjuvant chemotherapy because the residual tumor may exhibit extremely low tumor cellularity and high immune cell population cellularity as part of the local tissue response to tumor cell death. In cases that fail to meet minimum specimen requirements, discussion with the patient's clinician may be merited to determine whether testing the pretreatment tumor specimen may be of clinical value, acknowledging that the functional HR status of that specimen may differ from the current residual posttreatment tumor.

MORPHOLOGIC PREDICTORS OF HRD STATUS

Pelvic HGSC in women with *BRCA1/2* germline or somatic mutation may frequently exhibit so-called SET features (solid, pseudo-endometrioid, transitional cell-like growth), tumor infiltrating lymphocytes, high mitotic index, necrosis, and/or pushing pattern of growth in metastatic sites (**Fig. 8**).[70–74] However, these features are not sensitive or specific enough to outright replace formal testing for *BRCA1/2* mutation. The literature on the correlation of BRCA 1 IHC and *BRCA1* mutational status remains controversial.[75] Studies on correlation between the morphology of pelvic HGSC and clinical HRD test result status, particularly in tumors that are HRD positive and wild type *BRCA1/2*, have yet to be reported. If sensitive enough morphologic predictors or HRD status can be identified in future studies, then microscopic examination of tumors might assist in triaging which pelvic HGSC merit HRD testing.

SUMMARY

Clinical HRD testing of pelvic HGSC is emerging as a potential tool to refine treatment planning, specifically eligibility for PARP inhibitor therapy. Because the biological foundation for PARP inhibitor therapy is based on molecular alterations to DNA damage repair mechanisms that are associated with pelvic HGSC, surgical pathologists play a vital role in treatment planning by ensuring accurate tumor typing. Thus, awareness of the potential challenges and pitfalls in the diagnosis of pelvic HGSC, as well as of the practical solutions to such diagnostic problems, will permit surgical pathologists to maximize the opportunity for patients to obtain personalized cancer care.

DISCLOSURE

Dr J.T. Rabban reports that his spouse receives salary and stock options from Merck & Co.

REFERENCES

1. Lord CJ, Ashworth A. PARP inhibitors: Synthetic lethality in the clinic. Science 2017;355(6330):1152–8.
2. Pennington KP, Walsh T, Harrell MI, et al. Germline and somatic mutations in homologous recombination genes predict platinum response and survival in ovarian, fallopian tube, and peritoneal carcinomas. Clin Cancer Res 2014;20(3):764–75.
3. National Comprehensive Cancer Network. NCCN Clinical Practice Guidelines in Oncology. Ovarian cancer, including fallopian tube cancer and primary peritoneal cancer. Version 3.2021. www.nccn.org. Accessed October 4, 2021.
4. Miller RE, Leary A, Scott CL, et al. ESMO recommendations on predictive biomarker testing for homologous recombination deficiency and PARP inhibitor benefit in ovarian cancer. Ann Oncol 2020;31(12): 1606–22.
5. Hoppe MM, Sundar R, Tan DSP, et al. Biomarkers for homologous recombination deficiency in cancer. J Natl Cancer Inst 2018;110(7):704–13.
6. Liu JF, Konstantinopoulos PA, Matulonis UA. PARP inhibitors in ovarian cancer: current status and future promise. Gynecol Oncol 2014;133(2):362–9.
7. Konstantinopoulos PA, Norquist B, Lacchetti C, et al. Germline and somatic tumor testing in epithelial ovarian cancer: ASCO guideline. J Clin Oncol 2020;38(11):1222–45.
8. Norquist BM, Brady MF, Harrell MI, et al. Mutations in homologous recombination genes and outcomes in ovarian carcinoma patients in GOG 218: an NRG oncology/gynecologic oncology group study. Clin Cancer Res 2018;24(4):777–83.
9. Stover EH, Fuh K, Konstantinopoulos PA, et al. Clinical assays for assessment of homologous recombination DNA repair deficiency. Gynecol Oncol 2020; 159(3):887–98.
10. Radhakrishnan SK, Jette N, Lees-Miller SP. Nonhomologous end joining: emerging themes and unanswered questions. DNA Repair (Amst) 2014; 17:2–8.
11. Watkins JA, Irshad S, Grigoriadis A, et al. Genomic scars as biomarkers of homologous recombination deficiency and drug response in breast and ovarian cancers. Breast Cancer Res 2014;16(3):211.
12. Nesic K, Wakefield M, Kondrashova O, et al. Targeting DNA repair: the genome as a potential biomarker. J Pathol 2018;244(5):586–97.
13. Fuh K, Mullen M, Blachut B, et al. Homologous recombination deficiency real-time clinical assays, ready or not? Gynecol Oncol 2020;159(3):877–86.
14. Lord CJ, Ashworth A. The DNA damage response and cancer therapy. Nature 2012;481(7381):287–94.
15. Pilie PG, Tang C, Mills GB, et al. State-of-the-art strategies for targeting the DNA damage response in cancer. Nat Rev Clin Oncol 2019;16(2):81–104.
16. Konstantinopoulos PA, Ceccaldi R, Shapiro GI, et al. Homologous recombination deficiency: exploiting the fundamental vulnerability of ovarian cancer. Cancer Discov 2015;5(11):1137–54.
17. Satoh MS, Lindahl T. Role of poly(ADP-ribose) formation in DNA repair. Nature 1992;356(6367):356–8.
18. Bryant HE, Schultz N, Thomas HD, et al. Specific killing of BRCA2-deficient tumours with inhibitors of poly(ADP-ribose) polymerase. Nature 2005; 434(7035):913–7.
19. Farmer H, McCabe N, Lord CJ, et al. Targeting the DNA repair defect in BRCA mutant cells as a therapeutic strategy. Nature 2005;434(7035):917–21.
20. Ashworth A, Lord CJ, Reis-Filho JS. Genetic interactions in cancer progression and treatment. Cell 2011;145(1):30–8.
21. Dobzhansky T. Genetics of natural populations; recombination and variability in populations of Drosophila pseudoobscura. Genetics 1946;31: 269–90.
22. Stover EH, Konstantinopoulos PA, Matulonis UA, et al. Biomarkers of response and resistance to DNA repair targeted therapies. Clin Cancer Res 2016;22(23):5651–60.
23. Alsop K, Fereday S, Meldrum C, et al. BRCA mutation frequency and patterns of treatment response in BRCA mutation-positive women with ovarian cancer: a report from the Australian Ovarian Cancer Study Group. J Clin Oncol 2012;30(21):2654–63.
24. Walsh T, Casadei S, Lee MK, et al. Mutations in 12 genes for inherited ovarian, fallopian tube, and peritoneal carcinoma identified by massively parallel

sequencing. Proc Natl Acad Sci U S A 2011; 108(44):18032–7.

25. Norquist BM, Harrell MI, Brady MF, et al. Inherited Mutations in Women With Ovarian Carcinoma. JAMA Oncol 2016;2(4):482–90.

26. Cancer Genome Atlas Research Network. Integrated genomic analyses of ovarian carcinoma. Nature 2011;474(7353):609–15.

27. Noordermeer SM, van Attikum H. PARP inhibitor resistance: a tug-of-war in BRCA-Mutated cells. Trends Cell Biol 2019;29(10):820–34.

28. Wang Y, Bernhardy AJ, Cruz C, et al. The BRCA1-Delta11q alternative splice isoform bypasses germline mutations and promotes therapeutic resistance to PARP inhibition and cisplatin. Cancer Res 2016; 76(9):2778–90.

29. Abkevich V, Timms KM, Hennessy BT, et al. Patterns of genomic loss of heterozygosity predict homologous recombination repair defects in epithelial ovarian cancer. Br J Cancer 2012;107(10): 1776–82.

30. Popova T, Manie E, Rieunier G, et al. Ploidy and large-scale genomic instability consistently identify basal-like breast carcinomas with BRCA1/2 inactivation. Cancer Res 2012;72(21):5454–62.

31. Birkbak NJ, Wang ZC, Kim JY, et al. Telomeric allelic imbalance indicates defective DNA repair and sensitivity to DNA-damaging agents. Cancer Discov 2012;2(4):366–75.

32. Timms KM, Abkevich V, Hughes E, et al. Association of BRCA1/2 defects with genomic scores predictive of DNA damage repair deficiency among breast cancer subtypes. Breast Cancer Res 2014;16(6): 475.

33. Swisher EM, Lin KK, Oza AM, et al. Rucaparib in relapsed, platinum-sensitive high-grade ovarian carcinoma (ARIEL2 Part 1): an international, multicentre, open-label, phase 2 trial. Lancet Oncol 2017;18(1):75–87.

34. Coleman RL, Fleming GF, Brady MF, et al. Veliparib with first-line chemotherapy and as maintenance therapy in ovarian cancer. N Engl J Med 2019; 381(25):2403–15.

35. Moore KN, Secord AA, Geller MA, et al. Niraparib monotherapy for late-line treatment of ovarian cancer (QUADRA): a multicentre, open-label, single-arm, phase 2 trial. Lancet Oncol 2019;20(5):636–48.

36. Mirza MR, Monk BJ, Herrstedt J, et al. Niraparib maintenance therapy in platinum-sensitive, recurrent ovarian cancer. N Engl J Med 2016;375(22): 2154–64.

37. Ledermann J, Harter P, Gourley C, et al. Olaparib maintenance therapy in platinum-sensitive relapsed ovarian cancer. N Engl J Med 2012;366(15): 1382–92.

38. Moore K, Colombo N, Scambia G, et al. Maintenance olaparib in patients with newly diagnosed advanced ovarian cancer. N Engl J Med 2018; 379(26):2495–505.

39. Pujade-Lauraine E, Ledermann JA, Selle F, et al. Olaparib tablets as maintenance therapy in patients with platinum-sensitive, relapsed ovarian cancer and a BRCA1/2 mutation (SOLO2/ENGOT-Ov21): a double-blind, randomised, placebo-controlled, phase 3 trial. Lancet Oncol 2017;18(9):1274–84.

40. Ray-Coquard I, Pautier P, Pignata S, et al. Olaparib plus bevacizumab as first-line maintenance in ovarian cancer. N Engl J Med 2019;381(25): 2416–28.

41. Gonzalez-Martin A, Pothuri B, Vergote I, et al. Niraparib in patients with newly diagnosed advanced ovarian cancer. N Engl J Med 2019;381(25): 2391–402.

42. Ledermann JA, Oza AM, Lorusso D, et al. Rucaparib for patients with platinum-sensitive, recurrent ovarian carcinoma (ARIEL3): post-progression outcomes and updated safety results from a randomised, placebo-controlled, phase 3 trial. Lancet Oncol 2020;21(5):710–22.

43. Coleman RL, Oza AM, Lorusso D, et al. Rucaparib maintenance treatment for recurrent ovarian carcinoma after response to platinum therapy (ARIEL3): a randomised, double-blind, placebo-controlled, phase 3 trial. Lancet 2017;390(10106):1949–61.

44. Kristeleit R, Shapiro GI, Burris HA, et al. A phase I-II study of the oral PARP inhibitor rucaparib in patients with germline BRCA1/2-mutated ovarian carcinoma or other solid tumors. Clin Cancer Res 2017; 23(15):4095–106.

45. Kobel M, Kalloger SE, Huntsman DG, et al. Differences in tumor type in low-stage versus high-stage ovarian carcinomas. Int J Gynecol Pathol 2010; 29(3):203–11.

46. WHO Classification of Tumours Editorial Board. Female genital tumours. Lyon (France): International Agency for Research on Cancer; 2020. (WHO classification of tumours series, 5th ed.; vol. 4).

47. Kobel M, Rahimi K, Rambau PF, et al. An immunohistochemical algorithm for ovarian carcinoma typing. Int J Gynecol Pathol 2016;35(5):430–41.

48. Kobel M, Luo L, Grevers X, et al. Ovarian carcinoma histotype: strengths and limitations of integrating morphology with immunohistochemical predictions. Int J Gynecol Pathol 2019;38(4):353–62.

49. Lee S, Piskorz AM, Le Page C, et al. Calibration and Optimization of p53, WT1, and napsin A Immunohistochemistry Ancillary Tests for Histotyping of Ovarian Carcinoma: Canadian Immunohistochemistry Quality Control (CIQC) Experience. Int J Gynecol Pathol 2016;35(3):209–21.

50. Wright AA, Bohlke K, Armstrong DK, et al. Neoadjuvant chemotherapy for newly diagnosed, advanced ovarian cancer: society of gynecologic oncology and American society of clinical oncology clinical

practice guideline. Gynecol Oncol 2016;143(1): 3–15.

51. Bansal A, Srinivasan R, Rohilla M, et al. Morphologic and immunocytochemical features of high-grade serous carcinoma of ovary in ascitic fluid effusion and fine-needle aspiration cytology. Am J Clin Pathol 2020;154(1):103–14.

52. Stewart CJR, Crum CP, McCluggage WG, et al. Guidelines to aid in the distinction of endometrial and endocervical carcinomas, and the distinction of independent primary carcinomas of the endometrium and adnexa from metastatic spread between these and other sites. Int J Gynecol Pathol 2019; 38(Suppl 1):S75–92.

53. Leskela S, Romero I, Rosa-Rosa JM, et al. Molecular heterogeneity of endometrioid ovarian carcinoma: an analysis of 166 cases using the endometrial cancer subrogate molecular classification. Am J Surg Pathol 2020;44(7):982–90.

54. Parra-Herran C, Lerner-Ellis J, Xu B, et al. Molecular-based classification algorithm for endometrial carcinoma categorizes ovarian endometrioid carcinoma into prognostically significant groups. Mod Pathol 2017;30(12):1748–59.

55. D'Alessandris N, Travaglino A, Santoro A, et al. TCGA molecular subgroups of endometrial carcinoma in ovarian endometrioid carcinoma: A quantitative systematic review. Gynecol Oncol 2021; 163(2):427–32.

56. DeLair D, Oliva E, Kobel M, et al. Morphologic spectrum of immunohistochemically characterized clear cell carcinoma of the ovary: a study of 155 cases. Am J Surg Pathol 2011;35(1):36–44.

57. Kobel M, Kalloger SE, Carrick J, et al. A limited panel of immunomarkers can reliably distinguish between clear cell and high-grade serous carcinoma of the ovary. Am J Surg Pathol 2009;33(1): 14–21.

58. Chui MH, Momeni Boroujeni A, Mandelker D, et al. Characterization of TP53-wildtype tubo-ovarian high-grade serous carcinomas: rare exceptions to the binary classification of ovarian serous carcinoma. Mod Pathol 2021;34(2):490–501.

59. McCluggage WG, Lyness RW, Atkinson RJ, et al. Morphological effects of chemotherapy on ovarian carcinoma. J Clin Pathol 2002;55(1):27–31.

60. Chew I, Soslow RA, Park KJ. Morphologic changes in ovarian carcinoma after neoadjuvant chemotherapy: report of a case showing extensive clear cell changes mimicking clear cell carcinoma. Int J Gynecol Pathol 2009;28(5):442–6.

61. Miller K, Price JH, Dobbs SP, et al. An immunohistochemical and morphological analysis of post-chemotherapy ovarian carcinoma. J Clin Pathol 2008;61(5):652–7.

62. Espinosa I, Gallardo A, D'Angelo E, et al. Simultaneous carcinomas of the breast and ovary: utility of Pax-8, WT-1, and GATA3 for distinguishing independent primary tumors from metastases. Int J Gynecol Pathol 2015;34(3):257–65.

63. Kobel M, Ronnett BM, Singh N, et al. Interpretation of P53 immunohistochemistry in endometrial carcinomas: toward increased reproducibility. Int J Gynecol Pathol 2019;38(Suppl 1):S123–31.

64. Kobel M, Piskorz AM, Lee S, et al. Optimized p53 immunohistochemistry is an accurate predictor of TP53 mutation in ovarian carcinoma. J Pathol Clin Res 2016;2(4):247–58.

65. Rabban JT, Garg K, Ladwig NR, et al. Cytoplasmic Pattern p53 immunoexpression in pelvic and endometrial carcinomas with TP53 mutation involving nuclear localization domains: an uncommon but potential diagnostic pitfall with clinical implications. Am J Surg Pathol 2021;45(11):1441–51.

66. Singh N, Piskorz AM, Bosse T, et al. p53 immunohistochemistry is an accurate surrogate for TP53 mutational analysis in endometrial carcinoma biopsies. J Pathol 2020;250(3):336–45.

67. Altman AD, Nelson GS, Ghatage P, et al. The diagnostic utility of TP53 and CDKN2A to distinguish ovarian high-grade serous carcinoma from low-grade serous ovarian tumors. Mod Pathol 2013; 26(9):1255–63.

68. FoundationOne CDx Specimen Instructions. Available at: https://www.foundationmedicine.com/test/foundationone-cdx.

69. Myriad myChoice CDx Specimen Instructions. Available at: https://myriad-oncology.com/mychoice-cdx/.

70. Fujiwara M, McGuire VA, Felberg A, et al. Prediction of BRCA1 germline mutation status in women with ovarian cancer using morphology-based criteria: identification of a BRCA1 ovarian cancer phenotype. Am J Surg Pathol 2012;36(8):1170–7.

71. Howitt BE, Hanamornroongruang S, Lin DI, et al. Evidence for a dualistic model of high-grade serous carcinoma: BRCA mutation status, histology, and tubal intraepithelial carcinoma. Am J Surg Pathol 2015;39(3):287–93.

72. Hussein YR, Ducie JA, Arnold AG, et al. Invasion patterns of metastatic extrauterine high-grade serous carcinoma with BRCA germline mutation and correlation with clinical outcomes. Am J Surg Pathol 2016;40(3):404–9.

73. Reyes MC, Arnold AG, Kauff ND, et al. Invasion patterns of metastatic high-grade serous carcinoma of ovary or fallopian tube associated with BRCA deficiency. Mod Pathol 2014;27(10):1405–11.

74. Soslow RA, Han G, Park KJ, et al. Morphologic patterns associated with BRCA1 and BRCA2 genotype in ovarian carcinoma. Mod Pathol 2012;25(4):625–36.

75. Bartosch C, Clarke B, Bosse T. Gynaecological neoplasms in common familial syndromes (Lynch and HBOC). Pathology 2018;50(2):222–37.

Update on Ovarian Sex Cord–Stromal Tumors

Zehra Ordulu, MD

KEYWORDS

- Ovary • Sex cord-stromal tumor • Microcystic stromal tumor • Adult granulosa cell tumor
- Sertoli–Leydig cell tumor • Gynandroblastoma • FOXL2 • DICER1 • Juvenile Granulosa cell tumor

Key points

- Molecular testing might be useful in the diagnosis of morphologically challenging tumors, as illustrated by the *FOXL2* mutation testing for the differential diagnosis of adult granulosa cell tumor.

- Although adult granulosa cell tumors are typically characterized by *FOXL2* mutation, a minor subset is *FOXL2* wild type and the latter may be enriched in tumors admixed with other sex cord–stromal tumor morphologies.

- Molecular subtypes of Sertoli–Leydig cell tumors include *DICER1*-mutated, *FOXL2*-mutated, and *DICER1* and *FOXL2* wild type.

- Increasing molecular data combined with clinical and morphologic findings may result in revisiting some of the historical concepts such as gynandroblastomas, a subset of which may represent Sertoli-Leydig cell tumors with juvenile granulosa-like follicles.

ABSTRACT

This article focuses on the recent advances in ovarian sex cord–stromal tumors, predominantly in the setting of their molecular underpinnings. The integration of genetic information with morphologic and immunohistochemical findings in this rare subset of tumors is of clinical significance from refining the diagnostic and prognostic stratifications to genetic counseling.

INTRODUCTION

More than one-half of a century after the publication of the fundamental book "Endocrine Pathology of the Ovary" mainly focusing on ovarian sex cord–stromal tumors (SCSTs) by Drs Morris and Scully,[1] these neoplasms remain to be diagnostically challenging to the practicing pathologist due to their rarity, which is disproportionate to the variety in their morphology.[2–4] Although staining with sex cord–stromal markers (*eg*, WT1, SF1, FOXL2, inhibin, calretinin) and the lack of EMA expression can ascertain the lineage, immunohistochemistry is of limited value in further distinguishing among the SCST categories.[5–7] As in any other tumor type, molecular advances in this field over the last decade can provide an additional layer of information that may be beneficial for their diagnosis and clinical management.[7–9] Herein, ovarian SCSTs with recent clinicopathologic and genetic updates are discussed in line with their 2020 World Health Organization classification.[10]

PURE STROMAL TUMORS

FIBROMA

Fibromas, the most common ovarian stromal tumors, show fascicular growth of bland spindled to ovoid cells with scant cytoplasm and varying degrees of intercellular collagen.[10,11] They typically present as a unilateral mass in patients older than 30 and may be associated with ascites and pleural effusion (Meigs' syndrome) (**Table 1**).[12]

Department of Pathology, Immunology and Laboratory Medicine, University of Florida, 1345 Center Drive, Box 100275, Gainesville, FL 32610, USA
E-mail address: mordulusahin@ufl.edu

Surgical Pathology 15 (2022) 235–258
https://doi.org/10.1016/j.path.2022.02.004
1875-9181/22/Published by Elsevier Inc.

Table 1
World Health Organization classification of pure stromal tumors and corresponding clinical and molecular features

Histologic Classification (Pure Stromal)	Presentation	Average Age (Range)[a]	Altered Gene(s)	Syndromic Association
Fibroma	Pelvic mass, ascites and pleural effusion (Meigs' syndrome)	48 (any age, typically >30)	*IDH1*, cellular fibroma: *STK11*[b] and *PTCH1*[b]	Gorlin (*SUFU*, *PTCH1*), Ollier (*IDH1*)
Thecoma	Endocrine (E > A)	49.6–59.5 (16–81)	Rarely *FOXL2*[b]	NA
LTSP	Bilateral pelvic masses, bowel obstruction, ascites	28 (10 mo to 85 y)	NA	NA
SST	Pelvic mass, endocrine (E > A), rarely Meigs' syndrome	26 (12–63)	*GLI2* fusions (*FHL2* most common partner)	Gorlin (*SUFU*, *PTCH1*)
MST	Pelvic mass	45 (23–71)	*CTNNB1*, *APC*	FAP (*APC*)
SRST	Pelvic mass	36 (21–83)	*CTNNB1*[b]	NA
LCT	Endocrine (A > E)	58 (32–82)	NA	NA
SCT	Endocrine (A > E > Cushing syndrome), pelvic mass	43 (rare before puberty, wide range)	NA	Von Hippel–Lindau syndrome (*VHL*)
Ovarian fibrosarcoma	Pelvic mass	Postmenopausal	NA	Gorlin (*SUFU*, *PTCH1*), Maffucci (*IDH1*)

Abbreviations: A, androgenic; E, estrogenic; FAP, familial adenomatous polyposis; LTSP, luteinized thecoma with sclerosing peritonitis; LCT, Leydig cell tumor; MST, microcystic stromal tumor; mo: months, NA, not available; SCT, steroid cell tumor, SRST, signet ring stromal tumor, SST, sclerosing stromal tumor, y: years.
[a] In years unless specified otherwise.
[b] Controversial, see relevant subtitle.

Bilateral fibromas in younger patients occur in the setting of Gorlin (nevoid basal cell carcinoma) syndrome.[13] Among the individuals with Gorlin syndrome, those with germline *SUFU* alterations are more likely to have ovarian fibromas than those with *PTCH1*.[14] In addition, a single cellular fibroma case was reported to have an *IDH1* mutation in a patient with Ollier disease.[15] Common somatic alterations in fibromas include imbalances of chromosomes 4, 9, 12, and 19.[16–21] Of note, a single study showed that 50% of cellular fibromas have concurrent 9q22.3 and 19p13.3 loss of heterozygosity (LOH).[19] While 19p13.3 LOH was seen in usual fibromas and other SCSTs (albeit less frequently), 9q22.3 LOH was not detected in these tumors.[18,19] One of the conclusions from this study[19] was the potential involvement of *PTCH1* (9q22.3) and *STK11* (19p13.3) in cellular fibromas. However, these results should be interpreted with caution because the specific microsatellite markers that were lost did not encompass either *PTCH1* or *STK11*, and they were only on the same respective chromosome arms.

The morphologic diagnosis of a fibroma is usually straightforward. However, cellular fibromas, especially those that are mitotically active (≥4 mitoses/10 high-power field) (MACFs), may be challenging to differentiate from their malignant counterparts (fibrosarcoma)[11,22] and adult granulosa cell tumors (AGCTs). Although fibrosarcoma (exceedingly rare) and MACF both have increased mitotic rate and cellularity, the former also has moderate to severe atypia as opposed to the bland cytology of MACFs. In addition, fibrosarcoma is typically more homogenously cellular, whereas MACF can have usual fibroma-like foci admixed with the more cellular component.[3,22] In contrast, the distinction of cellular fibroma from

AGCT can be extremely difficult based on just morphology. Reticulin staining around individual cells favors the diagnosis of a fibroma in this setting (**Fig. 1**A, B). However, the interpretation of this stain might be problematic, as illustrated by a study having an indeterminate reticulin pattern in about one-third of the analyzed SCSTs.[23] A more definitive approach is to perform *FOXL2* mutation analysis for the characteristic p.C134W variant seen in up to greater than 95% of AGCTs,[24] whereas it is negative in cellular fibromas.[25] Last, it is interesting to note that one

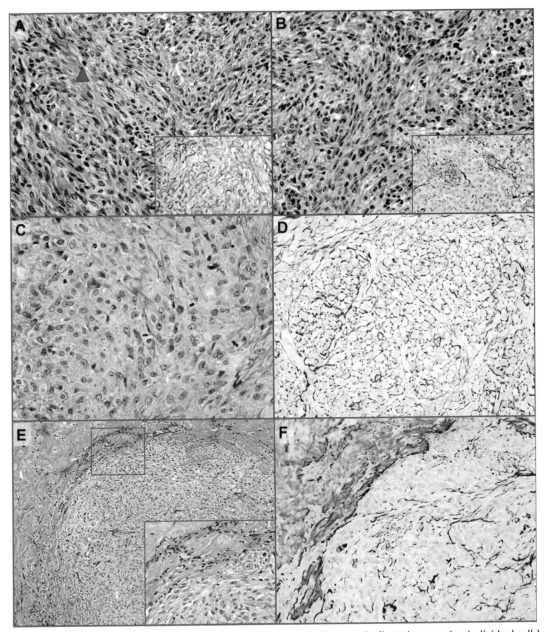

Fig. 1. (*A*) Mitotically active cellular fibroma (*arrowhead*, mitosis; *inset*, reticulin stain wrapping individual cells). (*B*) Diffuse AGCT (*inset*, reticulin stain showing nesting around tumor cell groups with loss of pericellular staining). (*C*) Thecoma with abundant pale gray cytoplasm. (*D*) Reticulin corresponding to the thecoma in (*C*), wrapping individual cells. (*E*) AGCT with thecoma-like foci (*inset*, high-power view to show the morphologic distinction between thecoma-like areas in the majority of the nodule and granulosa-like areas at the periphery of the nodule). (*F*) Reticulin corresponding to the tumor in (*E*) with nested pattern in both thecoma-like and granulosa-like areas.

case, classified by the authors as MACF, was shown to have a novel *FOXL2* mutation (p.R144W).[23]

DIAGNOSTIC PITFALL: CELLULAR FIBROMA VERSUS ADULT GRANULOSA CELL TUMORS

- Reticulin around individual cells favors fibroma

- Consider *FOXL2* mutation testing if reticulin is indeterminate

---

THECOMA

Thecomas have a diffuse to nodular growth pattern, occasionally with hyaline plaques, calcification, and sclerosis, and cells with bland nuclei, pale gray cytoplasm with indistinct cytoplasmic membranes.[26,27] They present with estrogenic symptoms in peri or postmenopausal women rather than symptoms of a pelvic mass.[28] Calcified thecomas tend to occur in younger women.[29] A unique molecular alteration specific for thecomas has not been identified; however, this may have been confounded by the single gene mutation based nature of the molecular assays used in the majority of relevant literature. A small subset of thecomas is reported to have the *FOXL2* mutation typical of AGCTs, which will be discussed further elsewhere in this article.[7,24,30–32]

It is well-established that thecomas have a morphologic overlap with fibromas. In tumors exhibiting both morphologies, the classification should be done based on predominant morphology, although some may also use the term fibrothecoma.[21] In contrast, AGCT represent a more challenging and clinically significant differential diagnosis, given its malignant potential. A recent series describing AGCTs with thecoma-like foci[33] reported that these tumors were usually nodular and had cells with moderately abundant pale-gray cytoplasm. The thecomatous versus granulosa nature of these cells were almost indistinguishable without the aid of a reticulin stain (**Fig. 1C–F**). In addition, the classic granulosa morphology with spindled to ovoid cells with scant cytoplasm was usually a minority of the tumor (typically at the periphery of the nodules) (see **Fig. 1E**). Therefore, based on hematoxylin and eosin staining alone, the granulosa component might be underestimated initially and, not surprisingly, 40% of the tumors in this series had the referral diagnosis as a thecoma. Overall, the authors highlighted the importance of reticulin staining particularly in the setting of thecomatous tumors with nodular architecture. These AGCTs with thecoma-like foci are

perhaps akin to the historical granulosa theca cell tumors[34,35] (further discussed under gynandroblastoma), which were shown to have the *FOXL2* mutation in 50% of the cases.[36] Taken together, the possibility of the previously mentioned rare thecomas with the *FOXL2* mutation actually representing an AGCT cannot be excluded. In fact, one of them was reported to have a minor granulosa cell component[24] and another study[31] reported an abdominal tumor with classic AGCT morphology in a woman who was diagnosed with a small ovarian thecoma 2 years prior. Both of these tumors had the same *FOXL2* mutation, suggesting that the initial thecoma was a misdiagnosed AGCT with thecoma-like foci.

DIAGNOSTIC PITFALL: ADULT GRANULOSA CELL TUMOR WITH THECOMA-LIKE FOCI

- Thecoma and AGCT morphology may look indistinguishable on hematoxylin and eosin staining, causing underestimation of the granulosa component

- Reticulin staining should be used liberally for nodular thecomatous tumors (loss of pericellular reticulin staining favoring AGCT)

SCLEROSING STROMAL TUMOR

Sclerosing stromal tumors (SSTs) have pseudolobulation, prominent ectatic vessels, and an admixture of lutein cells and fibroblasts.[37,38] They can show prominent luteinization during pregnancy[39] and rarely can be mitotically active.[38,40] They typically present with symptoms of a pelvic mass or are incidental. A single patient with Gorlin syndrome was reported to have SST.[41] Somatic alterations in SSTs include trisomy 12.[42,43] Recently, *GLI2* fusions have been detected in these tumors (most common partner: *FHL2*).[44]

Most SSTs are readily recognizable, but sometimes other SCSTs including fibromas, thecomas, luteinized thecoma with sclerosing peritonitis (**Fig 2A**), and steroid cell tumors (particularly in pregnant patients) enter in the differential diagnosis, as well as solitary fibrous tumors.[45,46] The unique combination of pseudolobulation, ectatic vessels, and the jumbled mixture of lutein cells and fibroblasts should prompt the diagnosis of SST[38] (**Fig. 2B–D**). For solitary fibrous tumors, STAT6 staining can provide additional reassurance given the rarity of these tumors at this site.

MICROCYSTIC STROMAL TUMOR AND SIGNET RING STROMAL TUMOR

Microcystic stromal tumors (MSTs) are rare and represent the most recently described SCST.[47]

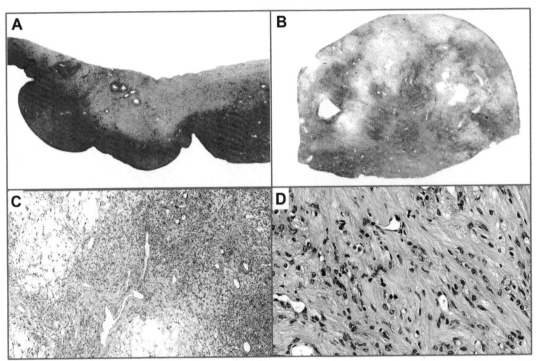

Fig. 2. (*A*) Luteinized thecoma with sclerosing peritonitis displays characteristic cerebriform hypercellularity at the periphery of the ovarian stroma. (*B–D*) SST is characterized by pseudolobulation at low power view (*B*), ectatic vessels and alternating hypocellular and hypercellular areas (*C*), and a mixture of luteinized cells and spindled cells (*D*).

The classic morphologic features include solid cellular zones with microcysts that may coalesce into larger channels, intersected by fibrous stroma with hyaline plaques (**Fig. 3**A–C). The tumor cells have pale or gray cytoplasm, sometimes vacuolated, as well as round, uniform nuclei with occasional bizarre atypia. On the other hand, MSTs with nonconventional morphology might have diffuse solid, corded, and/or nested architecture of cells with eosinophilic cytoplasm and variable intracytoplasmic vacuoles with only minimal or no microcysts (**Fig. 3**D).[48,131] Patients usually present with symptoms of a pelvic mass, typically unilateral. Bilateral ovarian involvement has been rarely reported.[50] MSTs may be seen in the setting of familial adenomatous polyposis with germline *APC* mutations and a second hit in the MST.[51,52] The most common somatic mutations involve *CTNNB1* and, less frequently, *APC*. They lack mutations in *FOXL2* and *DICER1*.[52–56] Although these tumors are generally considered benign, 2 cases with recurrence have been reported, one of which had variants of uncertain significance in *APC* and *KRAS*.[57,58] MSTs have a distinct immunohistochemical profile among the majority of SCSTs; as

beta catenin and cyclin D1 stains can be used as a surrogate for the activation of the WNT signaling pathway.[54] In addition, they are positive for CD10, WT1, SF1, and FOXL2, but negative for inhibin and calretinin.[48,54]

Signet ring stromal tumors (SRSTs)[59–61] are in the differential diagnosis of nonconventional MSTs. Both of these extremely rare tumors have cellular fibromatous stroma with signet ring cells, each featuring a single clear intracellular vacuole that is negative for lipid or mucin. Interestingly, testicular SRSTs have been shown to harbor *CTNNB1* mutations and express nuclear beta catenin postulating a potential link to MST.[62] One case described as ovarian SRST and showing nuclear beta catenin has been reported.[63] Moreover, a collusion tumor consisting of SRST and steroid cell tumor also showed nuclear beta catenin expression restricted to the SRST component.[64] However, it is possible that the reported ovarian SRSTs with *CTNNB1* mutations [63,64] may actually represent nonconventional MSTs based on the provided photomicrographs. A separate study documenting bilateral SRSTs showed lack of nuclear beta catenin expression,

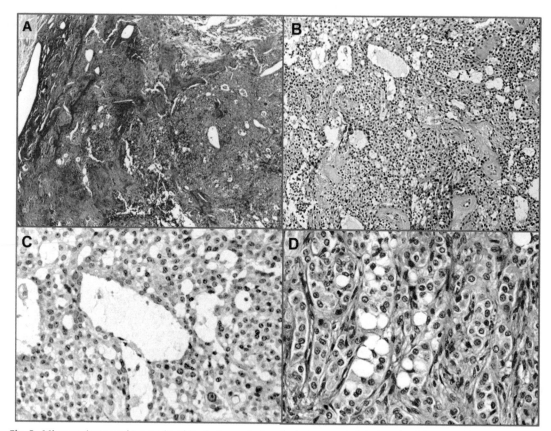

Fig. 3. Microcystic stromal tumor. (*A–C*) Typical morphology includes pseudolobulated architecture (*A*), microcysts and macrocysts with hyaline plaques in the background (*B*), and a monomorphic cell population with intracytoplasmic vacuoles and uniform round nuclei, forming microcysts (*C*). (*D*) Nonconventional morphology is sometimes seen, in this example featuring nests of cells with eosinophilic cytoplasm and intracytoplasmic vacuoles (Courtesy of Dr McCluggage).

as well as *CTNNB1* and *FOXL2* mutations,[65] a profile that is more in keeping with fibroma. Overall, it may be speculated that SRSTs represent a morphologic spectrum from fibromas with signet ring cells (*CTNNB1* wild-type) to non-conventional MSTs (*CTNNB1* mutated), and additional studies are warranted for better classification of these extremely rare tumors. With the currently available information, SRSTs usually show a signet ring cell component in a fibromatous background, whereas signet ring cells in MSTs are seen in a background of solid, nested and corded growth patterns separated by fibrous septae. MSTs do not always show the typical microcysts but when present, they help with the differential diagnosis. Of note, another rare neoplasm, solid pseudopapillary tumor of the ovary,[66,67] also has similar *CTNNB1* mutations and CD10 positivity, but should be differentiated based on morphologic features.

Another consideration for the differential of nonconventional MSTs and SRSTs is a Krukenberg tumor, which also exhibits signet ring cell morphology.[61,68–70] The mucinous nature of the vacuoles, as well as the atypia of the nuclei (which can be subtle, but often appreciable), should prompt the consideration of this possibility, which can be confirmed by histochemistry for mucicarmine and an immunostaining panel including the aforementioned markers and EMA (negative in SCSTs). Lastly, although a steroid cell tumor does not immediately come to mind as a mimicker, there is a case report of a steroid cell tumor in a patient with familial adenomatous polyposis,[71] where the photomicrographs may represent a nonconventional MST as pointed out by other authors.[52] The ancillary studies can also be used in this setting.

Molecular features and considerations for differential diagnosis of pure stromal tumors discussed herein are summarized in **BOX 1** and **BOX 2**, respectively.

Box 1
Molecular pathology features: pure stromal tumors

Fibroma

- Somatic: Chromosomal imbalances of 4, 9, 12 and 19, *IDH1* mutation

- Syndromic: Gorlin (*SUFU, PTCH1*), Ollier (*IDH1*) (single case report)

Thecoma

- Somatic: Small subset of cases described as harboring *FOXL2* mutation (may represent AGCT with thecoma-like foci)

Sclerosing stromal tumor

- Somatic: Trisomy 12, *GLI2* fusions (*FHL2* most common partner)

- Syndromic: Gorlin (*SUFU, PTCH1*) (single case report)

Microcystic stromal tumor

- Somatic: *CTNNB1* > *APC* mutations (mutually exclusive)

- Syndromic: Familial adenomatous polyposis (*APC*)

DIAGNOSTIC PITFALL: NONCONVENTIONAL MICROCYSTIC STROMAL TUMOR

- May be diffusely solid, nested, and corded (without obvious microcysts)

- Eosinophilic cytoplasm with occasional intra-cytoplasmic vacuoles

- Immunohistochemistry is helpful in confirming the diagnosis

PURE SEX CORD TUMORS

ADULT GRANULOSA CELL TUMOR

Accounting for 90% of malignant SCSTs of the ovary, AGCTs in their conventional form have scant cytoplasm and round to ovoid uniform nuclei with interspersed nuclear grooves. They show many architectural patterns (**Fig. 4**): diffuse,

---

Box 2
Differential diagnosis: pure stromal tumors

Mitotically active cellular fibroma

- Fibrosarcomas: Moderate to severe cytologic atypia

- AGCTs: Nested reticulin, *FOXL2* mutation

Thecoma

- Fibromas: If morphologic overlap, classify based on predominant morphology

- AGCTs with thecoma-like foci: Nested reticulin, *FOXL2* mutation

Sclerosing Stromal Tumor

- Other SCSTs: The unique constellation of pseudolobulation, ectatic vessels, and the jumbled mixture of lutein cells and fibroblasts separates SSTs from mimickers that may have 1 or 2 of these findings individually and focally.

- Solitary fibrous tumor: In addition to above-mentioned morphologic criteria, STAT6 expression in solitary fibrous tumors

Microcystic stromal tumor

- The morphologic spectrum recently expanded

- Those without microcysts can mimic SRST and Krukenberg

- Positive: Beta catenin (nuclear staining), cyclin D1, CD10, WT1, FOXL2, SF1

- Negative: Inhibin, calretinin, EMA

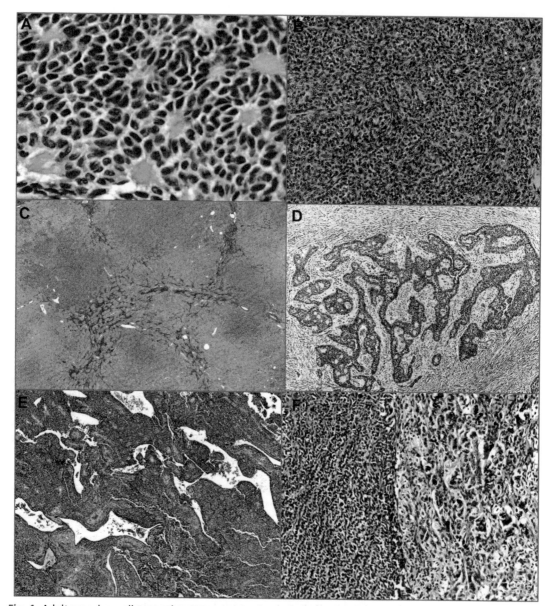

Fig. 4. Adult granulosa cell tumor shows a spectrum of morphologies. (*A*) Characteristic Call–Exner bodies (*rare*), (*B*) diffuse (most common), (*C*) fibrothecomatous nodules with more typical morphology at the periphery of the nodules, (*D*) trabeculated architecture in fibromatous stroma, (*E*) papillary architecture, and (*F*) high-grade transformation with a sharp demarcation between low-grade (*left*) and high-grade (*right*) components.

corded, trabecular, insular, and less frequently pseudopapillary, gyriform, and macrofollicular. The most distinctive morphology is microfollicular, which features with Call–Exner bodies (see **Fig. 4**A); however, this pattern is seen in a minority of cases. AGCTs typically present in perimenopausal women with abdominal pain and estrogenic symptoms (**Table 2**).[72] Although AGCTs are not recurrently associated with a syndrome, there is a single case with a germline *TP53* mutation showing multifocal intrafollicular AGCT.[73] Despite the variety in their morphology, AGCTs

are molecularly homogenous tumors showing a recurrent and relatively specific *FOXL2* mutation (c.C402G; p.C134W),[24,74] which can be used for diagnostic purposes. The frequency of this *FOXL2* mutation in AGCTs is reported as 90% or more in most studies,[23,24,30,74–76] with only few reports showing frequencies of 60% to 80%.[77–79] These discrepancies may be attributed to technical aspects of the sequencing (quality of the DNA, tumor percentage, etc); however, it is also important to note, at least for one of these series,[78] the nature of the cohort (being predominantly

Table 2
World Health Organization classification of pure sex-cord and mixed tumors and corresponding clinical and molecular features

Histologic Classification	Presentation	Average Age (Range)[a]	Altered Gene(s)	Syndromic Association
Pure sex cord				
AGCT	Solid and cystic pelvic mass, endocrine (E > A)	50 (any age, rare in first decade)	FOXL2, KMT2D High-grade: TP53 Recurrent: TERT	NA
JGCT	Solid and cystic pelvic mass, endocrine (prepubertal: isosexual pseudoprecocity, older: AUB)	13 (0–67)	Common: AKT1, GNAS, KMT2C, TERT rearrangement, DICER1 Rare: IDH1, FOXL2	DICER1-S, Ollier (IDH1) and Mafucci (IDH1)
Sertoli cell tumor	Pelvic mass, endocrine (E > A)	30 (any age)	Rarely DICER1	PJS (STK11)
SCTAT	Incidental, rarely progesterone	20–30 (<10->70)	NA	PJS (STK11)
Mixed				
SLCT	Endocrine (A) Endocrine (E > A)	24.5 (15–62) 79.5 (51–90) 51 (17–74)	DICER1 FOXL2 Non-DICER1/FOXL2	DICER1-S
SCST, NOS	NA	NA	Variable based on morphology	NA
Gynandroblastoma	Abdominal pain, endocrine	24.5 (14–80)	Variable based on morphology	DICER1-S

Abbreviations: A, androgenic; AGCT, adult granulosa cell tumor; AUB, abnormal uterine bleeding; E, estrogenic; JGCT, juvenile granulosa cell tumor; NA, not available; PJS, Peutz–Jeghers syndrome; S, syndrome; SCTAT, sex cord-tumor with annular tubules; SCST, NOS, sex cord–stromal tumor, not otherwise specified; SLCT, Sertoli-Leydig cell tumor.
[a] In years.

consult cases) implies these tumors were morphologically more challenging than a bona fide AGCT. In fact, one of the striking findings in this study was that the *FOXL2* wild-type AGCTs were enriched for other SCST elements (further discussed under Gynandroblastoma). Of note, a recent series using whole genome sequencing found *DICER1* mutations in 2/4 *FOXL2* wild-type AGCT.[76] FOXL2 is a transcription factor regulating ovarian granulosa and follicle cell development.[80] Germline *FOXL2* loss-of-function mutations may result in premature ovarian failure in the setting of autosomal dominant blepharophimoses, ptosis, and epicanthus syndrome.[81] Conversely, the *FOXL2* mutation in the AGCTs is presumed to be an oncogenic activation.[82] Of note, FOXL2 immunohistochemistry should not be used as a surrogate for *FOXL2* mutation, because it is also positive in other SCSTs in the absence of *FOXL2* aberrations.[31] Therefore, this stain is useful as a biomarker of sex cord–stromal lineage, but it is not specific for AGCT.

Unlike the majority of benign stromal tumors, AGCT are of low malignant potential with approximately a 20% recurrence rate, often decades after diagnosis, thus requiring close and long-term follow-up.[83–85] Recurrent tumors are predominantly enriched in *TERT* promoter variants.[76,86–88] A clinically significant recent advance is that *FOXL2* and *TERT* promoter mutations can be detected in circulating tumor DNA, which can be used as a biomarker for disease monitoring.[89,90] Other variants implied in recurrent tumors, but not consistently documented by multiple studies, include *KMT2D* (seen in approximately 10% of AGCT), *TP53*, and *MED12* mutations, and *CDKN2A*/B homozygous deletions.[88,91,92]

Recently, a rare subset of AGCTs with high-grade transformation have been described with relatively more aggressive behavior.[93,94] The high-grade areas of the tumor have an abrupt transition from the typical low-grade morphology (see **Fig. 4F**), and are characterized by marked atypia with multinucleated cells, a high mitotic count, and often a differential p53-mutated pattern staining, which is wild type in the low-grade areas. The high-grade areas may resemble juvenile granulosa cell tumor (JGCT) with abundant eosinophilic cytoplasm and intermediate sized follicles; however, both components have the typical *FOXL2* mutation indicating a clonal AGCT origin. The authors noted that these tumors may be similar to the previously reported AGCTs with sarcomatous transformation[95–97]; however, they are different than those with occasional bizarre nuclei with no significant mitotic activity.[98,99] In addition, an earlier series[32] reported an AGCT recurrence being misdiagnosed as a high-grade serous carcinoma due to pleomorphism and p53 staining,

which then was found to have the same *FOXL2* mutation with the primary AGCT tumor removed 2 years ago, thus evoking the phenomenon of high-grade transformation. Another similar report described an aggressive AGCT with rapid recurrence composed of low-grade and sarcomatoid components, the latter showing enlarged bizarre nuclei, increased mitosis, and mutated-pattern p53 expression, whereas the former with wild-type-pattern p53 staining.[97] Finally, a recent series with molecular analysis on AGCTs[76] identified a small subset (3/46) with *TP53* mutations, a high tumor mutational burden, and an increased mitotic index, recapitulating the findings of the aforementioned high-grade transformation study.[93]

DIAGNOSTIC PITFALL: ADULT GRANULOSA CELL TUMOR WITH HIGH-GRADE TRANSFORMATION

- High-grade transformation in AGCT may mimic other pleomorphic tumors, especially if tumor is not well-sampled or is the sole morphology in a recurrence

- Patient's clinical history and careful examination of the tumor for areas with typical morphology should alleviate this caveat, and prompt further ancillary studies if necessary

---

JUVENILE GRANULOSA CELL TUMOR

JGTCs have a nodular or diffuse growth pattern with interspersed follicles of various shapes and irregular contours, usually containing basophilic secretions and set in an edematous to myxoid stroma. The cells have abundant eosinophilic cytoplasm and hyperchromatic nuclei with variable atypia (**Fig. 5**).[100] Most lesions present as a unilateral solid and cystic mass in younger patients, with an average age of 13 (wide range, most commonly in the first decade). Most of the prepubertal patients affected show isosexual pseudoprecocity, whereas older patients can have symptoms of a pelvic mass and abnormal uterine bleeding.[100] These tumors can be seen in patients with Ollier disease, Maffucci syndrome (*IDH1*),[100–102] and *DICER1* syndrome.[103] Case reports of this tumor in a patient with tuberous sclerosis[104] and another with concurrent *TP53* and *PTEN* germline mutations, have been published.[105] Activating alterations of *AKT1* (60%) and *GNAS* (30%), as well as *DICER1* (10%) mutations are recurrently identified in JGCTs,[106,107] whereas *FOXL2* mutations are rare.[24,108–110] A recent comprehensive analysis of JGCTs reported *KMT2C* and other SWI/SNF complex gene mutations, as well as *TERT* rearrangements, in addition

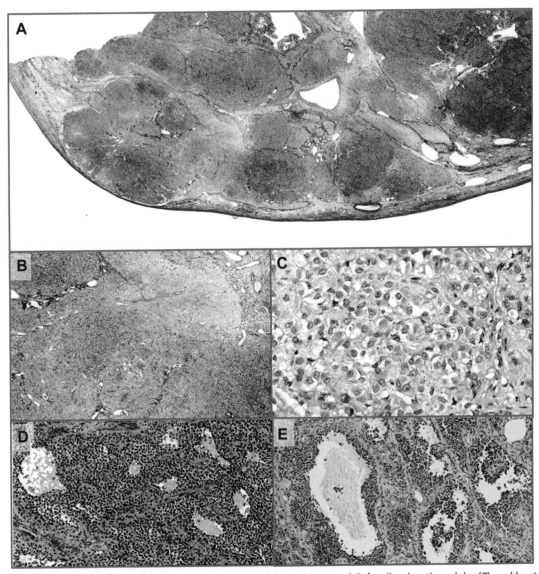

Fig. 5. (*A-C*) Juvenile granulosa cell tumor with multinodular architecture (*A*), focally sclerotic nodules (*B*), and (nests of cells with abundant cytoplasm and atypical nuclei *(C)*. (*D*) Juvenile granulosa cell tumor follicles have variable sizes and shapes and basophilic secretions. (*E*) Small cell carcinoma, hypercalcemic type is an important differential diagnosis, as it can form follicle-like spaces; these are lined by small round blue neoplastic cells without polarization.

to previously reported *AKT1* and *DICER1* mutations.[111]

The age group and the follicular growth seen in these tumors brings the differential consideration of small cell carcinoma, hypercalcemic type showing follicle-like spaces (see **Fig.** 5E) and, to a lesser extent, germ cell tumors, in particular yolk sac tumors forming cysts. However, the characteristic morphologic features and the lack of endocrine presentation in those tumors are usually enough to make a definitive diagnosis. For confirmatory purposes, EMA, and SMARCA4 can be performed to exclude small cell carcinoma, hypercalcemic type, and SALL4 for yolk sac tumors.

Molecular features and considerations for differential diagnosis of pure sex cord tumors discussed herein are summarized in **BOX 3** and **BOX 4**, respectively.

MIXED SEX CORD–STROMAL TUMORS

SERTOLI–LEYDIG CELL TUMOR

Sertoli–Leydig cell tumors (SLCTs) commonly have moderate to poorly and, less frequently, well-differentiated forms (usually seen in the pure

---

Box 3
Molecular pathology features: pure sex cord tumors

Adult granulosa cell tumor, somatic alterations:

- Most common (usually ≥90%): *FOXL2* c.C402G (p.C134W) mutation

- High-grade transformation: *TP53* mutations

- Recurrent: Predominantly *TERT* promoter mutations; however, *KMT2D* (seen in approximately 10% of AGCT), *TP53*, and *MED12* mutations, and *CDKN2A*/B homozygous deletions also anecdotally observed

Juvenile granulosa cell tumor

- Somatic: Commonly *AKT1, GNAS, KMT2C, TERT* rearrangements, *DICER1*; rarely *IDH1* and *FOXL2*

- Syndromic: Ollier (*IDH1*), Mafucci (*IDH1*), *DICER1* syndrome

---

Sertoli cell tumor setting). Differentiation depends on the presence and amount of tubular differentiation versus primitive gonadal stroma.[112] Well-differentiated forms have tubules showing no significant atypia. Moderately differentiated forms usually have a lobular pattern of Sertoli cells growing in nests (less often in tubules) with mild to moderate cytologic atypia. Leydig cells usually present at the periphery of the lobules. Poorly differentiated ones show a primitive and sarcomatoid stroma, sometimes admixed with moderately differentiated SLCT elements in the background. Retiform SLCTs have anastomosing spaces with papillary structures that are reminiscent of the rete testis. SLCTs can have heterologous elements in epithelial (carcinoid, intestinal glands) or mesenchymal (cartilage or skeletal muscle) forms.[113,114] They usually present with androgenic manifestations or symptoms of a pelvic mass (solid or solid cystic, less frequently cystic), but also can have estrogenic manifestations. Average age at presentation is 25 years with a wide range (1–84 years); those with a retiform morphology tend to occur in younger patients, whereas they are well-differentiated in older patients. SLCT has been reported in the setting of DICER1 syndrome.[103,115,116] Usually, these patients have a germline loss-of-function mutation and a somatic hotspot mutation in their tumors as a second hit. The risk of having a germline *DICER1* mutation after a diagnosis of ovarian SLCT can be as high as 69%.[117,118] In addition, this syndrome has low penetrance and, therefore, the lack of a family history or lack of other DICER1 syndrome related tumors in the patient might be misleading. Taken together, it is recommended that any woman with an SLCT should receive genetic counseling for DICER1 syndrome, unless screening for *DICER1* mutation in the tumor is possible as a first line approach (in which case, a negative result is reassuring, but a positive result should be followed by germline testing).

DICER1 mutations are common in SLCTs with moderate to poor differentiation.[117] Overall, they are present in approximately 65% of SLCTs,[9,108,109,117–121] a frequency that is slightly skewed upwards because of the studies with subject populations enriched in patients with DICER1

Box 4
Differential diagnosis: pure sex cord tumors

Adult granulosa cell tumor

- Fibrothecomatous tumors: Reticulin around individual cells

- Endometrioid carcinoma: EMA+

- FOXL2 immunostain: Not a surrogate for the mutation, but can be used for SCST lineage confirmation (also positive in other SCSTs)

- *FOXL2* mutation testing: Relatively sensitive and specific, but not definitive (particularly if differential includes SLCT in a postmenopausal women)

Juvenile granulosa cell tumor

- Small cell carcinoma, hypercalcemic type: Follicle-like spaces lined by small blue cells that lack polarization, EMA+, SMARCA4 lost

- Yolk sac tumor: Schiller Duval bodies, SALL4+

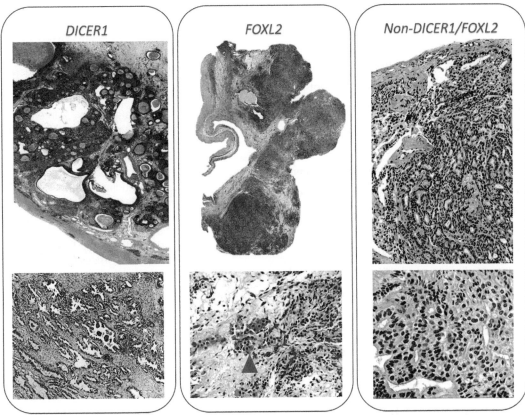

Fig. 6. Typical morphologic characteristics of the molecular SLCT subgroups. *DICER1*-mutated: Intermediate differentiation with heterologous elements in the form of intestinal epithelium (*top*). Retiform architecture mimicking rete testis (*bottom*). *FOXL2*-mutated: intermediate differentiation with lobulated architecture and without heterologous elements (*top*). Leydig cell clusters (arrowhead) at the periphery of the nodules (*bottom*). Non-*DICER1/FOXL2* mutated: well-differentiated SLCT (*top*). Leydig cells intermixed with the well-formed tubules (*bottom*).

syndrome (up to 97%).[118] Recently, a more inclusive study in terms of patient demographics has proposed that SLCTs have 3 molecular subgroups correlating with their clinicopathologic features[122]: *DICER1* (44%), *FOXL2* (19%), and non-*DICER1/FOXL2* (37%) mutated (**Fig. 6**, **Box 5**). Those with *DICER1* mutations were seen in the younger patients (median age, 24.5 years), whereas *FOXL2* occurs in older patients (median age, 79.5 years) and those wild type for both in between (median age, 51 years). *DICER1*-mutated cases had the typical clinical and morphologic features of SLCT with predominantly androgenic symptoms and moderate to poor differentiation, as well as the presence of heterologous and retiform elements. In contrast, *FOXL2*-mutated ones were seen in postmenopausal patients with abnormal bleeding, which also had moderate to poor differentiation, but without heterologous elements. Of note, the authors performed a thorough morphologic assessment to make sure these did not represent luteinized AGCTs. In addition, another study

simultaneously also described *FOXL2* mutations in an SLCT,[23] supportive the concept of a *FOXL2*-mutated SLCT category. The third group (*FOXL2* and *DICER1* wild type) mostly included well-differentiated SLCTs. The prognostic significance of this classification is currently unclear owing to the limited number of cases; however, it still has immediate implications for genetic counseling in the setting of DICER1 syndrome (which should be considered at least in all SLCT of intermediate or poor differentiation, particularly if retiform or heterologous components are found).

Most of the mimickers of SLCTs are usually discernible by morphologic features (**Fig. 7**) with occasional help from ancillary studies. Among them, perhaps the most challenging one would be the differentiation of a luteinized AGCT from a *FOXL2*-mutated SLCT without heterologous elements, as ancillary testing including mutational profile would not be useful. Morphologically, SLCT usually does not have a fibromatous stroma like AGCT, and rather has a lobulated architecture

---

Box 5
Molecular pathology features: Sertoli-Leydig cell tumors

DICER1-mutated

- If syndromic: Germline loss of function + somatic hotspot mutations

- Nonsyndromic: Usually somatic hotspot mutations

- Younger patients (mean, 24.5 years; range, 15–62 years)

- Androgenic manifestations

- Intermediate to poorly differentiated histology

- Retiform or heterologous elements common

- *DICER1* somatic alterations can be used to differentiate from AGCT

FOXL2-mutated

- Older patients (mean, 79.5 years; range, 51–90 years)

- Estrogenic > androgenic manifestations

- Intermediate to poorly differentiated histology

- No retiform or heterologous elements

- Distinction from AGCT should be done based on morphology

DICER1 and *FOXL2* wild type

- Intermediate age (mean 51, years; range, 17–74 years)

- Includes well-differentiated SLCTs

---

in an edematous stroma. The Leydig cells usually are clustered at the periphery of the sertoliform lobules, whereas in AGCT the luteinized cells are scattered throughout the stroma usually in a single-cell manner (see **Fig. 7**C, D). However, especially after *FOXL2* mutation status is established, perhaps the distinction of these 2 entities is of uncertain clinical significance. Overall, the similar clinical presentation and mutation profiles may indicate a spectrum of the same pathophysiology and additional studies are warranted.

CLINICS CARE POINTS

- Currently, any woman with a diagnosis of ovarian SLCT should be considered for genetic counseling for DICER1 syndrome.
- In an ideal scenario, an initial screening of tumor DNA for *DICER1* alterations can eliminate *DICER1*-wild type cases and capture the high-risk population of *DICER1*-mutated tumors for genetic counseling.

SEX CORD–STROMAL TUMOR, NOT OTHERWISE SPECIFIED AND GYNANDROBLASTOMA

SCST, not otherwise specified, does not have any definitive characteristic of a specific SCST

category (pure stromal, pure sex cord, or SLCT as listed in **Tables 1** and **2**), but has a morphologic and immunohistochemical clues of a sex cord-stromal lineage.[10] A recent series of challenging SCSTs showed that molecular analysis for *FOXL2*, *DICER1*, and *STK11* can help with the diagnosis in approximately 85% of the cases (42/50).[8] Another smaller series had 30% (6/20) of the cases resolved as AGCT based on *FOXL2* analysis.[32] These studies highlight the usefulness of molecular studies in the classification of morphologically-ambiguous SCSTs (**Box 6**).

Gynandroblastomas are presumed mixed tumors with components resembling both female (gyn-) and male (andro-) sex cord differentiation with varying stromal elements,[1,123] with an arbitrary cut off of having at least 10% of each morphology.[124] Overall, they are relatively indolent with only 2 recurrences in the literature.[125,126] Historically, SCST, not otherwise specified, and gynandroblastomas have been recognized as 2 different entities; however, in practice it may be difficult to make a definitive distinction depending on the percentage of each morphology and presence of their defining features. Not surprisingly, both terms have been used for tumors having overlapping characteristics in the literature. An additional challenge is to discern a true mixed SCST with collision of different tumor types from

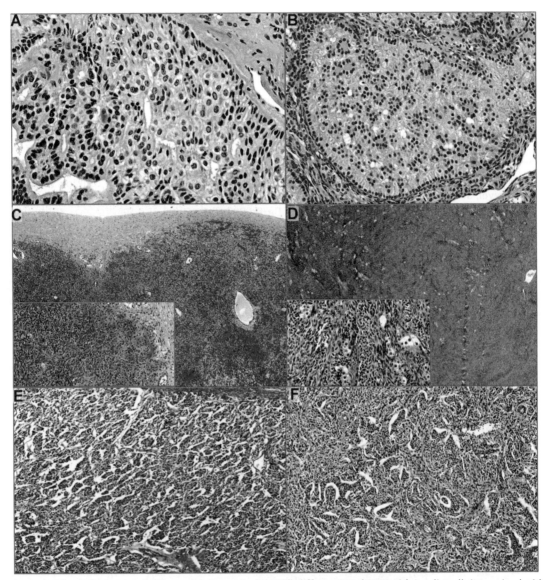

Fig. 7. SLCT morphology and differential diagnosis. (*A*) Well-differentiated SLCT with Leydig cells intermixed with sertoliform tubules. (*B*) Sex cord tumor with annular tubules with antipolar distribution of nuclei around basement membrane-like material. (*C*) SLCT with intermediate differentiation (*inset,* clusters of Leydig cells prominent at the periphery of the lobules). (*D*) AGCT with luteinization and fibromatous stroma (*inset,* scattered lutein cells throughout the stroma). (*E*) Retiform SLCT with somewhat papillary configuration of the Sertoli cells. (*F*) AGCT forming a trabeculated architecture with peculiar clefting mimicking the small papillae seen in retiform SLCT.

a rare morphologic variant of a single entity having areas resembling to another SCST. Given the rarity of these scenarios, currently it is difficult to speculate the clinical significance of separating or further defining SCST, not otherwise specified, from gynandroblastoma. For now, a clear and consistent nomenclature should be followed as much as possible for future accumulation of data and better stratification of patients. Of note, the subcategories discussed in the following paragraphs are not included in the 2020 World Health Organization classification[10] and are only used for better organization of the existing literature.

TUMORS WITH SERTOLI AND ADULT GRANULOSA MORPHOLOGY

A single study looking at individual components of gynandroblastomas[127] showed that *FOXL2* or *DICER1* mutations were absent in all tumors with

> **Box 6**
> **Molecular pathology features: SCST not otherwise specified and gynandroblastoma**
>
> - Tumors with overlapping fibrothecomatous and adult granulosa cell morphology are difficult to classify morphologically. A reticulin stain and/or *FOXL2* mutation testing can be extremely helpful in this setting.
>
> - Tumors with Sertoli and JGCT-like morphology may represent a morphologic variant of *DICER1*-mutated SLCTs with juvenile granulosa-like differentiation.
>
> - Tumors with adult granulosa cell and well-differentiated Sertoli morphology seem to be most frequently *DICER1*-and *FOXL2*-wild type, linking them with the group of SLCTs that is also well differentiated and lacks mutations in these genes.
>
> - Tumors with true biphasic morphology may exist (gynandroblastomas and true collision tumors); however, at least some gynandroblastomas have been shown to be tumors with morphologic ambiguity mimicking a collision phenomenon and have been re-classified as a specific SCST entity (for instance, SLCT with JGCT-like growth).

adult granulosa morphology with an accompanying Sertoli cell morphology (6/6).[127] It was interesting to note the majority of these cases had a well-differentiated Sertoli component (**Fig. 8**). In fact, none of the gynandroblastomas with well-differentiated Sertoli morphology in this study (7/7) showed either *FOXL2* or *DICER1* mutations, akin to the *FOXL2* and *DICER1* wild-type SLCTs

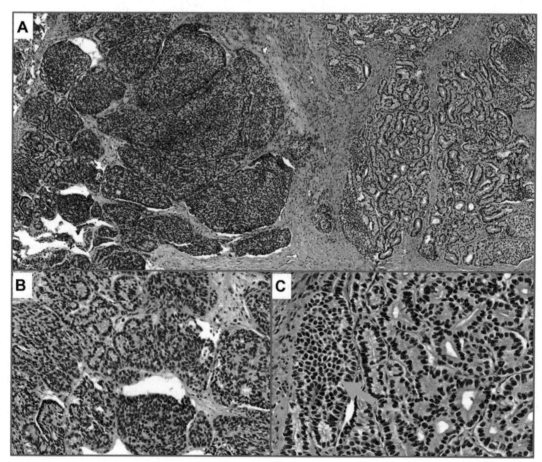

Fig. 8. (*A*). Tumor with adult granulosa (*left*) and well-differentiated Sertoli cell (*right*) morphology. (*B*) Sertoliform tubules intermixed with the adult granulosa background. (*C*) Well-differentiated Sertoli cell tubules transitioning into adult granulosa-like areas (*arrow*).

that are enriched in well-differentiated morphology.[122] Another study with 3 tumors with Sertoli cell and AGCT morphology also had wild type *FOXL2* in either component.[128] Another case of an AGCT and sex cord stromal tumor with annular tubules morphologies did not demonstrate either *DICER1* or *FOXL2* mutations.[8] In addition, the previously mentioned consult series of AGCTs with 70% *FOXL2* mutations[78] pointed out that many of the *FOXL2*-wild type cases had additional sex cord-stromal components. Overall, these findings indicate that the small subset of *FOXL2*-negative AGCTs are often enriched in other sex cord elements and suggest that they may have a morphologic and presumably undiscovered molecular continuum with FOXL2/ DICER1-wild type well-differentiated SLCT that may occasionally mimic a mixed tumor (see **Fig. 8**). Additional studies analyzing the clonality of each component for other molecular markers maybe of interest to support this hypothesis.

TUMORS WITH SERTOLI CELL AND JUVENILE GRANULOSA MORPHOLOGY

The previously mentioned study looking at individual components of gynandroblastomas[127] reported 40% (3/8) of tumors with moderate to poorly differentiated Sertoli cell component showed *DICER1* mutations, all of which also had additional juvenile granulosa morphology also showing the same mutations. Although this is the only report with the analysis of each component, multiple additional studies documented moderate to poorly differentiated Sertoli cell with juvenile granulosa morphology (the majority of them referred to as gynandroblastomas) having *DICER1* alterations,[110,117,121] including those seen in patients with DICER1 syndrome.[117,118,126] As mentioned previously in this article, *DICER1* relatively are a hallmark change in SLCT, and are in turn rare in JGCT. In addition, a recent study showed that SLCTs with JGCT-like follicles have (1) clinical features more akin to SLCT rather than JGCT, and (2) a predominant SLCT morphology where JGCT-like follicles gradually arise from the lobules of SLCT (**Fig. 9**).[129] Overall, these findings suggest that so-called gynandroblastomas with Sertoli cell and juvenile granulosa morphology likely represent a morphologic variant of *DICER1*-mutated SLCTs that shows JGCT-like differentiation and the subset of JGCTs with *DICER1* mutations may represent a continuum of these tumors.

An alternative but rare consideration in this morphologic spectrum is the high-grade transformation of an SLCT, which is exemplified by a single case of SLCT demonstrating *DICER1* and *TP53* mutations,[8] akin to the AGCTs with high-grade transformation having *FOXL2* and *TP53* mutations.

TUMORS WITH ADULT AND JUVENILE GRANULOSA MORPHOLOGY

Other than personal anecdotes of expert pathologists, there is only a single example of a combined AGCT and JGCT in the literature, which also has a Sertoli cell tumor component.[130] However, the authors of the AGCT with high-grade differentiation study[93] made a valid point in their discussion that perhaps a subset of these can be misinterpreted as mixed SCST with AGCT and JGCT components owing to pleomorphic and focally cystic morphology of the high-grade component. The authors of this study found *FOXL2* mutations in both AGCT and high-grade components, excluding this possibility and, in turn, suggesting a common clonal origin of the AGCT with JGCT-like elements in those cases with high-grade transformation.

FIBROTHECOMATOUS TUMORS WITH ADULT GRANULOSA MORPHOLOGY (SO-CALLED GRANULOSA–THECA CELL TUMORS)

Fibrothecomatous tumors with less than 10% sex cord elements have been referred to as stromal tumors with minor sex cord elements, and they are considered benign in nature.[132] Some pathologists use the term granulosa-theca cell tumors for those with 10% to 50% granulosa cells in a fibrothecomatous background,[34,35] whereas others call any tumor with a granulosa component beyond 10% as AGCTs. When called AGCTs, these tumors will be in the spectrum of AGCTs with thecoma-like foci and AGCT with extensive fibromatous background (see **Figs. 1E,F and 4C, D**).

In the previously mentioned series of challenging SCSTs,[8] the most common dilemma (29/50) was AGCTs with overlapping features with thecomas and cellular fibromas (and an additional cystic AGCT with a differential diagnosis of follicle cyst not included in this discussion but characterized further in a recent series[131]). Given that reticulin is not always conclusive,[23] *FOXL2* mutation analysis can be more sensitive in this setting. In this study, 15 of 29 tumors with the above differential were classified as AGCT based on morphologic features and the presence of *FOXL2* mutation, whereas only 1 in 29 cases was diagnosed as an AGCT despite the lack of *FOXL2* mutation based on morphologic clues only. In contrast, 13 of the 29 tumors were diagnosed as thecoma or cellular fibroma due to lack of *FOXL2* mutation. Overall, *FOXL2* mutation testing was helpful in 28 of the 29 cases with this differential,

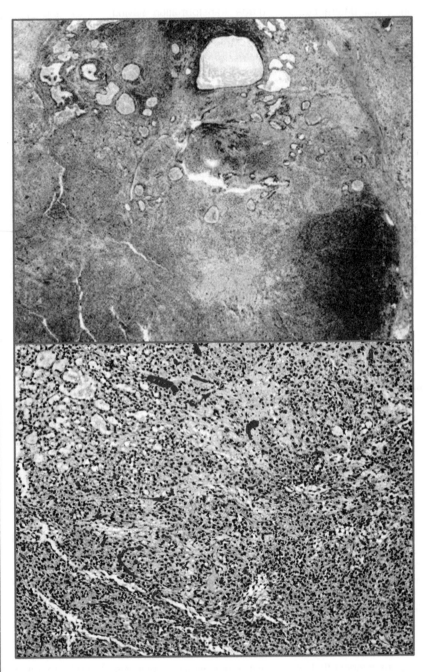

Fig. 9. SLCT with juvenile granulosa-like follicular differentiation: Follicles arising from the SLCT of intermediate differentiation lobules (*top*) and loosening of the pale stroma yielding to follicle-like structures (*bottom*).

where only in one AGCT the authors deferred to the morphologic impression, despite the lack of FOXL2 mutation. Four of these 29 cases had minor sex cord elements. Among those, only one had a FOXL2 mutation and was therefore reassigned as an AGCT. Of interest, this case had a fibromathecomatous background; therefore, the AGCT component might have been underestimated. Related to this point, in a separate small series, 3

ovarian fibromas with minor sex cord elements were not found to have the FOXL2 mutation,[25] which is supportive of the overall benign notion of these cases.

A separate study documenting tumors classified as granulosa theca cell tumors of the ovary[36] reported FOXL2 mutation in 6 of 12 tumors. The mutation was found in both fibromathecomatous and granulosa components in all 5 of 6 FOXL2-positive tumors that underwent microdissection and sequencing of both components. This finding may be analogous to the morphologic illusion seen in the AGCT with thecoma-like foci, where even though on the hematoxylin and eosin staining alone the classic morphology is limited (see **Fig. 1**E), reticulin stain highlights the majority of the tumor nodules being nested (see **Fig. 1**F). This phenomenon is important because it may cause underestimation of the AGCT component based on morphology alone. Overall, the data presented herein further question the existence of thecomas with *FOXL2* mutations. Particularly in the setting of a previously discussed example of a thecoma with a *FOXL2* mutation relapsing in 2 years with a classical AGCT morphology,[31] perhaps any thecoma with a *FOXL2* mutation should be interpreted with caution regarding their malignancy potential.

COLLISION TUMOR

A true collision tumor with both morphologic and molecular evidence is extremely rare to come across among these exceedingly rare tumors. However, there is at least one example in the literature describing a steroid cell tumor and SRST in the same ovary,[64] with only the latter tumor having a beta catenin nuclear localization. In addition, the 2 morphologies seemed to have an abrupt change without any intermingling between the 2 components. Therefore, in this particular case, the morphologic and molecular features suggest different clonality of each component in keeping with a collision tumor. Of note, as previously discussed, the SRST in this tumor may represent a nonconventional MST (see **Fig. 3**D) based on the provided image. Currently, this distinction is difficult to make and requires further studies for a more definitive categorization.

CLINICS CARE POINTS

- Reticulin staining and *FOXL2* mutation analysis are helpful diagnostic tools in separating AGCTs from thecomas with nodular morphology and mitotically active cellular fibromas.

- *FOXL2* and *TERT* promoter mutations can be detected as biomarkers in cell-free AGCT DNA for disease monitoring.

- Sex cord–stromal tumor, not otherwise specified, diagnoses can further be screened for *DICER1*, *FOXL2*, and/or *STK11* mutation status depending on the scenario for better categorization of these tumors.

- Molecular subtypes of SLCTs (*FOXL2, DICER1,* non-*FOXL2/DICER1*) have overlap in clinical presentation and molecular features with AGCTs (*FOXL2,* as well as non-*FOXL2/DICER1*), JGCTs (*DICER1*), and so-called gynandroblastomas (*DICER1,* as well as non-*FOXL2/DICER1*).

- The diagnosis of an SLCT should prompt genetic counseling, given that tumor *DICER1* mutation testing is not routinely offered, *DICER1* syndrome has low penetrance and therefore, lack of personal and family history of *DICER1* related tumors may be misleading.

ACKNOWLEDGMENTS

The author thanks to Dr Robert Henry Young for sharing his consultation files, which were used for the majority of the photomicrographs herein and Dr McCluggage for providing the nonconventional MST image.

DISCLOSURE

The author has no disclosures to make.

REFERENCES

1. Morris JM, Scully RE. Endocrine pathology of the ovary. St. Louis: The C. V. Mosby Company; 1958.
2. Young RH. Ovarian sex cord-stromal tumors: reflections on a 40-year experience with a fascinating group of tumors, including comments on the seminal observations of Robert E. Scully, MD. Arch Pathol Lab Med 2018;142(12):1459–84.
3. Young RH. Ovarian sex cord-stromal tumours and their mimics. Pathology 2018;50(1):5–15.
4. Hanley KZ, Mosunjac MB. Practical Review of Ovarian Sex Cord-Stromal Tumors. Surg Pathol Clin 2019;12(2):587–620.
5. McCluggage WG, Young RH. Immunohistochemistry as a diagnostic aid in the evaluation of ovarian tumors. Semin Diagn Pathol 2005;22(1):3–32.
6. Rabban JT, Zaloudek CJ. A practical approach to immunohistochemical diagnosis of ovarian germ cell tumours and sex cord-stromal tumours. Histopathology 2013;62(1):71–88.
7. Lim D, Oliva E. Ovarian sex cord-stromal tumours: an update in recent molecular advances. Pathology 2018;50(2):178–89.
8. Stewart CJR, Amanuel B, De Kock L, et al. Evaluation of molecular analysis in challenging ovarian sex cord-stromal tumours: a review of 50 cases. Pathology 2020;52(6):686–93.
9. Rabban JT, Karnezis AN, Devine WP. Practical roles for molecular diagnostic testing in ovarian adult granulosa cell tumour, Sertoli-Leydig cell

tumour, microcystic stromal tumour and their mimics. Histopathology 2020;76(1):11–24.

10. WHO classification of tumours: female genital tumours. 5th edition. vol. 4. Lyon (France): International Agency for Research on Cancer; 2020.

11. Prat J, Scully RE. Cellular fibromas and fibrosarcomas of the ovary: a comparative clinicopathologic analysis of seventeen cases. Cancer 1981; 47(11):2663–70.

12. Meigs JV. Fibroma of the ovary with ascites and hydrothorax; Meigs' syndrome. Am J Obstet Gynecol 1954;67(5):962–85.

13. Gorlin RJ. Nevoid basal-cell carcinoma syndrome. Medicine (Baltimore) 1987;66(2):98–113.

14. Evans DG, Oudit D, Smith MJ, et al. First evidence of genotype-phenotype correlations in Gorlin syndrome. J Med Genet 2017;54(8):530–6.

15. Kenny SL, Patel K, Humphries A, et al. Ovarian cellular fibroma harbouring an isocitrate dehydrogenase 1 (1DH1) mutation in a patient with Ollier disease: evidence for a causal relationship. Histopathology 2013;62(4):667–70.

16. Shashi V, Golden WL, von Kap-Herr C, et al. Interphase fluorescence in situ hybridization for trisomy 12 on archival ovarian sex cord-stromal tumors. Gynecol Oncol 1994;55(3 Pt 1):349–54.

17. Tsuji T, Kawauchi S, Utsunomiya T, et al. Fibrosarcoma versus cellular fibroma of the ovary: a comparative study of their proliferative activity and chromosome aberrations using MIB-1 immunostaining, DNA flow cytometry, and fluorescence in situ hybridization. Am J Surg Pathol 1997;21(1):52–9.

18. Kato N, Romero M, Catasus L, et al. The STK11/LKB1 Peutz-Jegher gene is not involved in the pathogenesis of sporadic sex cord-stromal tumors, although loss of heterozygosity at 19p13.3 indicates other gene alteration in these tumors. Hum Pathol 2004;35(9):1101–4.

19. Tsuji T, Catasus L, Prat J. Is loss of heterozygosity at 9q22.3 (PTCH gene) and 19p13.3 (STK11 gene) involved in the pathogenesis of ovarian stromal tumors? Hum Pathol 2005;36(7):792–6.

20. Streblow RC, Dafferner AJ, Nelson M, et al. Imbalances of chromosomes 4, 9, and 12 are recurrent in the thecoma-fibroma group of ovarian stromal tumors. Cancer Genet Cytogenet 2007;178(2):135–40.

21. Hunter SM, Dall GV, Doyle MA, et al. Molecular comparison of pure ovarian fibroma with serous benign ovarian tumours. BMC Res Notes 2020; 13(1):349.

22. Irving JA, Alkushi A, Young RH, et al. Cellular fibromas of the ovary: a study of 75 cases including 40 mitotically active tumors emphasizing their distinction from fibrosarcoma. Am J Surg Pathol 2006;30(8):929–38.

23. Buza N, Wong S, Hui P. FOXL2 mutation analysis of ovarian sex cord-stromal tumors: genotype-phenotype correlation with diagnostic considerations. Int J Gynecol Pathol 2018;37(4):305–15.

24. Shah SP, Kobel M, Senz J, et al. Mutation of FOXL2 in granulosa-cell tumors of the ovary. N Engl J Med 2009;360(26):2719–29.

25. McCluggage WG, Singh N, Kommoss S, et al. Ovarian cellular fibromas lack FOXL2 mutations: a useful diagnostic adjunct in the distinction from diffuse adult granulosa cell tumor. Am J Surg Pathol 2013;37(9):1450–5.

26. Loeffler EP A. Bindegewebige Gewächse des Eierstockes von besonderer Bauart (Fibroma thecocellulare xanthomatodes ovarii). Beitr Path Anat 1932; 90:199–221.

27. Burandt E, Young RH. Thecoma of the ovary: a report of 70 cases emphasizing aspects of its histopathology different from those often portrayed and its differential diagnosis. Am J Surg Pathol 2014;38(8):1023–32.

28. Bjorkholm E, Silfversward C. Theca-cell tumors. Clinical features and prognosis. Acta Radiol Oncol 1980;19(4):241–4.

29. Young RH, Clement PB, Scully RE. Calcified thecomas in young women. A report of four cases. Int J Gynecol Pathol 1988;7(4):343–50.

30. Kim MS, Hur SY, Yoo NJ, et al. Mutational analysis of FOXL2 codon 134 in granulosa cell tumour of ovary and other human cancers. J Pathol 2010; 221(2):147–52.

31. Al-Agha OM, Huwait HF, Chow C, et al. FOXL2 is a sensitive and specific marker for sex cord-stromal tumors of the ovary. Am J Surg Pathol 2011;35(4): 484–94.

32. Kommoss S, Anglesio MS, Mackenzie R, et al. FOXL2 molecular testing in ovarian neoplasms: diagnostic approach and procedural guidelines. Mod Pathol 2013;26(6):860–7.

33. Stall JN, Young RH. Granulosa cell tumors of the ovary with prominent thecoma-like foci: a report of 16 cases emphasizing the ongoing utility of the reticulin stain in the modern era. Int J Gynecol Pathol 2019;38(2):143–50.

34. Stage AH, Grafton WD. Thecomas and granulosatheca cell tumors of the ovary: an analysis of 51 tumors. Obstet Gynecol 1977;50(1):21–7.

35. Norris HJ, Taylor HB. Prognosis of granulosa-theca tumors of the ovary. Cancer 1968;21(2):255–63.

36. Nolan A, Joseph NM, Sangoi AR, et al. FOXL2 mutation status in granulosa theca cell tumors of the ovary. Int J Gynecol Pathol 2017;36(6):568–74.

37. Chalvardjian A, Scully RE. Sclerosing stromal tumors of the ovary. Cancer 1973;31(3):664–70.

38. Devins KM, Young RH, Watkins JC. Sclerosing stromal tumour: a clinicopathological study of 100 cases of a distinctive benign ovarian stromal tumour typically occurring in the young. Histopathology 2021. https://doi.org/10.1111/his.14554.

39. Bennett JA, Oliva E, Young RH. Sclerosing stromal tumors with prominent luteinization during pregnancy: a report of 8 cases emphasizing diagnostic problems. Int J Gynecol Pathol 2015;34(4): 357–62.

40. Goebel EA, McCluggage WG, Walsh JC. Mitotically active sclerosing stromal tumor of the ovary: report of a case series with parallels to mitotically active cellular fibroma. Int J Gynecol Pathol 2016;35(6): 549–53.

41. Grechi G, Clemente N, Tozzi A, et al. Laparoscopic treatment of sclerosing stromal tumor of the ovary in a woman with Gorlin-Goltz syndrome: a case report and review of the literature. J Minim Invasive Gynecol 2015;22(5):892–5.

42. Kostopoulou E, Moulla A, Giakoustidis D, et al. Sclerosing stromal tumors of the ovary: a clinicopathologic, immunohistochemical and cytogenetic analysis of three cases. Eur J Gynaecol Oncol 2004;25(2):257–60.

43. Kawauchi S, Tsuji T, Kaku T, et al. Sclerosing stromal tumor of the ovary: a clinicopathologic, immunohistochemical, ultrastructural, and cytogenetic analysis with special reference to its vasculature. Am J Surg Pathol 1998;22(1):83–92.

44. Kim SH, Da Cruz Paula A, Basili T, et al. Identification of recurrent FHL2-GLI2 oncogenic fusion in sclerosing stromal tumors of the ovary. Nat Commun 2020;11(1):44.

45. Devins KM, Young RH, Croce S, et al. Solitary fibrous tumors of the female genital tract: a study of 27 cases emphasizing nonvulvar locations, variant histology, and prognostic factors. Am J Surg Pathol 2021;8. https://doi.org/10.1097/PAS.0000000000001829.

46. Yang EJ, Howitt BE, Fletcher CDM, et al. Solitary fibrous tumour of the female genital tract: a clinicopathological analysis of 25 cases. Histopathology 2018;72(5):749–59.

47. Irving JA, Young RH. Microcystic stromal tumor of the ovary: report of 16 cases of a hitherto uncharacterized distinctive ovarian neoplasm. Am J Surg Pathol 2009;33(3):367–75.

48. McCluggage WG, Chong AS, Attygalle AD, et al. Expanding the morphological spectrum of ovarian microcystic stromal tumour. Histopathology 2019; 74(3):443–51.

49. Parra-Herran C, McCluggage WG. Ovarian microcystic stromal tumour: from morphological observations to syndromic associations. Histopathology. 2022 Jan 12. https://doi.org/10.1111/his.14616. Epub ahead of print. PMID: 35020947.

50. Parra-Herran C. Endometrioid tubal intraepithelial neoplasia and bilateral ovarian microcystic stromal tumors harboring APC mutations: report of a case. Int J Gynecol Pathol 2021. https://doi.org/10.1097/PGP.0000000000000814.

51. Lee SH, Koh YW, Roh HJ, et al. Ovarian microcystic stromal tumor: a novel extracolonic tumor in familial adenomatous polyposis. Genes Chromosomes Cancer 2015;54(6):353–60.

52. McCluggage WG, Irving JA, Chong AS, et al. Ovarian microcystic stromal tumors are characterized by alterations in the beta-catenin-APC pathway and may be an extracolonic manifestation of familial adenomatous polyposis. Am J Surg Pathol 2018;42(1):137–9.

53. Maeda D, Shibahara J, Sakuma T, et al. beta-catenin (CTNNB1) S33C mutation in ovarian microcystic stromal tumors. Am J Surg Pathol 2011;35(10): 1429–40.

54. Irving JA, Lee CH, Yip S, et al. Microcystic Stromal Tumor: A Distinctive Ovarian Sex Cord-Stromal Neoplasm Characterized by FOXL2, SF-1, WT-1, Cyclin D1, and beta-catenin Nuclear Expression and CTNNB1 Mutations. Am J Surg Pathol 2015;39(10): 1420–6.

55. Bi R, Bai QM, Yang F, et al. Microcystic stromal tumour of the ovary: frequent mutations of beta-catenin (CTNNB1) in six cases. Histopathology 2015;67(6):872–9.

56. Meurgey A, Descotes F, Mery-Lamarche E, et al. Lack of mutation of DICER1 and FOXL2 genes in microcystic stromal tumor of the ovary. Virchows Arch 2017;470(2):225–9.

57. Zhang Y, Tao L, Yin C, et al. Ovarian microcystic stromal tumor with undetermined potential: case study with molecular analysis and literature review. Hum Pathol 2018;78:171–6.

58. Man X, Wei Z, Wang B, et al. Ovarian microcystic stromal tumor with omental metastasis: the first case report and literature review. J Ovarian Res 2021;14(1):73.

59. Ramzy I. Signet-ring stromal tumor of ovary. Histochemical, light, and electron microscopic study. Cancer 1976;38(1):166–72.

60. Dickersin GR, Young RH, Scully RE. Signet-ring stromal and related tumors of the ovary. Ultrastruct Pathol 1995;19(5):401–19.

61. Vang R, Bague S, Tavassoli FA, et al. Signet-ring stromal tumor of the ovary: clinicopathologic analysis and comparison with Krukenberg tumor. Int J Gynecol Pathol 2004;23(1):45–51.

62. Michalova K, Michal M Jr, Kazakov DV, et al. Primary signet ring stromal tumor of the testis: a study of 13 cases indicating their phenotypic and genotypic analogy to pancreatic solid pseudopapillary neoplasm. Hum Pathol 2017;67:85–93.

63. Kopczynski J, Kowalik A, Chlopek M, et al. Oncogenic activation of the Wnt/beta-catenin signaling pathway in signet ring stromal cell tumor of the ovary. Appl Immunohistochem Mol Morphol 2016; 24(5):e28–33.

64. McGregor SM, Schoolmeester JK, Lastra RR. Collision signet-ring stromal tumor and steroid cell tumor of the ovary: report of the first case. Int J Gynecol Pathol 2017;36(3):261–4.

65. Chen PH, Hui P, Buza N. Bilateral signet-ring stromal tumor of the ovary: a case report with next-generation sequencing analysis and FOXL2 mutation testing. Int J Gynecol Pathol 2020;39(2):193–8.

66. Deshpande V, Oliva E, Young RH. Solid pseudopapillary neoplasm of the ovary: a report of 3 primary ovarian tumors resembling those of the pancreas. Am J Surg Pathol 2010;34(10):1514–20.

67. Singh K, Patel N, Patil P, et al. Primary ovarian solid pseudopapillary neoplasm with CTNNB1 c.98C>G (p.S33C) point mutation. Int J Gynecol Pathol 2018; 37(2):110–6.

68. Choi Y, Choi H, Kim HS, et al. Signet-ring stromal cell tumour of the ovary confused with Krukenberg's tumour; a case report. J Obstet Gynaecol 2021;41(1):155–7.

69. Kiyokawa T, Young RH, Scully RE. Krukenberg tumors of the ovary: a clinicopathologic analysis of 120 cases with emphasis on their variable pathologic manifestations. Am J Surg Pathol 2006; 30(3):277–99.

70. Bennett JA, Young RH, Chuang AY, et al. Ovarian metastases of breast cancers with signet ring cells: a report of 17 cases including 14 Krukenberg tumors. Int J Gynecol Pathol 2018;37(6):507–15.

71. Hu PJ, Knoepp SM, Wu R, et al. Ovarian steroid cell tumor with biallelic adenomatous polyposis coli inactivation in a patient with familial adenomatous polyposis. Genes Chromosomes Cancer 2012; 51(3):283–9.

72. Lee IH, Choi CH, Hong DG, et al. Clinicopathologic characteristics of granulosa cell tumors of the ovary: a multicenter retrospective study. J Gynecol Oncol 2011;22(3):188–95.

73. Nogales FF, Musto ML, Saez AI, et al. Multifocal intrafollicular granulosa cell tumor of the ovary associated with an unusual germline p53 mutation. Mod Pathol 2004;17(7):868–73.

74. Jamieson S, Butzow R, Andersson N, et al. The FOXL2 C134W mutation is characteristic of adult granulosa cell tumors of the ovary. Mod Pathol 2010;23(11):1477–85.

75. Kim T, Sung CO, Song SY, et al. FOXL2 mutation in granulosa-cell tumours of the ovary. Histopathology 2010;56(3):408–10.

76. Roze J, Monroe G, Kutzera J, et al. Whole genome analysis of ovarian granulosa cell tumors reveals tumor heterogeneity and a high-grade TP53-specific subgroup. Cancers (Basel) 2020;12(5):1308.

77. Oseto K, Suzumori N, Nishikawa R, et al. Mutational analysis of FOXL2 p.C134W and expression of bone morphogenetic protein 2 in Japanese patients with granulosa cell tumor of ovary. J Obstet Gynaecol Res 2014;40(5):1197–204.

78. D'Angelo E, Mozos A, Nakayama D, et al. Prognostic significance of FOXL2 mutation and mRNA expression in adult and juvenile granulosa cell tumors of the ovary. Mod Pathol 2011;24(10):1360–7.

79. Rosario R, Wilson M, Cheng WT, et al. Adult granulosa cell tumours (GCT): clinicopathological outcomes including FOXL2 mutational status and expression. Gynecol Oncol 2013;131(2):325–9.

80. Caburet S, Georges A, L'Hote D, et al. The transcription factor FOXL2: at the crossroads of ovarian physiology and pathology. Mol Cell Endocrinol 2012;356(1–2):55–64.

81. Crisponi L, Deiana M, Loi A, et al. The putative forkhead transcription factor FOXL2 is mutated in blepharophimosis/ptosis/epicanthus inversus syndrome. Nat Genet 2001;27(2):159–66.

82. Pilsworth JA, Todeschini AL, Neilson SJ, et al. FOXL2 in adult-type granulosa cell tumour of the ovary: oncogene or tumour suppressor gene? J Pathol 2021;255(3):225–31.

83. Mangili G, Ottolina J, Gadducci A, et al. Long-term follow-up is crucial after treatment for granulosa cell tumours of the ovary. Br J Cancer 2013; 109(1):29–34.

84. Miller K, McCluggage WG. Prognostic factors in ovarian adult granulosa cell tumour. J Clin Pathol 2008;61(8):881–4.

85. Sun HD, Lin H, Jao MS, et al. A long-term follow-up study of 176 cases with adult-type ovarian granulosa cell tumors. Gynecol Oncol 2012;124(2):244–9.

86. Pilsworth JA, Cochrane DR, Xia Z, et al. TERT promoter mutation in adult granulosa cell tumor of the ovary. Mod Pathol 2018;31(7):1107–15.

87. Alexiadis M, Rowley SM, Chu S, et al. Mutational landscape of ovarian adult granulosa cell tumors from whole exome and targeted TERT promoter sequencing. Mol Cancer Res 2019;17(1):177–85.

88. Da Cruz Paula A, da Silva EM, Segura SE, et al. Genomic profiling of primary and recurrent adult granulosa cell tumors of the ovary. Mod Pathol 2020;33(8):1606–17.

89. Groeneweg JW, Roze JF, Peters EDJ, et al. FOXL2 and TERT promoter mutation detection in circulating tumor DNA of adult granulosa cell tumors as biomarker for disease monitoring. Gynecol Oncol 2021;162(2):413–20.

90. Farkkila A, McConechy MK, Yang W, et al. FOXL2 402C>G mutation can be identified in the circulating tumor DNA of patients with adult-type granulosa cell tumor. J Mol Diagn 2017;19(1):126–36.

91. Pilsworth JA, Cochrane DR, Neilson SJ, et al. Adult-type granulosa cell tumor of the ovary: a FOXL2-centric disease. J Pathol Clin Res 2021;7(3):243–52.

92. Hillman RT, Celestino J, Terranova C, et al. KMT2D/MLL2 inactivation is associated with recurrence in adult-type granulosa cell tumors of the ovary. Nat Commun 2018;9(1):2496.

93. Fashedemi Y, Coutts M, Wise O, et al. Adult granulosa cell tumor with high-grade transformation: report of a series With FOXL2 mutation analysis. Am J Surg Pathol 2019;43(9):1229–38.

94. Mubeen A, Martin I, Dhall D. High-grade Transformation in Adult Granulosa Cell Tumor: Potential Diagnostic Challenges and the Utility of Molecular Testing. Int J Surg Pathol. 2022 Feb 4:10668969221076553. https://doi.org/10.1177/10668969221076553. Epub ahead of print. PMID: 35118890.

95. McNeilage J, Alexiadis M, Susil BJ, et al. Molecular characterization of sarcomatous change in a granulosa cell tumor. Int J Gynecol Cancer 2007;17(2):398–406.

96. Susil BJ, Sumithran E. Sarcomatous change in granulosa cell tumor. Hum Pathol 1987;18(4):397–9.

97. Sonoyama A, Kanda M, Ojima Y, et al. Aggressive granulosa cell tumor of the ovary with rapid recurrence: a case report and review of the literature. Kobe J Med Sci 2015;61(4):E109–14.

98. Young RH, Scully RE. Ovarian sex cord-stromal tumors with bizarre nuclei: a clinicopathologic analysis of 17 cases. Int J Gynecol Pathol 1983;1(4):325–35.

99. Gaffey MJ, Frierson HF Jr, Iezzoni JC, et al. Ovarian granulosa cell tumors with bizarre nuclei: an immunohistochemical analysis with fluorescence in situ hybridization documenting trisomy 12 in the bizarre component [corrected]. Mod Pathol 1996;9(3):308–15.

100. Young RH, Dickersin GR, Scully RE. Juvenile granulosa cell tumor of the ovary. A clinicopathological analysis of 125 cases. Am J Surg Pathol 1984;8(8):575–96.

101. Velasco-Oses A, Alonso-Alvaro A, Blanco-Pozo A, et al. Ollier's disease associated with ovarian juvenile granulosa cell tumor. Cancer 1988;62(1):222–5.

102. Tanaka Y, Sasaki Y, Nishihira H, et al. Ovarian juvenile granulosa cell tumor associated with Maffucci's syndrome. Am J Clin Pathol 1992;97(4):523–7.

103. Schultz KA, Pacheco MC, Yang J, et al. Ovarian sex cord-stromal tumors, pleuropulmonary blastoma and DICER1 mutations: a report from the International Pleuropulmonary Blastoma Registry. Gynecol Oncol 2011;122(2):246–50.

104. Guo H, Keefe KA, Kohler MF, et al. Juvenile granulosa cell tumor of the ovary associated with tuberous sclerosis. Gynecol Oncol 2006;102(1):118–20.

105. Plon SE, Pirics ML, Nuchtern J, et al. Multiple tumors in a child with germ-line mutations in TP53 and PTEN. N Engl J Med 2008;359(5):537–9.

106. Bessiere L, Todeschini AL, Auguste A, et al. A hotspot of in-frame duplications activates the Oncoprotein AKT1 in juvenile granulosa cell tumors. EBioMedicine 2015;2(5):421–31.

107. Kalfa N, Ecochard A, Patte C, et al. Activating mutations of the stimulatory g protein in juvenile ovarian granulosa cell tumors: a new prognostic factor? J Clin Endocrinol Metab 2006;91(5):1842–7.

108. Heravi-Moussavi A, Anglesio MS, Cheng SW, et al. Recurrent somatic DICER1 mutations in nonepithelial ovarian cancers. N Engl J Med 2012;366(3):234–42.

109. Goulvent T, Ray-Coquard I, Borel S, et al. DICER1 and FOXL2 mutations in ovarian sex cord-stromal tumours: a GINECO Group study. Histopathology 2016;68(2):279–85.

110. Baillard P, Genestie C, Croce S, et al. Rare DICER1 and Absent FOXL2 mutations characterize ovarian juvenile granulosa cell tumors. Am J Surg Pathol 2021;45(2):223–9.

111. Vougiouklakis T, Zhu K, Vasudevaraja V, Serrano J, Shen G, Linn RL, Feng X, Chiang S, Barroeta JE, Thomas KM, Schwartz LE, Shukla PS, Malpica A, Oliva E, Cotzia P, DeLair DF, Snuderl M, Jour G. Integrated Analysis of Ovarian Juvenile Granulosa Cell Tumors Reveals Distinct Epigenetic Signatures and Recurrent TERT Rearrangements. Clin Cancer Res. 2022 Jan 14. https://doi.org/10.1158/1078-0432.CCR-21-3394. Epub ahead of print. PMID: 35031544.

112. Young RH, Scully RE. Ovarian Sertoli-Leydig cell tumors. A clinicopathological analysis of 207 cases. Am J Surg Pathol 1985;9(8):543–69.

113. Young RH, Prat J, Scully RE. Ovarian Sertoli-Leydig cell tumors with heterologous elements. I. Gastrointestinal epithelium and carcinoid: a clinicopathologic analysis of thirty-six cases. Cancer 1982;50(11):2448–56.

114. Prat J, Young RH, Scully RE. Ovarian Sertoli-Leydig cell tumors with heterologous elements. II. Cartilage and skeletal muscle: a clinicopathologic analysis of twelve cases. Cancer 1982;50(11):2465–75.

115. Hill DA, Ivanovich J, Priest JR, et al. DICER1 mutations in familial pleuropulmonary blastoma. Science 2009;325(5943):965.

116. Rio Frio T, Bahubeshi A, Kanellopoulou C, et al. DICER1 mutations in familial multinodular goiter with and without ovarian Sertoli-Leydig cell tumors. JAMA 2011;305(1):68–77.

117. de Kock L, Terzic T, McCluggage WG, et al. DICER1 mutations are consistently present in moderately and poorly differentiated Sertoli Leydig cell tumors. Am J Surg Pathol 2017;41(9):1178–87.

118. Schultz KAP, Harris AK, Finch M, et al. DICER1-related Sertoli-Leydig cell tumor and gynandroblastoma: Clinical and genetic findings from the International Ovarian and Testicular Stromal Tumor Registry. Gynecol Oncol 2017;147(3):521–7.

119. Conlon N, Schultheis AM, Piscuoglio S, et al. A survey of DICER1 hotspot mutations in ovarian and testicular sex cord-stromal tumors. Mod Pathol 2015;28(12):1603–12.

120. Kato N, Kusumi T, Kamataki A, et al. DICER1 hotspot mutations in ovarian Sertoli-Leydig cell tumors: a potential association with androgenic effects. Hum Pathol 2017;59:41–7.

121. Witkowski L, Mattina J, Schonberger S, et al. DICER1 hotspot mutations in non-epithelial gonadal tumours. Br J Cancer 2013;109(10): 2744–50.

122. Karnezis AN, Wang Y, Keul J, et al. DICER1 and FOXL2 mutation status correlates with clinicopathologic features in ovarian Sertoli Leydig cell tumors. Am J Surg Pathol 2019;43(5):628–38.

123. Meyer R. Tubuläre (testiculäre) und solide Formen des Andreiblastoma ovarii und ihre Beziehung zur Vermännlichung. Beith Path Anat 1930;84: 485–520.

124. Novak ER. Gynandroblastoma of the ovary: review of 8 cases from the ovarian tumor registry. Obstet Gynecol 1967;30(5):709–15.

125. Chivukula M, Hunt J, Carter G, et al. Recurrent gynandroblastoma of ovary-A case report: a molecular and immunohistochemical analysis. Int J Gynecol Pathol 2007;26(1):30–3.

126. Mercier AM, Zorn KK, Quick CM, et al. Recurrent gynandroblastoma of the ovary with germline DICER1 mutation: a case report and review of the literature. Gynecol Oncol Rep 2021;37:100806.

127. Wang Y, Karnezis AN, Magrill J, et al. DICER1 hotspot mutations in ovarian gynandroblastoma. Histopathology 2018;73(2):306–13.

128. Oparka R, Cassidy A, Reilly S, et al. The C134W (402 C>G) FOXL2 mutation is absent in ovarian gynandroblastoma: insights into the genesis of an unusual tumour. Histopathology 2012;60(5): 838–42.

129. Ordulu Z, Young RH. Sertoli-Leydig cell tumors of the ovary with follicular differentiation often resembling juvenile granulosa cell tumor: a report of 38 cases including comments on sex cord-stromal tumors of mixed forms (So-called Gynandroblastoma). Am J Surg Pathol 2021; 45(1):59–67.

130. Jarzembowski JA, Lieberman RW. Pediatric sex cord-stromal tumor with composite morphology: a case report. Pediatr Dev Pathol 2005;8(6):680–4.

131. Young RH, Scully RE. Ovarian stromal tumors with minor sex cord elements: a report of seven cases. Int J Gynecol Pathol 1983;2(3):227–34.

132. Boyraz B, Watkins JC, Soubeyran I, Bonhomme B, Croce S, Oliva E, Young RH. Cystic Granulosa Cell Tumors of the Ovary. Arch Pathol Lab Med. 2022 Mar 30. https://doi.org/10.5858/arpa.2021-0385-OA. Epub ahead of print. PMID: 35353158.

Peritoneal Pathology Review
Mullerian, Mucinous and Mesothelial Lesions

Takako Kiyokawa, MD, PhD*

KEYWORDS

• Endometriosis • Endosalpingiosis • Pseudomyxoma peritonei • Mesothelial tumors

Key points

- Endometriosis mostly occurs in women of reproductive age and is histologically often underdiagnosed. Its glands and stroma can show various changes as seen in the eutopic endometrium. Malignant neoplasms may develop in association with endometriosis.

- Other non-neoplastic glandular lesions of the Müllerian type aside from endometriosis include endosalpingiosis and endocervicosis. The former is relatively common, and the latter is rare.

- Pseudomyxoma peritonei (PMP) is a clinical term to describe the grossly evident intra-abdominal accumulation of gelatinous mucoid material due to a disseminated mucinous neoplasm, mostly low-grade appendiceal mucinous neoplasm

- Most peritoneal mesotheliomas in women are of epithelioid type. The association with asbestos is uncommon and the prognosis is better than that of its pleural counterpart.

ABSTRACT

This review provides an overview of the pathology of selected benign and malignant lesions of the female peritoneum and their often-encountered differential diagnoses. It includes endometriosis and its related lesions, endosalpingiosis, pseudomyxoma peritonei (PMP) and related ovarian/appendiceal pathology, and malignant and benign mesothelial tumors. The current terminology associated with PMP is also discussed.

ENDOMETRIOSIS AND RELATED LESIONS

INTRODUCTION

Endometriosis is defined as the presence of benign endometrioid glands surrounded by endometrioid-type stroma outside the endometrium and myometrium. It occurs in up to 15% of women of reproductive age.[1] It is uncommon in adolescents and postmenopausal women. Typical symptoms include dysmenorrhea, lower abdominal or pelvic pain, back pain, dyspareunia, irregular bleeding, and infertility. The condition may be discovered as an incidental microscopic finding in tissues removed for other reasons. Endometriosis is usually seen in the pelvis, including the peritoneum and adnexae, and is less commonly seen in the colorectum, appendix, ureter, and abdominal scar from a cesarean section.[2–5] Rarely, endometriosis may be associated with ascites. Patients usually have elevated serum CA125 levels.

The majority of endometriosis cases are thought to result from the transtubal retrograde displacement of endometrial tissue that implants in the peritoneum and other distant sites of susceptible women.[6] In addition, a subset of cases results from the traumatic displacement of the

Department of Pathology, The Jikei University School of Medicine, 3-25-8 Nishishimbashi Minato-ku, Tokyo 105-8461, Japan
* Corresponding author.
E-mail address: kiyokawa@jikei.ac.jp

Surgical Pathology 15 (2022) 259–276
https://doi.org/10.1016/j.path.2022.02.005
1875-9181/22/© 2022 Elsevier Inc. All rights reserved.

endometrial tissue or vascular dissemination.[6] Migratory stem cells originating from the endometrial tissues or bone marrow have also been proposed to be the possible origin of endometriosis in some cases.[7] Endometriosis, particularly atypical endometriosis, has been reported to demonstrate somatic mutations of oncogenes and monoclonality, and a clonal relationship between endometriosis and associated cancers has been documented.[8–11] In particular, recent findings of mutations in *KRAS, PTEN, PPP2R1A,* or *ARID1A* in the epithelium of deep infiltrating endometriosis (with no evidence of malignant transformation), and even in histologically normal endometrium suggest that genomic "oncogenic" changes may be common events in eutopic and ectopic endometrial tissues, and that these are not obligatory events in the development of neoplastic transformation.[10,12]

GROSS FEATURES

Endometriosis of the peritoneum typically consists of punctate, blue, brown, or red patches or nodules with a puckered surface. Although endometriosis is often discovered in the setting of chronic pelvic pain or as an incidental microscopic finding, it can also form a mass as a result of cystic changes, associated muscle hypertrophy, fibrosis, and/or adhesion to the surrounding tissue. Polypoid endometriosis may present as an exophytic nodule, closely mimicking a neoplasm.

Ovarian endometriosis usually forms a cystic mass containing a fibrous cystic wall with brown to yellow shaggy lining and chocolate-colored cystic content.

MICROSCOPIC FEATURES

Endometriosis is composed of benign endometrioid glands and varying amounts of periglandular endometrioid-type stroma containing arterioles. The epithelium can show a variety of metaplastic changes, including ciliated, mucinous, hobnail, eosinophilic, squamous, and clear cells. Glandular cells with abundant eosinophilic cytoplasm and smudgy nuclei may be seen as reactive changes (**Fig. 1**). Hemorrhage or hemosiderin deposits and concurrent inflammatory changes are usually observed. Indeed, many accept two or three elements (Mullerian-type glands, endometrioid-type stroma, evidence of hemorrhage) as diagnostic of endometriosis. Importantly, the stroma may be subtle, or it may be the only component (stromal endometriosis). Stromal endometriosis is relatively common in the pelvic peritoneum, often forming microscopic nodules on the peritoneal surface,

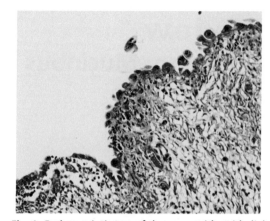

Fig. 1. Endometriotic cyst of the ovary with epithelial reactive atypia. The cyst is lined by a single layer of glandular cells, some with eosinophilic cytoplasm and enlarged hyperchromatic smudgy nuclei.

and is frequently underdiagnosed.[13,14] Endometrioid-type stromal cells can be highlighted by CD10, IFITM1, and estrogen receptor (ER) staining, if needed.[15,16] However, CD10 is nonspecific, and other mesenchymal cells in the female genital tract may be positive for ER.[14]

Both glands and stroma can show morphologic changes associated with endogenous or exogenous hormonal effects (**Fig. 2**). Decidualized stromal cells may contain cytoplasmic vacuoles that mimic signet-ring cells. The stroma can also show fibrosis, fibromuscular proliferation, pseudoxanthomatous nodules, and calcification. Peritoneal adhesions, peritoneal inclusion cysts, and mesothelial hyperplasia are commonly associated with endometriosis. Endometriosis can be intimately admixed with foci of peritoneal leiomyomatosis or gliosis.[17,18]

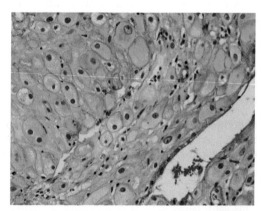

Fig. 2. Endometriosis found as a flat elevated lesion in the pelvic peritoneum at the time of cesarean section. The lesion shows prominent stromal decidualization and a gland lined by single-layered flat epithelial cells.

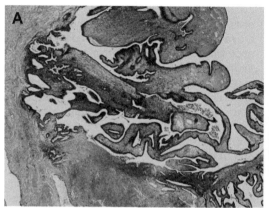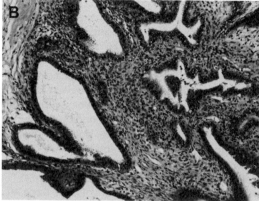

Fig. 3. Polypoid endometriosis in the pelvic peritoneum. Polypoid lesion protruding into cyst consisting of irregularly distributed glands and partly fibrous (upper part of the lesion) stroma (*A*). Glands are irregular in size and shape surrounded by endometrioid-type or fibrous stroma (*B*).

Polypoid endometriosis is endometriosis forming a polypoid lesion that may be histologically similar to an endometrial polyp (**Fig. 3**). Glands may show a variety of architectures and cytology, most commonly irregular cystic glands. Intraglandular stromal papillae may also be present focally. The stroma is variably fibrous and contains thick-walled blood vessels.[18,19]

Atypical endometriosis, as currently defined by the World Health Organization (WHO), is a term used for two types of morphology. One presents as crowded endometrioid glands with cytologic atypia resembling atypical hyperplasia/intraepithelial neoplasia in the eutopic endometrium, while the other is seen as stratification, disorganization, and prominent cytologic atypia in an architecturally simple glandular lining epithelium (**Fig. 4**). Atypical endometriosis is almost always located in the ovary, with fallopian tube and pelvic peritoneum being less common sites. The lesion may be associated with an endometriosis-related neoplasm.[14,20–23]

Endometriosis-associated neoplasms (EANs) are reported in about 1% of patients with endometriosis.[24,25] They are more likely to arise in the ovary than in extra-ovarian sites[26]. The two most common ovarian EANs are clear cell carcinoma and endometrioid carcinoma, and the least common types are seromucinous and endometrioid borderline tumors.[14] Other uncommon EANs include adenosarcoma, low-grade endometrioid stromal sarcoma (LGESS), and carcinosarcoma.[14,20,26,27]

DIFFERENTIAL DIAGNOSIS

Low-grade endometrioid stromal sarcoma: Stromal endometriosis can sometimes appear expansile and contain arterioles, thus resembling LGESS. However, LGESSs usually form masses, demonstrate invasive growth (including vascular invasion), and undergo mitoses, while stromal endometriosis lacks these features. The presence of uterine mass or a history of uterine LGESS may aid in the diagnosis of LGESS.

Adenosarcoma: This neoplasm is characterized by periglandular condensation, which is also seen in endometriosis, especially polypoid endometriosis. However, it also shows at least mild cytologic atypia and conspicuous mitoses in the mesenchymal cells, which should not be seen in polypoid

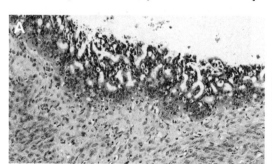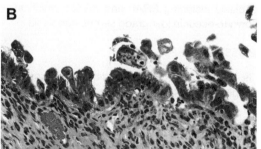

Fig. 4. Atypical endometriosis is characterized by glandular crowding and complexity confined to the epithelium (*A*). The term is also applied to endometriotic lesions with simple epithelial lining displaying nuclear enlargement, hyperchromasia, and loss of polarity (*B*); notice the morphologic overlap with **Fig. 1**.

endometriosis. Most importantly, the frond-like stromal papillae projecting into glandular spaces that are characteristic of an adenosarcoma are rare or focal in polypoid endometriosis.

Other non-neoplastic glandular lesions of the Müllerian-type: These include endosalpingiosis (see later in discussion) and endocervicosis. The latter is composed of endocervical-type mucinous glands and is rare. Periglandular endometrioid-type stroma is absent in these lesions. Both can involve the peritoneum and retroperitoneal lymph nodes and are usually incidental findings. However, they rarely form cystic masses mimicking neoplasm.[28,29] Lesions composed of two or more of these three lesions (endometriosis, endosalpingiosis, and endocervicosis) are referred to as Müllerianosis.[30]

Adenocarcinoma: The presence of glands in the peritoneum or in lymph nodes with sparse endometrioid-type stroma may potentially mislead the diagnosis of endometriosis as adenocarcinoma, particularly in small biopsy material. Adenocarcinoma is usually architecturally complex and shows cytologic atypia and mitoses.

ENDOSALPINGIOSIS

INTRODUCTION

Endosalpingiosis is defined as the presence of benign ciliated tubal-type epithelium outside the fallopian tube. It is relatively common in the serosa of uterus and tubes, cul-de-sac, omentum, and lymph nodes. Less common sites are the parietal pelvic peritoneum, serosa of the urinary bladder, and intestine. Those in lymph nodes are also referred to as Müllerian inclusion cysts, and similar glands in the ovary are by convention referred to as surface epithelial inclusion glands.

Endosalpingiosis of the peritoneum has been suggested to originate through metaplastic transformation, direct implantation of exfoliated tubal epithelium, or transit via lymphatics.[31] Similar to endometriosis, it has recently been demonstrated to harbor mutations typically attributed to Mullerian neoplasia including *BRAF* and *KRAS*, which are known to occur in low-grade serous neoplasia.[32]

GROSS FEATURES

It is usually an incidental finding. Occasionally, multiple tiny cysts (less than 5 mm in diameter) may be seen. Rarely, it forms cystic mass mimicking a neoplasm.[28,33,34]

MICROSCOPIC FEATURES

Glands with variable size and shape are lined by a single layer of tubal-type columnar cells including

ciliated cells, nonciliated secretory cells, and peg cells. Nuclear atypia is absent or mild, and mitoses are rare (**Fig. 5**). Small papillae or epithelial proliferation without cell detachment can be seen. Psammoma bodies are commonly present. The subepithelial stroma is absent or composed of loose or fibrous connective tissue. Rarely, serous borderline tumors (SBTs) and carcinomas arise from endosalpingiosis.[35–40]

Endosalpingiosis with mild cellular stratification and mild to moderate atypia has been referred to as *atypical endosalpingiosis*.[31] Some authors have used this term to describe lesions with changes suggestive of SBT or when there is no SBT in the adnexa. However, the distinction between the two is, at the moment, arbitrary. It is, for now, prudent to designate a lesion as serous borderline neoplasia if the epithelial proliferation shows hierarchical papillary, tufting, or detached cell clusters in the stroma morphologically resembling implants, even if the lesion is associated with conventional endosalpingiosis or there is no dominant mass[39].

DIFFERENTIAL DIAGNOSIS

The distinction between peritoneal serous cystadenoma and cystic endosalpingiosis is arbitrary. Other nonneoplastic glandular lesions of Müllerian-type (endometriosis, endocervicosis) and metastatic adenocarcinoma are discussed above.

PSEUDOMYXOMA PERITONEI AND RELATED OVARIAN/APPENDICEAL PATHOLOGY

INTRODUCTION

Pseudomyxoma peritonei is a clinical term used to describe a grossly evident intra-abdominal

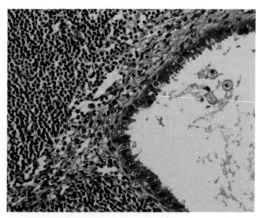

Fig. 5. Endosalpingiosis in a lymph node. A gland is lined by tubal-type columnar epithelium including ciliated and nonciliated cells without atypia and is surrounded by lymphocytic lymphoid tissue.

accumulation of gelatinous mucoid material due to disseminated mucinous neoplasm.[41,42] It is characterized by the redistribution phenomenon, wherein the mucinous material and neoplastic cells accumulate as they are redistributed through the peritoneal cavity by following the physiologic flow of peritoneal fluid to the site of reabsorption, such as the omentum, paracolic gutters, and inferior surface of the diaphragm.[43] The estimated incidence of PMP is approximately 1 to 3 per million people annually.[44] Most cases are secondary to an appendiceal mucinous neoplasm and are rarely secondary to mucinous neoplasms of the ovary, colon, pancreas, gallbladder, and urachus. Although it was believed in the past that PMP could rarely be derived from primary peritoneal tumors, we now know that primary peritoneal examples do not exist. Lymphatic and hematogenous metastases are uncommon, except in rare high-grade diseases.

Patients with PMP are typically middle-aged, with a mean age of 54 years (range 20–80) in one study.[45] They typically present with progressive abdominal distention, pain, or a palpable mass on abdominal or pelvic examination. They may also be asymptomatic and incidentally detected either intraoperatively or through imaging studies performed for other medical purposes. In addition, some patients may present with appendicitis.

Staging is based on the primary site of the neoplasm. For appendiceal primaries, the stage of PMP depends on the presence or absence of mucinous epithelium within the mucinous deposits. Cytoreductive surgery combined with hyperthermic intraperitoneal chemotherapy (HIPEC) is now considered a standard of care for PMPs.

PMP is a clinical term and should not be used as a final pathologic diagnosis, although it may be mentioned in the comment or description. In a pathology report, the histologic grade of peritoneal disease and information on whether peritoneal disease is derived from an appendiceal mucinous neoplasm or other types of tumors should be provided.

GROSS FEATURES

Light yellow to orange gelatinous mucoid material is present in the abdominal cavity. Typically, the appendix and one or both ovaries are involved. The appendix may be dilated due to abnormal accumulation of mucin or may show grossly evident perforation with mucin extrusion. The wall may be thickened with calcification foci. However, the appendix may be grossly unremarkable. Given that the majority of PMPs are derived from appendiceal mucinous neoplasms, the entire appendix should be submitted for histologic examination to exclude the possibility of an appendiceal primary, even if the appendix is macroscopically unremarkable.

When present, the associated ovarian tumor is typically large, multicystic with gelatinous content, and is often accompanied by mucin on the ovarian surface.

MICROSCOPIC FEATURES

Unlike other neoplasms, PMP has generally been classified according to the histology of the peritoneal disease rather than the primary tumor. The terminology and histologic classification of PMP and appendiceal mucinous neoplasms, which are the most common sources of PMP, have been contentious for many years owing to the low-grade features of neoplastic cells despite their malignant behavior. The Peritoneal Surface Oncology Group International (PSOGI) consensus on the terminology and classification of both peritoneal and appendiceal mucinous neoplasms was published in 2016[42] and formed the basis of the 5th edition of WHO classification. The POSGI recommends a 3-tiered system for grading neoplasms with an additional "acellular mucin" category in the peritoneal cavity.[42]

In PMP, by definition, at least 50% of the lesion must consist of mucin. Pools of mucin are typically dissecting in the fibrotic or often hyalinized stroma (dissecting mucin with fibrosis) (**Fig. 6**). Extracellular mucin may be acellular or may contain mucinous epithelial cells that may be forming glands or cysts. The extent of mucinous epithelial cells may vary between tumor regions. The 5th edition of WHO classification also recommends a 3-tiered system to grade peritoneal lesions based on tumor cellularity, cytologic features, and the presence of signet-ring cells[46] (**table 1**). Grade 1 tumors are composed of hypocellular mucinous deposits with scattered strips of mucinous epithelium embedded in the stroma or surrounding the periphery of the mucin pools, lacking stromal invasion. Epithelial cells are tall columnar with small nuclei with bland to mild cytologic atypia. Goblet cells may also be observed. Grade 2 tumors are composed of hypercellular mucinous deposits as observed at 20 × magnification, and more than 10% of tumor cells show high-grade cytologic features. Infiltrative-type invasion in a desmoplastic stroma, complex glandular growth, or a pattern of numerous mucin pools containing clusters of tumor cells may be observed. Grade 3 tumors are composed of signet-ring cells or sheets of tumor cells. Signet-ring cells may float in the mucin pools or infiltrate the stroma, and the latter may be prognostically more important. A lower limit for the

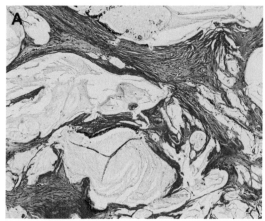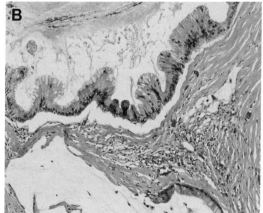

Fig. 6. Pseudomyxoma peritonei secondary to a low-grade appendiceal mucinous neoplasm. There is extensive mucin deposition dissecting fibroconnective tissue and associated with a relatively sparse tumor cell population (*A*). The latter is characterized by tall columnar mucinous cytoplasm and small, bland nuclei (*B*).

percentage of signet-ring cells was not set. Focal signet-ring cells floating in mucin should be distinguished from degenerated single cells (so-called pseudo-signet-ring cells) sloughed into mucin pools in an otherwise lower-grade tumor[46] In some cases whereby signet-ring cells are in the peritoneum, the primary appendiceal tumor may be a goblet cell adenocarcinoma. In the 5th edition of WHO classification, mucin in the peritoneal cavity without identifiable mucinous epithelial cells is designated as acellular mucin only, and grade is not applicable. Mucinous carcinoma peritonei is an acceptable terminology, while disseminated

peritoneal adenomucinosis and peritoneal mucinous carcinoma are not recommended.[46]

Appendiceal neoplasms as a primary lesion of pseudomyxoma peritonei

Appendiceal mucinous neoplasms that may be the source of PMPs include low-grade appendiceal mucinous neoplasm (LAMN), high-grade appendiceal mucinous neoplasm (HAMN), and mucinous adenocarcinoma, with LAMN being the most common and HAMN being the rarest. The vast majority of LAMNs have *KRAS* mutations, and most have

Table 1
Histological classification and grading of pseudomyxoma peritonei

WHO classification (2020)$	PSOGI classification#	Usual primary tumor
Acellular mucin only (grade not applicable)	Acellular mucin	Low-grade appendiceal mucinous neoplasm/Grade 1 mucinous adenocarcinoma of diverse sites
Pseudomyxoma peritonei, grade 1	Low-grade mucinous carcinoma, peritonei	Low-grade appendiceal mucinous neoplasm/Grade 1 mucinous adenocarcinoma of diverse sites
Pseudomyxoma peritonei, grade 2	High-grade mucinous carcinoma, peritonei	High-grade appendiceal mucinous neoplasm/Grade 2 mucinous adenocarcinoma of diverse sites
Pseudomyxoma peritonei, grade 3	High-grade mucinous carcinoma, peritonei with signet-ring cells	Signet-ring cell carcinoma of diverse sites. Appendiceal goblet cell adenocarcinoma

Data from The 5th edition of WHO classification of female genital tumours ($, Ref. 42) and Peritoneal Surface Oncology Group International (#, Ref. 46).

GNAS mutations.[47–49] High-grade tumors also have KRAS mutations but with greater frequency and are accompanied by mutations of other additional genes, including TP53, SMAD4, and MYC, while GNAS mutations are less common.[49–51]

LAMN is characterized by the replacement of the appendiceal mucosa with the filiform villous proliferation of neoplastic mucinous epithelial cells. The tumor cells are typically tall columnar with abundant cytoplasmic mucin that compresses the nucleus to create a cytologically bland appearance. The tumors may show an undulating or scalloped appearance with epithelial cells with nuclear pseudostratification. An attenuated or flattened monolayer of the mucinous epithelium is common. The lymphoid tissue of the appendix is usually absent, and varying degrees of fibrosis, hyalinization, and calcification tend to be present in the stroma. The gland-forming neoplastic epithelial cells may protrude into or through the appendiceal wall with a pushing pattern of invasion but lack destructive or infiltrative invasion. The mucin may dissect through the appendiceal wall and extend to the peritoneal surface or cause rupture of the appendix (**Fig. 7**).

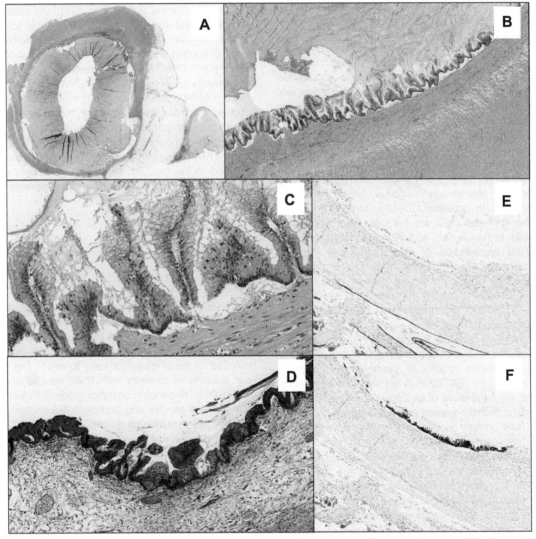

Fig. 7. Low-grade Appendiceal Mucinous Neoplasm (LAMN) with metastasis to the ovary. The appendiceal tumor (*A*) shows mucin accumulation with the distention of the lumen and dissection/thinning of the wall (best seen on lower aspect), as well as mucin deposition on the serosa (right lower corner). The neoplastic population is relatively simple (*B*) but shows evident scalloping (*C*), and comprised of tall, hypermucinous cells with preserved polarity and bland nuclear cytomorphology (*C*). The ovarian metastasis also shows a relatively simple architecture and bland cytomorphology highly resembling a primary ovarian mucinous borderline tumor (*D*). Lesional cells are negative for CK7 (*E*) and diffusely positive for CK20 (*F*), confirming an intestinal phenotype.

HAMNA is characterized by architectural features similar to those of LAMN, including a pushing pattern of invasion, but contains neoplastic epithelial cells with high-grade cytologic atypia, such as enlarged, hyperchromatic, and pleomorphic nuclei and frequent atypical mitoses.[42,52,53]

Appendiceal mucinous adenocarcinoma is characterized by focal infiltrative invasion with or without a signet-ring cell component. Lymphatic and hematogenous metastases are more likely to occur compared with LAMN or HAMN, and peritoneal metastases are still more common than nodal metastases.[54]

OVARIAN PATHOLOGY ASSOCIATED WITH PSEUDOMYXOMA PERITONEI

Synchronous ovarian and appendiceal mucinous neoplasms associated with PMPs should be assumed to have the primary in the appendix with metastasis to the ovary until proven otherwise clinically and pathologically. Rare exceptions include a primary ovarian mucinous neoplasm arising in a mature teratoma. Metastatic LAMNs are often bilateral and typically have mucin on the ovarian surface and pools of mucin dissecting through the ovarian stroma (pseudomyxoma ovarii), with or without hyaline stromal reaction. The epithelial cells are tall columnar with cytoplasmic mucin-rich and have nuclei showing a bland appearance or mild atypia (see **Fig. 7**). They characteristically form glands with a scalloped contour by multiple shallow outpouching and detachment from the underlying stroma due to artifacts.[55] Infiltrating-type invasion, vascular involvement, hilar involvement, and presence of signet-ring cells are features suggestive of metastatic mucinous adenocarcinoma rather than primary ovarian mucinous carcinoma. Moreover, positivity for SATB2+ in immunohistochemistry (IHC) is suggestive of an appendiceal origin rather than a primary ovarian mucinous tumor.[56]

Rare primary ovarian tumors that cause PMP are almost always mucinous ovarian tumors arising from teratomas, which can be histologically bland.[57] They typically have histologic features that more closely resemble those of metastatic LAMN (including tall columnar cells, scalloped contour of the glands, and detachment of epithelial cells from the underlying stroma) than those of ovarian mucinous tumors unassociated with teratoma.

DIFFERENTIAL DIAGNOSIS

Disseminated mucinous adenocarcinoma originating in various organs may have peritoneal mucin deposits; however, they tend to form solid masses without gelatinous mucoid material.

Ruptured primary mucinous ovarian tumor may result in peritoneal mucin deposits, but it lacks typical gross features of PMP. The mucin deposits are associated with a prominent lymphohistiocytic inflammatory response and granulation tissue (organized mucin), but they lack prominent stromal hyalinization, and epithelial cells are rare.

The differential diagnosis of appendiceal lesions associated with PMP includes ruptured diverticular disease, which often shows mucin extrusion on the appendiceal surface and mucosal hyperplastic changes but has maintained crypts separated by the lamina propria and lymphoid tissue, often accompanied by Schwann cell proliferation in the lamina propria.[58] Appendiceal sessile serrated lesions should also be considered in the differential. They are composed of columnar hypermucinous cells simulating LAMN. However, unlike LAMN, sessile serrated lesions have a retained crypt architecture; the crypts show basal dilatation and branching as well as a combination of goblet and nongoblet cells. More importantly, unlike LAMN a sessile serrated lesion is entirely confined to the mucosa: the muscularis mucosa, submucosa, and muscularis propria are spared.[59]

PROGNOSIS

PMP is associated with a protracted clinical course. The prognosis depends on the histologic grade of the peritoneal disease, extent of disease, and completeness of cytoreduction of macroscopically visible lesions within the abdomen. Generally, the grade of both appendiceal and peritoneal tumors is concordant. The grade of the peritoneal tumor seems to have a greater effect on the prognosis than that of appendiceal primary tumor.[45] The 5-year survival of patients with PMP ranges from 44% to 86%, depending on tumor grade.[60] Patients with grade 1 tumors and complete cytoreduction have a median survival time of 59 to 170 months, whereas those with grade 2 and 3 tumors have median survival times of 45 to 59 months and 18.9 to 26 months, respectively.[44,61–63]

 Differential Diagnosis

- Mucinous adenocarcinoma spreading to the peritoneum (solid mass without gelatinous mucoid material)

- Ruptured primary mucinous ovarian tumor unassociated with teratoma (absence of gelatinous mucoid material and prominent stromal hyalinization, a paucity of epithelial cells)

- Ruptured appendiceal diverticular disease (appendix with retained crypts separated by the lamina propria and lymphoid tissue)

MESOTHELIOMA

INTRODUCTION

Mesothelioma is a malignant tumor arising from the mesothelium. Peritoneal mesothelioma accounts for approximately 20% of all mesotheliomas in female patients.[64] Patients range widely in age (3–85 years) with a mean age of 50 years and a median age of 52 years at diagnosis.[65] Most patients present with abdominal distension/bloating or abdominal pain, but some may be asymptomatic, and the tumor may be an incidental intraoperative finding.[64–66] Association with asbestos is uncommon in women with peritoneal mesothelioma.[65] Approximately 10% of the patients are estimated to have an association with germline BRCA-1 related protein 1 gene (BAP1) mutations (BAP1 tumor predisposition syndrome).[67] Approximately 40% to 80% of patients harbor somatic biallelic mutations or homozygous deletion of BAP1, and less frequently cyclin-dependent kinase inhibitor 2A (CDKN2A9, coding p16 and p14) homozygous deletion, and mutations in NF2, SETD2, and DDX3X genes.[47,68–70]

GROSS FEATURES

The gross appearance of mesothelioma is variable, and its characteristics include granular, nodular, plaque-like, or papillary involvement of the visceral or parietal peritoneum.

MICROSCOPIC FEATURES

Mesothelioma is characterized by a proliferation of malignant mesothelial cells invading the underlying tissue. Most peritoneal mesotheliomas are epithelioid. The typical architectural patterns are tubular, papillary solid, cord-like, small nests, or single cells; admixtures of several patterns are common (**Fig. 8**). Papillae are often coalescent, complex, and lack hierarchical branching. Tubules and papillae are lined by single-layered tumor cells with minimal stratification and cell budding. Tumor cells are polygonal, cuboidal, or low columnar, with a moderate amount of

eosinophilic cytoplasm and occasional cytoplasmic vacuoles. Notably, nuclear atypia is usually mild to moderate, and mitoses are rarely observed. Areas resembling adenomatoid tumor or well-differentiated papillary mesothelial tumor (WDPMT) may be present.[65,66] Rarely, tumor cells have abundant cytoplasm, simulating decidual cells. The stroma varies from hyalinized to fibrous, desmoplastic, or myxoid. Infiltrating lymphocytes, plasma cells, and foamy histiocytes may be observed. While psammoma bodies are common, sarcomatoid and biphasic mesotheliomas are rare in the peritoneum.

Immunohistochemically, epithelioid mesotheliomas are positive for calretinin, D2-40, CK5/6, WT-1, mesothelin, thrombomodulin, CK7, and PAX-8; uniformly negative for claudin-4; and usually negative for BerEP4, MOC31, ER, and progesterone receptor (PR).[65,71–75] Sarcomatoid mesothelioma may not show calretinin and D2-40 expression, but the spindle tumor cells are positive for AE1/AE3, CK18, or CAM 5.2[76]. Recent studies have revealed that loss of nuclear BAP1 expression in IHC correlates with BAP1 mutations and that it is a reliable marker of malignancy, including mesothelioma, with a sensitivity of 65% and specificity of 100% in the setting of a peritoneal mesothelial proliferation.[77,78] Loss of BAP1 is more frequent in epithelioid than in biphasic or sarcomatoid peritoneal mesotheliomas.[70,72,79] Homozygous deletion of CDKN2A9 is much less frequent in peritoneal mesothelioma than in its pleural counterpart.[70,80] Methylthioadenosine phosphorylase (MTAP) is frequently codeleted with CDKN2A,[81] and loss of cytoplasmic MTAP and deletion of CDKN2A, as evidenced by IHC and FISH, respectively, are seen in 74% to 82% of the patients.[80,82,83] It is noteworthy that as various nonmesothelial malignant tumors may show loss of BAP 1 or MTAP expression, or CDKN2A deletion, these tests must be applied to lesions that were first established to be mesothelial in nature.

Recently, cases of malignant mesothelioma in situ, including one in the female peritoneum have been described.[84] They were diagnosed based on a single layer of slightly reactive-appearing mesothelial cells that showed loss of BAP1 expression, and seven of 10 patients developed invasive mesothelioma at a median time of 60 months.

DIFFERENTIAL DIAGNOSIS

Carcinoma: Like mesothelioma, both low-grade and high-grade serous carcinomas (SCs) have papillary, tubular, and solid patterns, as well as

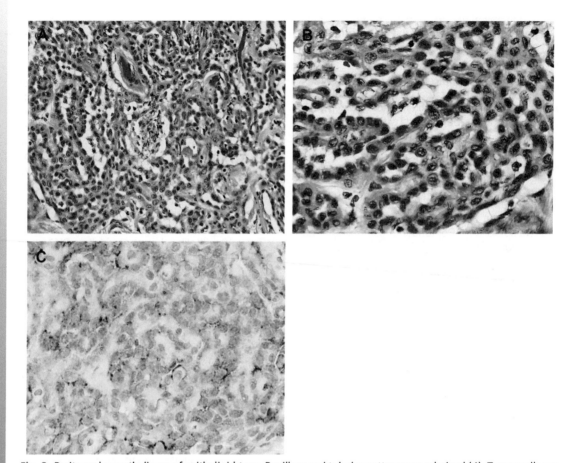

Fig. 8. Peritoneal mesothelioma of epithelioid-type. Papillary and tubular patterns are admixed (*A*). Tumor cells are cuboidal with eosinophilic cytoplasm and mild to moderate nuclear atypia. Mitoses are absent (*B*). Tumor cells are diffusely positive for D2-40 (*C*).

WT-1 expression. Clear cell carcinoma (CCC) of the peritoneum, though rare, shares with mesothelioma papillary or tubular patterns, cytoplasmic clearing, and negativity for ER and PR. In challenging cases, an expanded IHC panel is required to confirm the diagnosis. Carcinomas are frequently positive for claudin-4, while mesothelioma is uniformly negative for it.[73,76,85] Both SCs and CCC are usually positive for PAX8, MOC-31, and Ber-EP4.[86,87] SCs are typically positive for ER and PR[65,88] and most CCCs are positive for HNF1-B and napsin-A.[87,89] A subset of peritoneal mesotheliomas may be positive for PAX8, ER, or PR.[71,90] Loss of BAP-1 is seen in approximately 65% of peritoneal mesotheliomas but is rare in SC.[69,83,91] *CDKN2A* deletions are found in almost half of peritoneal mesotheliomas; however, none are found in ovarian carcinomas.[92] Lastly, the severe nuclear pleomorphism and brisk proliferation of high-grade SC would be highly unusual in peritoneal mesothelioma.

Serous Borderline Tumor (primary peritoneal or implants of ovarian SBT): It shares with mesothelioma a distinctive papillary architecture, but its papillae characteristically show hierarchical branching and typically contain ciliated cells admixed with nonciliated cells (except in the micropapillary variant), whereas ciliated cells are absent in mesothelioma. Although SBT can have microinvasion, it lacks destructive stromal invasion of greater than 5 mm. While SBT shows positivity for ER and PR, diffuse positivity for calretinin, D2-40, and cytokeratin 5/6, and negativity for Claudin-4 establishes the mesothelial nature of the lesion.[65,73,93]

Mesothelial hyperplasia: Florid mesothelial hyperplasia is usually related to chronic effusions, inflammation, endometriosis, and abdominal neoplasms.[94,95]

Florid mesothelial hyperplasia may have increased cellularity, cytologic atypia, mitotic activity, lymphovascular involvement, and

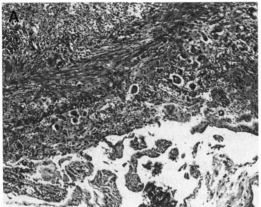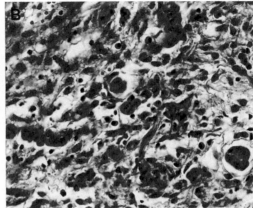

Fig. 9. Mesothelial hyperplasia associated with an ovarian endometriotic cyst. Small nests of mesothelial cells are entrapped within fibrous stroma simulating invasive growth; however, the nests are confined to the adhesions, being arranged parallel to the surface of the cyst without invasive growth (*A*). Mesothelial cells are arranged in small nests, show only mild cytologic atypia, and are surrounded by inflammatory stroma (*B*).

entrapment of mesothelial cells within the fibrous stroma of the peritoneum or ovarian surface may simulate invasive growth (**Fig. 9**). The cords of mesothelial cells in fibrous stroma are often arranged parallel to the surface, and the extent of involvement is limited in a reactive process. In challenging cases, analysis of BAP-1 and *CDKN2A* deletion by IHC and FISH, respectively, may help distinguish the mesothelial hyperplasia from mesothelioma.[65,76]

PROGNOSIS

The prognosis of peritoneal mesothelioma is better than that of its pleural counterpart, with a median overall survival time of approximately 50 months.[96] Factors associated with a better outcome include epithelioid subtype, age younger than 40 years, cytoreductive surgery and HIPEC, absence of extraperitoneal spread, and absence of lymph node metastasis.[65,96–98]

Pathologic key features

- Proliferation of neoplastic mesothelial cells invading the underlying tissue.

- Appropriate IHC is needed

- BAP1 loss by ICH and/or *CDKN2A* homozygous deletion by FISH confirms the diagnosis but is not present in all cases; loss of MTAP by IHC is also helpful.

Pitfalls

! Various nonmesothelial malignant tumors may show loss of nuclear BAP 1 or cytoplasmic MTAP expression by IHC, or CDKN2A deletion by FISH.

! Retained BAP1 by IHC or absence of CDKN2A deletion does not exclude the diagnosis of mesothelioma.

WELL-DIFFERENTIATED PAPILLARY MESOTHELIAL TUMOR (WDPMT)

INTRODUCTION

WDPMT is a rare, benign, papillary neoplasm of mesothelial origin, formerly known as "Well-differentiated papillary mesothelioma." The change in nomenclature acknowledges the indolent nature of this lesion and hopes to provide a clearer separation from malignant mesothelioma. WDPMT predominantly affects the female peritoneum, although cases in men and in the pleura have been reported.[99,100] Patients ranged in age from 23 to 75 years, with a median age of 47 years.[99,101] It is usually an incidental finding but may cause abdominal pain in rare cases.[101,102] The etiology of this condition is unknown, and there is no proven association with asbestos exposure.[101,102] WDPMTs demonstrate either somatic missense *TRAF7* or *CDC42* mutations, but lack mutations in *BAP1*, *NF2*, *CDKN2A*, *DDX3X*, *SETD2*, and *ALK*, which are frequent in mesothelioma.[103]

GROSS FEATURES

The tumors are usually solitary but may be multiple. They are gray to white papillary or nodular lesions, usually a few millimeters to a few centimeters in diameter.[101]

MICROSCOPIC FEATURES

WDPMT is an exophytic papillary lesion with a broad fibrous core lined by single-layered flattened or cuboidal mesothelial cells without stromal invasion (**Fig. 10**). Areas of tubulo-papillary, branching cords, or adenomatoid-like arrangements may be present. The tumor cells contain nuclei of bland appearance with or without occasional mild atypia. Mitoses are absent or at most rare.

DIFFERENTIAL DIAGNOSIS

Mesothelioma: Papillary architecture of mesothelioma is common and may even have a focal WDPMT-like pattern. However, stromal invasion, solid growth, coalescent and complex papillae, extensive nuclear stratification, nuclei with more than mild atypia, and increased mitoses are not features of WDPMT and are instead more in keeping with mesothelioma. Additionally, BAP1 expression may be lost in mesothelioma, unlike WDPMT which is always retained. Accurate clinical and radiological correlation is required to ensure that the tissue available for microscopic examination is representative, including the tissue underlying the lesion which should be carefully examined to rule out the presence of invasion before making a diagnosis of WDPMT.[101]

Mesothelial hyperplasia: Like WDPMT, mesothelial hyperplasia lacks invasion into the underlying stroma and can sometimes have a papillary

architecture, but its papillae are very small and composed exclusively of mesothelial cells or contain very thin fibrous cores, in contrast to the broad fibrous core of WDPM. Mesothelial hyperplasia is associated with reactive/inflammatory changes in the adjacent serosa, which are absent in WDPMT.[101]

Serous borderline tumors: This lesion features papillae with a fibrous core lined by cuboidal to columnar neoplastic cells with mild cytologic atypia and can mimic WDPMT. However, neoplastic cells of SBT are characteristically stratified with hierarchical epithelial tufting and more often columnar with fewer cuboidal cells. In challenging cases, IHC leads to a correct diagnosis.

PROGNOSIS

Although recurrent disease can occur, WDPMT has an excellent prognosis. Occasional cases with an aggressive course may represent misclassified mesotheliomas.

Differential diagnosis

- Mesothelioma, epithelioid type (presence of stromal invasion, solid growth, coalescent and complex papillae, extensive nuclear pseudostratification, nuclei with more than mild atypia, increased mitoses, loss of nuclear BAP1 expression homozygous *p16* deletions by FISH).

- Mesothelial hyperplasia (discreet papillary projections composed exclusively of mesothelial cells or with very thin fibrous cores, reactive/inflammatory changes in the adjacent serosa)

- SBT (stratified columnar cells with less cuboidal cells, presence of occasional ciliated cells, positivity for ER, and PR)

ADENOMATOID TUMOR

INTRODUCTION

Adenomatoid tumor is a benign mesothelial tumor. In women, most cases occur in the uterus (subserosal or intramural) and the tubes (usually subserosal). It rarely affects extragenital peritoneum and may be multiple.[104–106] Lesions in the small intestine mesentery, ileocecal region, and hernia sac has been reported.[104,107,108] The patients are usually asymptomatic, and the tumor is incidentally found during surgeries for other conditions.

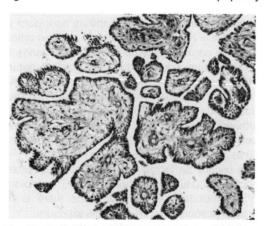

Fig. 10. Well-differentiated papillary mesothelial tumor. The lesion is papillary with broad fibrous cores and lined by single-layered bland cuboidal mesothelial cells without stromal invasion.

Adenomatoid tumors in immunocompromised patients have been reported. Recent studies have shown mutations in *somatic necrosis factor-associated factor 7 (TRAF7)*, which may regulate immunomodulatory signal pathways, in adenomatoid tumors possibly explain the association between these tumors and immunosuppression.[109]

GROSS FEATURES

Most tumors have relatively ill-defined borders and cut surfaces are typically greyish-white, firm, and nodular. Some tumors are partially or totally cystic.

MICROSCOPIC FEATURES

Typically, tumor shows variable combinations of slit-like, tubular, or microcystic branching spaces lined by flat or cuboidal cells (**Fig. 11**). The surrounding fibrous of fibromuscular tissue can be quite prominent, and the epithelial elements can be easily missed at scanning magnification. Solid areas or short papillae may be seen. Invasion into the adjacent tissue is absent. The neoplastic cells have scant eosinophilic cytoplasm and nuclear atypia is mild to moderate. Mitoses are absent or rare. Signet-ring cells, vacuolated cells may be seen. Adenomatoid tumor may contain papillary structures on its surface, focally mimicking WDPMT.

Tumor cells are positive for calretinin, WT1, D2-40, cytokeratin AE1/AE3, and CAM5.2, but IHC is not necessary for the diagnosis in most cases. BAP 1 expression is retained.[68,104,110]

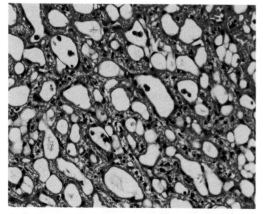

Fig. 11. Adenomatoid tumor of the peritoneum. Proliferation of slit-like, tubular, and microcystic branching spaces lined by flat cells. The neoplastic cells have scant eosinophilic cytoplasm and nuclear atypia is mild. Note some neoplastic cells show signet-ring type appearance due to intracytoplasmic vacuoles.

DIFFERENTIAL DIAGNOSIS

Mesothelioma: Mesothelioma should always be included in the differential diagnosis unless the lesion appears to be small with typical histology. This malignant tumor can show adenomatoid patterns focally or diffusely. Invasion into the underlying tissue, increased cytologic atypia, prominent nucleoli and mitotic activity, loss of BAP 1 expression by IHC are distinguishing features of mesothelioma.

Multilocular peritoneal inclusion cyst: Predominantly cystic adenomatoid tumors can be misdiagnosed as inclusion cysts. Mesothelial inclusion cysts tend to have inflammation in the stroma and occasional squamous metaplasia in contrast to adenomatoid tumor, which is not associated with these findings. Most patients have a history of a prior abdominal operation, pelvic inflammatory disease, or endometriosis.[111,112] Though it has been known under various names including inflammatory peritoneal cysts, postoperative peritoneal cyst, and benign multicystic mesothelioma, now it is considered as nonneoplastic and the term "cystic mesothelioma" is not recommended.[111]

PROGNOSIS

Adenomatoid tumors are benign. Up to 50% of cases can recur.[111]

CLINICS CARE POINTS

- Benign glandular lesions of the Müllerian type include endometriosis, endosalpingiosis and endocervicosis. In the peritoneum or in lymph nodes, these glands may potentially be interpreted as adenocarcinoma, particularly in small biopsy material.

- The stroma of endometriosis may be subtle, or it may be the only component (stromal endometriosis). Stromal endometriosis is relatively common in the pelvic peritoneum and is frequently underdiagnosed.

- Most cases of PMP are secondary to an appendiceal mucinous neoplasm with rare exceptions including a primary ovarian mucinous neoplasm arising in a mature teratoma.

- Florid mesothelial hyperplasia shares histological features (increased cellularity, cytologic atypia, mitotic activity, lymphovascular involvement, and entrapment of mesothelial cells within the fibrous stroma simulating invasive growth) with mesothelioma. In challenging cases, analysis of BAP-1 and CDKN2A deletion by IHC and FISH, respectively, may help distinguish it from mesothelioma.

DISCLOSURE

The author has nothing to disclose.

REFERENCES

1. Bougie O, Yap MI, Sikora L, et al. Influence of race/ethnicity on prevalence and presentation of endometriosis: a systematic review and meta-analysis. Bjog 2019;126(9):1104–15.
2. Ross WT, Newell JM, Zaino R, et al. Appendiceal Endometriosis: Is Diagnosis Dependent on Pathology Evaluation? A Prospective Cohort Study. J Minim Invasive Gynecol 2020;27(7):1531–7.
3. Gadducci A, Zannoni GF. Endometriosis-associated Extraovarian Malignancies: A Challenging Question for the Clinician and the Pathologist. Anticancer Res 2020;40(5):2429–38.
4. Audebert A, Petousis S, Margioula-Siarkou C, et al. Anatomic distribution of endometriosis: A reappraisal based on series of 1101 patients. Eur J Obstet Gynecol Reprod Biol 2018;230:36–40.
5. Charatsi D, Koukoura O, Ntavela IG, et al. Gastrointestinal and Urinary Tract Endometriosis: A Review on the Commonest Locations of Extrapelvic Endometriosis. Adv Med 2018;2018:3461209.
6. Wang Y, Nicholes K, Shih IM. The Origin and Pathogenesis of Endometriosis. Annu Rev Pathol 2020;15:71–95.
7. Hufnagel D, Li F, Cosar E, et al. The Role of Stem Cells in the Etiology and Pathophysiology of Endometriosis. Semin Reprod Med 2015;33(5):333–40.
8. Jiang X, Morland SJ, Hitchcock A, et al. Allelotyping of endometriosis with adjacent ovarian carcinoma reveals evidence of a common lineage. Cancer Res 1998;58(8):1707–12.
9. Wiegand KC, Shah SP, Al-Agha OM, et al. ARID1A mutations in endometriosis-associated ovarian carcinomas. N Engl J Med 2010;363(16):1532–43.
10. Lac V, Nazeran TM, Tessier-Cloutier B, et al. Oncogenic mutations in histologically normal endometrium: the new normal? J Pathol 2019;249(2):173–81.
11. Ayhan A, Mao TL, Seckin T, et al. Loss of ARID1A expression is an early molecular event in tumor progression from ovarian endometriotic cyst to clear cell and endometrioid carcinoma. Int J Gynecol Cancer 2012;22(8):1310–5.
12. Anglesio MS, Papadopoulos N, Ayhan A, et al. Cancer-Associated Mutations in Endometriosis without Cancer. N Engl J Med 2017;376(19):1835–48.
13. Boyle DP, McCluggage WG. Peritoneal stromal endometriosis: a detailed morphological analysis of a large series of cases of a common and under-recognised form of endometriosis. J Clin Pathol 2009;62(6):530–3.
14. McCluggage WG. Endometriosis-related pathology: a discussion of selected uncommon benign, premalignant and malignant lesions. Histopathology 2020;76(1):76–92.
15. Sumathi VP, McCluggage WG. CD10 is useful in demonstrating endometrial stroma at ectopic sites and in confirming a diagnosis of endometriosis. J Clin Pathol 2002;55(5):391–2.
16. Sun H, Fukuda S, Hirata T, et al. IFITM1 is a Novel, Highly Sensitive Marker for Endometriotic Stromal Cells in Ovarian and Extragenital Endometriosis. Reprod Sci 2020;27(8):1595–601.
17. Dworák O, Knöpfle G, Varchmin-Schultheiss K, et al. Gliomatosis peritonei with endometriosis externa. Gynecol Oncol 1988;29(2):263–6.
18. Zotalis G, Nayar R, Hicks DG. Leiomyomatosis peritonealis disseminata, endometriosis, and multicystic mesothelioma: an unusual association. Int J Gynecol Pathol 1998;17(2):178–82.
19. Parker RL, Dadmanesh F, Young RH, et al. Polypoid endometriosis: a clinicopathologic analysis of 24 cases and a review of the literature. Am J Surg Pathol 2004;28(3):285–97.
20. Matias-Guiu X, Stewart CJR. Endometriosis-associated ovarian neoplasia. Pathology 2018;50(2):190–204.
21. Seidman JD. Prognostic importance of hyperplasia and atypia in endometriosis. Int J Gynecol Pathol 1996;15(1):1–9.
22. Czernobilsky B, Morris WJ. A histologic study of ovarian endometriosis with emphasis on hyperplastic and atypical changes. Obstet Gynecol 1979;53(3):318–23.
23. Fukunaga M, Nomura K, Ishikawa E, et al. Ovarian atypical endometriosis: its close association with malignant epithelial tumours. Histopathology 1997;30(3):249–55.
24. Taniguchi F. New knowledge and insights about the malignant transformation of endometriosis. J Obstet Gynaecol Res 2017;43(7):1093–100.
25. Gadducci A, Lanfredini N, Tana R. Novel insights on the malignant transformation of endometriosis into ovarian carcinoma. Gynecol Endocrinol 2014;30(9):612–7.
26. Stern RC, Dash R, Bentley RC, et al. Malignancy in endometriosis: frequency and comparison of ovarian and extraovarian types. Int J Gynecol Pathol 2001;20(2):133–9.
27. Masand RP, Euscher ED, Deavers MT, et al. Endometrioid stromal sarcoma: a clinicopathologic study of 63 cases. Am J Surg Pathol 2013;37(11):1635–47.
28. Clement PB, Young RH. Florid cystic endosalpingiosis with tumor-like manifestations: a report of four cases including the first reported cases of transmural endosalpingiosis of the uterus. Am J Surg Pathol 1999;23(2):166–75.
29. Clement PB, Young RH. Endocervicosis of the urinary bladder. A report of six cases of a benign müllerian lesion that may mimic adenocarcinoma. Am J Surg Pathol 1992;16(6):533–42.

30. Young RH, Clement PB. Müllerianosis of the urinary bladder. Mod Pathol 1996;9(7):731–7.

31. Talia KL, Fiorentino L, Scurry J, et al. A Clinicopathologic Study and Descriptive Analysis of "Atypical Endosalpingiosis. Int J Gynecol Pathol 2020;39(3):254–60.

32. Chui MH, Shih IM. Oncogenic BRAF and KRAS mutations in endosalpingiosis. J Pathol 2020;250(2): 148–58.

33. Morales-Roselló J, Pamplona-Bueno L, Montero-Balaguer B, et al. Florid Cystic Endosalpingiosis (Müllerianosis) in Pregnancy. Case Rep Obstet Gynecol 2016;2016:8621570.

34. Rosenberg P, Nappi L, Santoro A, et al. Pelvic mass-like florid cystic endosalpingiosis of the uterus: a case report and a review of literature. Arch Gynecol Obstet 2011;283(3):519–23.

35. Sah S, Fulmali R, McCluggage WG. Low-grade Serous Carcinoma Arising in Inguinal Nodal Endosalpingiosis: Report of 2 Cases and Literature Review. Int J Gynecol Pathol 2020;39(3):273–8.

36. Djordjevic B, Malpica A. Ovarian serous tumors of low malignant potential with nodal low-grade serous carcinoma. Am J Surg Pathol 2012;36(7): 955–63.

37. Djordjevic B, Clement-Kruzel S, Atkinson NE, et al. Nodal endosalpingiosis in ovarian serous tumors of low malignant potential with lymph node involvement: a case for a precursor lesion. Am J Surg Pathol 2010;34(10):1442–8.

38. Fadare O. Recent developments on the significance and pathogenesis of lymph node involvement in ovarian serous tumors of low malignant potential (borderline tumors). Int J Gynecol Cancer 2009;19(1):103–8.

39. Bell DA, Scully RE. Serous borderline tumors of the peritoneum. Am J Surg Pathol 1990;14(3):230–9.

40. McCoubrey A, Houghton O, McCallion K, et al. Serous adenocarcinoma of the sigmoid mesentery arising in cystic endosalpingiosis. J Clin Pathol 2005;58(11):1221–3.

41. Carr NJ, Bibeau F, Bradley RF, et al. The histopathological classification, diagnosis and differential diagnosis of mucinous appendiceal neoplasms, appendiceal adenocarcinomas and pseudomyxoma peritonei. Histopathology 2017;71(6):847–58.

42. Carr NJ, Cecil TD, Mohamed F, et al. A Consensus for Classification and Pathologic Reporting of Pseudomyxoma Peritonei and Associated Appendiceal Neoplasia: The Results of the Peritoneal Surface Oncology Group International (PSOGI) Modified Delphi Process. Am J Surg Pathol 2016; 40(1):14–26.

43. Sugarbaker PH. Pseudomyxoma peritonei. A cancer whose biology is characterized by a redistribution phenomenon. Ann Surg 1994;219(2): 109–11.

44. Govaerts K, Lurvink RJ, De Hingh I, et al. Appendiceal tumours and pseudomyxoma peritonei: Literature review with PSOGI/EURACAN clinical practice guidelines for diagnosis and treatment. Eur J Surg Oncol 2021;47(1):11–35.

45. Carr NJ, Finch J, Ilesley IC, et al. Pathology and prognosis in pseudomyxoma peritonei: a review of 274 cases. J Clin Pathol 2012;65(10):919–23.

46. Misdraji J, Carr NJ, Pai RK, et al. Pseudomyxoma peritonei. In: WHO Classification of Tumours Editorial Board. Female genital tumours. Lyon (France): International Agency for Research on Cancer; 2020. p. 211, (WHO classification of tumours series, 5th ed.; vol. 4).

47. Alakus H, Yost SE, Woo B, et al. BAP1 mutation is a frequent somatic event in peritoneal malignant mesothelioma. J Transl Med 2015;13:122.

48. Nishikawa G, Sekine S, Ogawa R, et al. Frequent GNAS mutations in low-grade appendiceal mucinous neoplasms. Br J Cancer 2013;108(4):951–8.

49. Singhi AD, Davison JM, Choudry HA, et al. GNAS is frequently mutated in both low-grade and high-grade disseminated appendiceal mucinous neoplasms but does not affect survival. Hum Pathol 2014;45(8):1737–43.

50. Pengelly RJ, Rowaiye B, Pickard K, et al. Analysis of Mutation and Loss of Heterozygosity by Whole-Exome Sequencing Yields Insights into Pseudomyxoma Peritonei. J Mol Diagn 2018;20(5):635–42.

51. Liu X, Mody K, de Abreu FB, et al. Molecular profiling of appendiceal epithelial tumors using massively parallel sequencing to identify somatic mutations. Clin Chem 2014;60(7):1004–11.

52. Misdraji J, Carr NJ, Pai RK, et al. Appendiceal mucinous neoplasms. In: WHO Classification of Tumours Editorial Board. Digestive system tumours. Lyon (France): International Agency for Research on Cancer; 2018. pp. 144-146. (WHO classification of tumours series, 5th ed.).

53. Liao X, Vavinskaya V, Sun K, et al. Mutation profile of high-grade appendiceal mucinous neoplasm. Histopathology 2020;76(3):461–9.

54. Mehta A, Mittal R, Chandrakumaran K, et al. Peritoneal Involvement Is More Common Than Nodal Involvement in Patients With High-Grade Appendix Tumors Who Are Undergoing Prophylactic Cytoreductive Surgery and Hyperthermic Intraperitoneal Chemotherapy. Dis Colon Rectum 2017;60(11): 1155–61.

55. Misdraji J, Carr NJ, Pai RK. Appendiceal mucinous neoplasms. In: WHO Classification of Tumours Editorial Board. Digestive system tumours. Lyon (France): International Agency for Research on Cancer; 2018. p. 144-6, (WHO classification of tumours series, 5th ed.).

56. Strickland S, Wasserman JK, Giassi A, et al. Immunohistochemistry in the Diagnosis of Mucinous

Neoplasms Involving the Ovary: The Added Value of SATB2 and Biomarker Discovery Through Protein Expression Database Mining. Int J Gynecol Pathol 2016;35(3):191–208.

57. Vang R, Gown AM, Zhao C, et al. Ovarian Mucinous Tumors Associated With Mature Cystic Teratomas: Morphologic and Immunohistochemical Analysis Identifies a Subset of Potential Teratomatous Origin That Shares Features of Lower Gastrointestinal Tract Mucinous Tumors More Commonly Encountered as Secondary Tumors in the Ovary. Am J Surg Pathol 2007;31(6):854–69.

58. Hsu M, Young RH, Misdraji J. Ruptured appendiceal diverticula mimicking low-grade appendiceal mucinous neoplasms. Am J Surg Pathol 2009; 33(10):1515–21.

59. Hissong E, Yantiss RK. The Frontiers of Appendiceal Controversies: Mucinous Neoplasms and Pseudomyxoma Peritonei. Am J Surg Pathol 2022;46(1):e27–42.

60. Misdraji J, Yantiss RK, Graeme-Cook FM, et al. Appendiceal mucinous neoplasms: a clinicopathologic analysis of 107 cases. Am J Surg Pathol 2003;27(8):1089–103.

61. Narasimhan V, Wilson K, Britto M, et al. Outcomes Following Cytoreduction and HIPEC for Pseudomyxoma Peritonei: 10-Year Experience. J Gastrointest Surg 2020;24(4):899–906.

62. Ihemelandu C, Sugarbaker PH. Clinicopathologic and Prognostic Features in Patients with Peritoneal Metastasis from Mucinous Adenocarcinoma, Adenocarcinoma with Signet Ring Cells, and Adenocarcinoid of the Appendix Treated with Cytoreductive Surgery and Perioperative Intraperitoneal Chemotherapy. Ann Surg Oncol 2016;23(5):1474–80.

63. Munoz-Zuluaga C, Sardi A, King MC, et al. Outcomes in Peritoneal Dissemination from Signet Ring Cell Carcinoma of the Appendix Treated with Cytoreductive Surgery and Hyperthermic Intraperitoneal Chemotherapy. Ann Surg Oncol 2019;26(2): 473–81.

64. Pavlisko EN, Liu B, Green C, et al. Malignant Diffuse Mesothelioma in Women: A Study of 354 Cases. Am J Surg Pathol 2020;44(3):293–304.

65. Malpica A, Euscher ED, Marques-Piubelli ML, et al. Malignant Mesothelioma of the Peritoneum in Women: A Clinicopathologic Study of 164 Cases. Am J Surg Pathol 2021;45(1):45–58.

66. Baker PM, Clement PB, Young RH. Malignant peritoneal mesothelioma in women: a study of 75 cases with emphasis on their morphologic spectrum and differential diagnosis. Am J Clin Pathol 2005; 123(5):724–37.

67. Panou V, Gadiraju M, Wolin A, et al. Frequency of Germline Mutations in Cancer Susceptibility Genes in Malignant Mesothelioma. J Clin Oncol 2018; 36(28):2863–71.

68. Joseph NM, Chen YY, Nasr A, et al. Genomic profiling of malignant peritoneal mesothelioma reveals recurrent alterations in epigenetic regulatory genes BAP1, SETD2, and DDX3X. Mod Pathol 2017;30(2):246–54.

69. Leblay N, Leprêtre F, Le Stang N, et al. BAP1 Is Altered by Copy Number Loss, Mutation, and/or Loss of Protein Expression in More Than 70% of Malignant Peritoneal Mesotheliomas. J Thorac Oncol 2017;12(4):724–33.

70. Singhi AD, Krasinskas AM, Choudry HA, et al. The prognostic significance of BAP1, NF2, and CDKN2A in malignant peritoneal mesothelioma. Mod Pathol 2016;29(1):14–24.

71. Chapel DB, Husain AN, Krausz T, et al. PAX8 Expression in a Subset of Malignant Peritoneal Mesotheliomas and Benign Mesothelium has Diagnostic Implications in the Differential Diagnosis of Ovarian Serous Carcinoma. Am J Surg Pathol 2017;41(12):1675–82.

72. Tandon R, Jimenez-Cortez Y, Taub R, et al. Immunohistochemistry in peritoneal mesothelioma: a single-center experience of 244 cases. Arch Pathol Lab Med 2018;142(2):236–42.

73. Ordonez NG. Value of claudin-4 immunostaining in the diagnosis of mesothelioma. Am J Clin Pathol 2013;139(5):611–9.

74. Ordonez NG. Value of immunohistochemistry in distinguishing peritoneal mesothelioma from serous carcinoma of the ovary and peritoneum: a review and update. Adv Anat Pathol 2006;13(1): 16–25.

75. Ordóñez NG. Application of immunohistochemistry in the diagnosis of epithelioid mesothelioma: a review and update. Hum Pathol 2013;44(1):1–19.

76. Husain AN, Colby TV, Ordonez NG, et al. Guidelines for Pathologic Diagnosis of Malignant Mesothelioma 2017 Update of the Consensus Statement From the International Mesothelioma Interest Group. Arch Pathol Lab Med 2018;142(1):89–108.

77. Churg A, Naso JR. The Separation of Benign and Malignant Mesothelial Proliferations: New Markers and How to Use Them. Am J Surg Pathol 2020; 44(11):e100–12.

78. Wang LM, Shi ZW, Wang JL, et al. Diagnostic accuracy of BRCA1-associated protein 1 in malignant mesothelioma: a meta-analysis. Oncotarget 2017; 8(40):68863–72.

79. Hwang HC, Pyott S, Rodriguez S, et al. BAP1 Immunohistochemistry and p16 FISH in the Diagnosis of Sarcomatous and Desmoplastic Mesotheliomas. Am J Surg Pathol 2016;40(5):714–8.

80. Berg KB, Dacic S, Miller C, et al. Utility of Methylthioadenosine Phosphorylase Compared With BAP1 Immunohistochemistry, and CDKN2A and NF2 Fluorescence In Situ Hybridization in Separating Reactive Mesothelial Proliferations From

Epithelioid Malignant Mesotheliomas. Arch Pathol Lab Med 2018;142(12):1549–53.

81. Krasinskas AM, Bartlett DL, Cieply K, et al. CDKN2A and MTAP deletions in peritoneal mesotheliomas are correlated with loss of p16 protein expression and poor survival. Mod Pathol 2010; 23(4):531–8.

82. Hida T, Hamasaki M, Matsumoto S, et al. Immunohistochemical detection of MTAP and BAP1 protein loss for mesothelioma diagnosis: Comparison with 9p21 FISH and BAP1 immunohistochemistry. Lung Cancer 2017;104:98–105.

83. Chapel DB, Schulte JJ, Berg K, et al. MTAP immunohistochemistry is an accurate and reproducible surrogate for CDKN2A fluorescence in situ hybridization in diagnosis of malignant pleural mesothelioma. Mod Pathol 2020;33(2):245–54.

84. Churg A, Galateau-Salle F, Roden AC, et al. Malignant mesothelioma in situ: morphologic features and clinical outcome. Mod Pathol 2020;33(2): 297–302.

85. Boylan KL, Misemer B, De Rycke MS, et al. Claudin 4 Is differentially expressed between ovarian cancer subtypes and plays a role in spheroid formation. Int J Mol Sci 2011;12(2):1334–58.

86. Laury AR, Hornick JL, Perets R, et al. PAX8 reliably distinguishes ovarian serous tumors from malignant mesothelioma. Am J Surg Pathol 2010;34(5):627–35.

87. Iwamoto M, Nakatani Y, Fugo K, et al. Napsin A is frequently expressed in clear cell carcinoma of the ovary and endometrium. Hum Pathol 2015; 46(7):957–62.

88. Ordonez NG. Value of estrogen and progesterone receptor immunostaining in distinguishing between peritoneal mesotheliomas and serous carcinomas. Hum Pathol 2005;36(11):1163–7.

89. Fadare O, Zhao C, Khabele D, et al. Comparative analysis of Napsin A, alpha-methylacyl-coenzyme A racemase (AMACR, P504S), and hepatocyte nuclear factor 1 beta as diagnostic markers of ovarian clear cell carcinoma: an immunohistochemical study of 279 ovarian tumours. Pathology 2015; 47(2):105–11.

90. Chua TC, Yao P, Akther J, et al. Differential expression of Ki-67 and sex steroid hormone receptors between genders in peritoneal mesothelioma. Pathol Oncol Res 2009;15(4):671–8.

91. Andrici J, Jung J, Sheen A, et al. Loss of BAP1 expression is very rare in peritoneal and gynecologic serous adenocarcinomas and can be useful in the differential diagnosis with abdominal mesothelioma. Hum Pathol 2016;51:9–15.

92. Ito T, Hamasaki M, Matsumoto S, et al. p16/CDKN2A FISH in Differentiation of Diffuse Malignant Peritoneal Mesothelioma From Mesothelial Hyperplasia and Epithelial Ovarian Cancer. Am J Clin Pathol 2015;143(6):830–8.

93. Glavind K, Grove A. Estrogen and progesterone receptors in epithelial ovarian tumours. Apmis 1990; 98(10):916–20.

94. Clement PB, Young RH. Florid mesothelial hyperplasia associated with ovarian tumors: a potential source of error in tumor diagnosis and staging. Int J Gynecol Pathol 1993;12(1):51–8.

95. Baker PM, Clement PB, Young RH. Selected topics in peritoneal pathology. Int J Gynecol Pathol 2014; 33(4):393–401.

96. Enomoto LM, Shen P, Levine EA, et al. Cytoreductive surgery with hyperthermic intraperitoneal chemotherapy for peritoneal mesothelioma: patient selection and special considerations. Cancer Manag Res 2019;11:4231–41.

97. Cerruto CA, Brun EA, Chang D, et al. Prognostic significance of histomorphologic parameters in diffuse malignant peritoneal mesothelioma. Arch Pathol Lab Med 2006;130(11):1654–61.

98. Yan TD, Brun EA, Cerruto CA, et al. Prognostic indicators for patients undergoing cytoreductive surgery and perioperative intraperitoneal chemotherapy for diffuse malignant peritoneal mesothelioma. Ann Surg Oncol 2007;14(1):41–9.

99. Kim M, Kim HS. Clinicopathological Characteristics of Well-differentiated Papillary Mesothelioma of The Peritoneum: A Single-institutional Experience of 12 Cases. Vivo 2019;33(2):633–42.

100. Galateau-Salle F, Vignaud JM, Burke L, et al. Well-differentiated papillary mesothelioma of the pleura: a series of 24 cases. Am J Surg Pathol 2004;28(4):534–40.

101. Malpica A, Sant'Ambrogio S, Deavers MT, et al. Well-differentiated papillary mesothelioma of the female peritoneum: a clinicopathologic study of 26 cases. Am J Surg Pathol 2012;36(1):117–27.

102. Daya D, McCaughey WT. Well-differentiated papillary mesothelioma of the peritoneum. A clinicopathologic study of 22 cases. Cancer 1990;65(2):292–6.

103. Stevers M, Rabban JT, Garg K, et al. Well-differentiated papillary mesothelioma of the peritoneum is genetically defined by mutually exclusive mutations in TRAF7 and CDC42. Mod Pathol 2019;32(1):88–99.

104. Karpathiou G, Hiroshima K, Peoc'h M. Adenomatoid Tumor: A Review of Pathology With Focus on Unusual Presentations and Sites, Histogenesis, Differential Diagnosis, and Molecular and Clinical Aspects With a Historic Overview of Its Description. Adv Anat Pathol 2020;27(6):394–407.

105. Hayes SJ, Clark P, Mathias R, et al. Multiple adenomatoid tumours in the liver and peritoneum. J Clin Pathol 2007;60(6):722–4.

106. Yeh CJ, Chuang WY, Chou HH, et al. Multiple extragenital adenomatoid tumors in the mesocolon and omentum. Apmis 2008;116(11):1016–9.

107. Craig JR, Hart WR. Extragenital adenomatoid tumor: Evidence for the mesothelial theory of origin. Cancer 1979;43(5):1678–81.

108. Ruiz-Tovar J, Santos J, Lopez-Delgado A, et al. Transmural peritoneal adenomatoid tumour in the ileocaecal region causing massive haemoperitoneum and low gastrointestinal bleeding: differential diagnosis with capillary haemangiomas. Ann R Coll Surg Engl 2011;93(4):e3–5.

109. Goode B, Joseph NM, Stevers M, et al. Adenomatoid tumors of the male and female genital tract are defined by TRAF7 mutations that drive aberrant NF-kB pathway activation. Mod Pathol 2018;31(4): 660–73.

110. Erber R, Warth A, Muley T, et al. BAP1 Loss is a Useful Adjunct to Distinguish Malignant Mesothelioma Including the Adenomatoid-like Variant From Benign Adenomatoid Tumors. Appl Immunohistochem Mol Morphol 2020; 28(1):67–73.

111. Rapisarda AMC, Cianci A, Caruso S, et al. Benign multicystic mesothelioma and peritoneal inclusion cysts: are they the same clinical and histopathological entities? A systematic review to find an evidence-based management. Arch Gynecol Obstet 2018;297(6):1353–75.

112. Vallerie AM, Lerner JP, Wright JD, et al. Peritoneal inclusion cysts: a review. Obstet Gynecol Surv 2009;64(5):321–34.

Endometrial Cancer
An Update on Prognostic Pathologic Features and Clinically Relevant Biomarkers

Joshua J.X. Li, MBChB, FHKCPath[a],
Philip P.C. Ip, MBChB, FRCPath[b],*

KEYWORDS

- Endometrial carcinoma • Molecular classification • Biomarkers

Key points

- Molecular classification of endometrial cancer improves prognostication, identifies high-risk groups, and selects patients for targeted therapy and/or de-escalation of therapy.
- Applying diagnostic surrogate algorithms using immunohistochemistry and adopting a sequential approach for molecular classification can alleviate time and resource barriers.
- Potential issues such as the limitations of different assays and presence of tumor heterogeneity/subclones should be recognized to avoid pitfalls in interpretation.

ABSTRACT

The prognosis of endometrial cancers has historically been determined by the evaluation of histologic typing, grading, and staging. Recently, molecular classification, pioneered by the 4 prognostic categories from The Cancer Genome Atlas Research Network, has been shown to independently predict the outcome, correlate with biomarker expression, and predict response to adjuvant chemotherapy. In modern-day pathology practice, it has become necessary to integrate the time-honored prognostic pathologic features with molecular classification to optimize patient management. In this review, the significance of the molecular classification of endometrioid carcinomas, the application of practical diagnostic surrogate algorithms, and interpretation of test results will be addressed. Histologic features and theragnostic biomarkers will also be discussed in relation to the molecular subtypes of endometrial cancers.

OVERVIEW

The pathologic assessment of endometrial cancers has largely been based on the assessment of morphologic features, grading, and staging and the management of patients, to a certain degree, has historically been based on Bokhman's dualistic classification in which carcinomas are either considered as type I (low-grade, indolent) or type II (high-grade, aggressive).[1] Through integrated genomic characterization, The Cancer Genome Atlas (TCGA) Research Network described 4 prognostic categories for endometrial cancers: POLE ultramutated, microsatellite instability (MSI) hypermutated, copy-number low, and copy-number high.[2] Building on the TCGA classification, clinically practical algorithms using immunohistochemistry and POLE mutation analysis to identify the 4 prognostic categories have been proposed.[3,4] At the same time, the application of theragnostic markers on endometrial cancers, including HER2, programmed death-1/programmed death ligand-1

---

[a] Department of Anatomical and Cellular Pathology, Prince of Wales Hospital, The Chinese University of Hong Kong, Hong Kong SAR; [b] Department of Pathology, School of Clinical Medicine, The University of Hong Kong, Queen Mary Hospital, 102 Pok Fu Lam Road, Hong Kong SAR
* Corresponding author.
E-mail address: philipip@pathology.hku.hk

Surgical Pathology 15 (2022) 277–299
https://doi.org/10.1016/j.path.2022.02.006
1875-9181/22/© 2022 Elsevier Inc. All rights reserved.

(PD-1/PD-L1) and to a lesser degree, ER/PR (estrogen (ER) receptor/progesterone (PR) receptor), have garnered research interest and are now under active investigations. This review aims to summarize the recent developments in prognostic features of endometrial cancers, focusing on the application of the molecular classification of endometrial cancers in clinical practice, the interpretation of necessary immunostains and molecular tests, and introducing biomarkers more readily available to practicing pathologists and clinicians.

PROGNOSTIC HISTOLOGIC FEATURES

Despite the advances in ancillary and molecular methods, histology remains an indispensable cornerstone of pathologic assessment of malignancies. Recently, there has been no major changes made in the staging of endometrial cancers, except for a few modifications and refinements.[5] These include withdrawal of peritoneal cytology as a component of the International Federation of Gynecology and Obstetrics (FIGO) staging system,[6] the increased practice of sentinel lymph node biopsy for endometrial carcinomas,[7] and the inclusion of isolated tumor cells and micrometastasis in the 8th edition of the American Joint Committee on Cancer (AJCC) cancer staging.[8] It has been shown that when time-tested histologic features are combined with staging and molecular subtyping, patients may be better stratified into different risk profiles and treatments are more refined.[9–11]

In the current World Health Organization Classification of Tumors of Female Genital Organs,[12] endometrial cancers are classified microscopically into endometrioid, serous, clear cell, and mixed carcinomas, carcinosarcoma, and other novel types such as mesonephric-like adenocarcinoma and gastric-type mucinous carcinoma. Endometrial mucinous carcinoma is now regarded as a subtype of endometrioid carcinoma rather than a distinct entity. Undifferentiated/dedifferentiated carcinoma has been included as a distinct tumor type.

The significance and pathologic assessment of tumor-infiltrating lymphocytes (TILs) has extensively been studied in melanoma, breast, colorectal, and other cancers.[12–15] TILs in endometrial cancers have demonstrated some association with outcome[16,17] and TCGA molecular classification.[18,19]

Lymphovascular space invasion (LVSI) is another histologic feature used in prognosticating endometrial cancers.[20–22] Continued efforts in standardizing assessment and reporting of LVSI concluded that not only the presence, but the amount of LVSI (focal vs extensive) correlates with loco-regional recurrence. To this end, a semiquantitative approach, both prognostically significant and reproducible, has been recently developed.[20,23] This approach separates LVSI as absent, focal (less than 4 vessels containing tumor emboli), and substantial (4 vessels containing tumor emboli or more).[20] Estimation of LVSI following this schema is now recognized as a core element in the endometrial cancer histopathology reporting guide by the International Collaboration on Cancer Reporting.[5] In evaluating LVSI, the pathologist first needs to exclude, to the best of their ability, foci of artificial tumor displacement into vascular spaces.

MOLECULAR CLASSIFICATION OF ENDOMETRIAL CARCINOMA

The TCGA laid a foundation for the current molecular classification of endometrial cancers, with prognostic correlations described in the initial cohort,[2] and validated by subsequent studies.[24] Copy-number high tumors are associated with the worst prognosis, POLE ultramutated tumors carry the best outcome, whereas MSI hypermutated and copy-number low tumors are intermediate between the 2 groups.[2,24]

When correlating with morphologic features, the copy-number high group had a high representation of serous or serous-like endometrioid carcinomas,[2] in keeping with the high rate of TP53 mutations seen in these tumor types. MSI hypermutated tumors, similar to cancers in patients with Lynch syndrome,[25] are more often endometrioid type, feature prominent TILs and peritumoral Crohn's-like lymphocytic infiltrates.[26] Despite these associations, it is now acknowledged that histology alone is insufficient as a surrogate for the molecular subtyping of endometrial cancer,[26,27] owing to the morphologic overlap between TCGA molecular groups. For example, a significant proportion of POLE ultramutated tumors are high-grade with the atypia approaching that of serous carcinomas.[28] Also, neither TILs nor peritumoral lymphocytes are histologic features unique to MSI hypermutated tumors as they may also be seen in POLE ultramutated tumors.[28]

Although the initial cohort of TCGA molecular classification did not include any clear cell, undifferentiated/dedifferentiated carcinomas, neuroendocrine carcinomas, or carcinosarcomas,[2] subsequent studies on these histologic types have discovered that each may also be categorized into the 4 TCGA subgroups[29–43] (**Tables 1**

Table 1
Summary of the 4 molecular subgroups of endometrial cancer according to the TCGA classification

	POLE Ultramutated	MSI Hypermutated	Copy Number Low	Copy Number High
Frequency				
TCGA	7%	28%	39%	26%
ProMisE	20%–29%	8%–9%	44%–45%	11%–27%
PORTEC	9%–16%	12%–26%	38%–59%	6%–34%
Mutational burden	> 100 mutations/Mb	10–100 mutations/Mb	< 10 mutations/Mb	< 10 mutations/Mb
Somatic copy-number alterations	Very low	Low	Low	High
Histologic features	High-grade Ambiguous morphology Tumor giant cells High TILs	High-grade Mucinous differentiation MELF pattern invasion LVI High TILs Crohn's like reaction Lower segment involvement	Low-grade Squamous differentiation TILs absent	High-grade Glandular and solid patterns Diffuse marked cytologic atypia LVI
Clinical features	Lower BMI Younger age Presents at the early stage	Higher BMI Lynch syndrome	Higher BMI	Older age Presents at the later stage
Prognosis	Best	Middling	Middling	Worst
Surrogate groups				
ProMisE	POLE EDM	MMR deficient	p53 wild-type	p53 abnormal
TransPORTEC	POLE mutant	Microsatellite instable	NSMP	p53 mutant
Testing methods	POLE EDM sequencing Tumor mutational burden SNV NGS	MSI PCR MMR immunostain Tumor mutational burden	By exclusion of other molecular subtypes	TP53 sequencing p53 immunostain
Related biomarkers	PD-L1 ER/PR	PD-L1 ER/PR	ER/PR NHEJ H2AX Beta-catenin L1CAM	HER2

Abbreviations: BMI, body mass index; EDM, exonuclease domain mutations; ER, estrogen receptor; H2AX, histone protein H2AX; HER2, human epidermal growth factor receptor 2; LVI, lymphovascular invasion; Mb, megabase; MELF, microcystic, elongated, and fragmented; MMR, mismatch repair protein; MSI, microsatellite instability; NGS, next-generation sequencing; NHEJ, nonhomologous end joining; NSMP, no specific molecular profile; PD-L1, programmed death ligand 1; PR, progesterone receptor; SNV, single-nucleotide variant; TIL, tumor-infiltrating lymphocyte.

Adapted from[54,181] McAlpine J, Leon-Castillo A, Bosse T. The rise of a novel classification system for endometrial carcinoma; integration of molecular subclasses. *The Journal of Pathology.* 2018;244(5):538-549, Alexa M, Hasenburg A, Battista MJ. The TCGA Molecular Classification of Endometrial Cancer and Its Possible Impact on Adjuvant Treatment Decisions. *Cancers (Basel).* 2021;13(6).

and 2). Despite the genetic heterogeneity among these histotypes, tumors that harbored POLE mutations in morphologic clear cell and undifferentiated/dedifferentiated carcinomas also had better outcomes when compared with tumors of the same histotypes without these mutations.[29,44] This highlights the independent prognostic power of molecular classification in endometrial cancers.

Table 2
Summary of the 4 molecular subgroups of endometrial cancer in clear cell and undifferentiated/dedifferentiated carcinomas

	POLE Ultramutated	MSI Hypermutated	Copy Number Low	Copy Number High
Clear cell carcinoma				
Frequency	2%–16%[32,33]	0%–10%[32,33]	54%–59%[32,33]	24%–35%[32,33]
Clinical features: Older/postmenopausal age, advanced-stage presentation, and poor survival compared with endometrioid carcinoma				
Related biomarkers: PDL1: 15%–75%[34,35], HER2 (3+): 22%–23%[36,37], ER: 5%–9%[34,38], PR: 10%–45%[34,38]				
Dedifferentiated/undifferentiated carcinoma				
Frequency	11%–29%[39,44]	33%–57%[39,40,44]	14%–17%[39,44]	22%–24%[39,44]
Clinical features: Advanced-stage presentation and poor survival compared with endometrioid and clear cell carcinoma				
Related biomarkers: PDL1: 15%–75%[34,35], HER2 (3+): 22%–23%[36,37], ER: 5%–9%[34,38], PR: 10%–45%[34,38,182]				
Neuroendocrine carcinoma				
Frequency	7%[43]	43%[43]	36%[43]	14%[43]
Clinical features: May indicate aggressive behavior, but case number limited[183]				
Related biomarkers: ER: 33%[183], PR: 17%[183], no data on PDL1 and HER2 (3+)				

In view of the poor interobserver reproducibility in high-grade endometrial carcinomas,[45] and emerging evidence that histotyping may not be an independent predictor of survival,[26,29,44] there is a need to incorporate molecular classification in the pathologic assessment of endometrial cancers.

SURROGATE MARKERS AND ALGORITHMS FOR MOLECULAR CLASSIFICATION

The integrated genomic analysis performed in the TCGA classification required resources that may not be available in standard clinical laboratories. In view of this, surrogate markers and algorithms have been subsequently explored. Surrogate markers included mismatch repair proteins (MMR) (to identify tumors with a hypermutated/microsatellite unstable profile) and p53 immunohistochemistry (to identify tumors with a copy number high profile), in addition to POLE mutational analysis. Two algorithmic approaches using these markers have been proposed: the ProMisE (Proactive Molecular Risk Classifier for Endometrial Cancer) algorithm, based on the Vancouver cohorts,[4,10,46] and the classification system from the TransPORTEC consortium, based on the PORTEC trials.[3,9,47] These surrogate markers and algorithms are reproducible between pathologists and between independent laboratories; they may also be readily integrated with clinicopathological factors,[9,10] and can be applied to preoperative biopsies and hysterectomies.[48–50] In addition to

the demonstration of independent prognostic significance, these surrogate markers and algorithms are also validated for the prognostication of endometrial carcinomas of uncommon histotypes not initially included in the TCGA study such as clear cell and undifferentiated carcinomas[32,46,47,51] (Fig. 1).

The TransPORTEC classification system adopts a parallel testing method whereby p53 immunostain (or TP53 mutation if p53 stain was not evaluable), MMR immunostains, and POLE sequencing are performed simultaneously.[47] In the studies involving the PORTEC-1 and -2 trials, polymerase chain reaction (PCR) for microsatellite status defined the MSI hypermutated group,[9,47] but MMR immunostain was subsequently adopted for the more recent PORTEC-3 trial.[52] Tumors without any abnormality in the above assays are considered no specific molecular profile (NSMP). On the other hand, when multiple abnormalities are present, the tumor is considered as a "multiple-classifier" endometrial carcinoma (n = 27/861%, 3%)[9] (see "Tumors with multiple classifying alterations" section later in discussion). The ProMisE algorithm eliminates the dilemma of detecting multiple abnormalities through a stepwise, one test at-a-time approach.[53] POLE sequencing, MMR protein immunostains, and p53 immunostain are performed in sequence. The presence of POLE pathogenic variants classifies the tumor as ultramutated/POLE mutated. Tumors without POLE alterations then are tested for MMR. Loss of MMR immunoexpression then identifies the MMR-

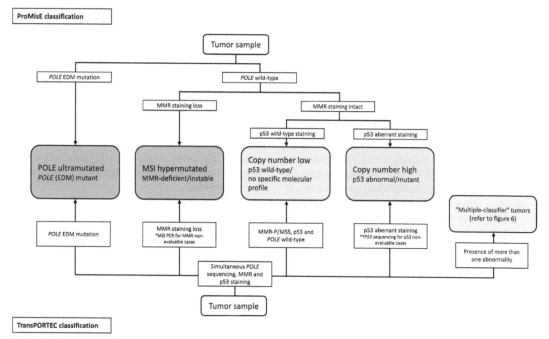

Fig. 1. The ProMisE and TransPORTEC classification systems. * indicates "notes/disclaimer".

deficient (MMR-D) group (hypermutated/microsatellite unstable). If no abnormality is detected by MMR immunostains and *POLE* sequencing, p53 immunohistochemistry separates p53 wild-type from p53 abnormal tumors.[10] It is important to note that the original iteration of the ProMisE algorithm placed *MMR* testing before *POLE* testing.[4,10,46] However, more recent studies by the proposing group.[32] have switched this order to place *POLE* as the first step in the process, likely in response to the growing evidence that *POLE* alterations prevail over MMR deficiency in double-classifier tumors that have both alterations (see "Tumors with multiple classifying alterations" section later in discussion). Tumors in the ProMisE system are regarded "unclassifiable" if any of the testing components are missing (n = 2/143%, 1%).[10] Adoption of any algorithm into clinical practice is dependent on the availability of resources. The ProMisE algorithm has been claimed to be useful in resource-limited settings. Nonetheless, it also requires *POLE* sequencing from the start, which is to date the least accessible test within the algorithm. Moreover, tumors with multiple molecular abnormalities will not be identified using this approach.

In addition to these surrogate markers, the TransPORTEC initiative recently published a refinement to the NSMP and p53 abnormal groups by adding immunohistochemical assessment of proteins involved in DNA damage (γ-H2AX) and regulators of error-prone nonhomologous end joining (DNA-dependent protein kinase (DNA-pk), FANCD2) for high-risk endometrial cancers.[3] The techniques available, interpretation and prognostic implications of *TP53*/p53, MSI/MMR, and *POLE* status, which are at the core of the molecular classification, will be discussed in detail.

TP53 AND P53 IMMUNOHISTOCHEMISTRY

TP53 mutated endometrial cancers have the highest somatic copy-number alterations among all molecular subgroups[54] and are aggressive tumors with poor clinical outcome.[2,10,47] *TP53* alterations are observed at a rate of 20.5% in endometrial cancers.[55] Serous carcinoma has the highest prevalence (88%), followed by undifferentiated, clear cell, and high-grade endometrial carcinomas (range 30%–40%),[42,56–58] while the frequencies are lowest in low-grade endometrioid carcinomas (grade I, 3%, grade II, 11%).[56] Regardless of the histotype, carcinomas with underlying *TP53* mutations demonstrate inferior prognosis compared with the *TP53* wild-type counterparts.[58–60] Even among low-grade endometrioid cancers, *TP53* mutation identifies a subgroup with shorter progression-free and overall survival.[59] It is, therefore, of clinical importance to demonstrate the presence of *TP53* mutations.

In endometrial cancer, immunostaining for the p53 protein is highly accurate as a surrogate for

TP53 sequencing,[61] and its staining pattern reflects the different types of TP53 mutation.[62] The wild-type p53 protein has a short half-life and is constantly degraded,[63] resulting in the nuclear staining of heterogeneous/variable intensity within normal tissues and tumors with wild-type TP53[64] (Fig. 2A). Abnormal staining patterns encompass diffuse nuclear overexpression, complete absence, or cytoplasmic with variable nuclear staining[64,65] (Fig. 2B, C). TP53 missense mutations generally lead to nuclear p53 overexpression in greater than 99% of cases.[62,66] Null mutations (frameshift, nonsense, and splicing junction) result in negative staining.[62] The cytoplasmic pattern is the rarest of the 4 patterns, caused by mutations truncating the nuclear localization domain of the p53 protein[64,65] (Fig. 2D, E). Missense mutations are the most common in endometrioid, serous, and clear cell endometrial carcinomas[56] and the majority are sporadic (43). Interpretation of what constitutes diffuse p53 expression has been a subject of debate. In addition to complete expression, various cut-offs which ranged from 50% to 90% have been proposed.[57,61,67] The International Society of Gynecologic Pathologists Endometrial Cancer Project endorses strong nuclear positivity in at least 80% of tumor cells as the definition of p53 immunohistochemical overexpression.[64,68]

As a pitfall, approximately one out of 20 tumors shows discordance between p53 immunoexpression and TP53 mutation,[69] and some studies report a lower rate of detection by immunostaining compared with sequencing.[70,71] Another critical issue is the intratumoral heterogeneity of p53 staining. There is a reported discordance rate of p53 staining between tumor blocks at 6.1%.[72] This is partly related to artifacts induced from suboptimal or prolonged fixation that caused loss of tissue antigenicity.[73] Such loss leads to a false-negative staining pattern, which can be erroneously interpreted as a p53 null pattern. Attention should be paid to internal and external, negative and positive controls. In case of doubt, it may be advisable to repeat staining and consider using another tissue block.[74]

It is important to emphasize the importance of clarity in reporting p53 immunohistochemistry results. The stain should not be reported simply as positive or negative, but rather, as abnormal or wild-type. Abnormal p53 staining can be further reported as overexpression ($\geq$80%), complete absence of staining, or cytoplasmic staining.[64,65]

Passenger TP53 mutations may be seen in POLE ultramutated or MSI hypermutated endometrial cancers. It has been shown that the secondary TP53 mutations are acquired during tumor progression and do not confer the same poor prognosis as seen in copy-number high endometrial cancers.[75] These tumors usually contain subclones that display abnormal p53 staining patterns[64] (Fig. 2F). In the setting of heterogeneous or difficult to classify p53 staining results, the background tumor needs to be reviewed for potential histologic features of TP53 mutant/copy-number high groups (serous-like features), and staining should be repeated on another section from the tumor. In cases with unresolved staining patterns, analysis in light of pathogenic POLE mutational status and MMR expression is recommended.

MICROSATELLITE INSTABILITY AND MISMATCH REPAIR PROTEIN

Microsatellites are short tandem repeats distributed throughout the human genome.[76] Aberrations during DNA replication results in insertions and deletions of the repeating microsatellites.[77] MMR proteins are responsible for correcting DNA mismatch generated in the process of DNA replication and recombination, including errors involving microsatellites.[78] Defective MMR proteins cause accumulation of mismatches, insertions, and deletions, and usually results in genomic instability and predisposition to cancer development.[78,79] Germline MMR gene mutation in Lynch syndrome is the classical example.[80] MSI status serves as an indicator for genomic instability[81] and is defined as the presence of repeat DNA sequence of different lengths compared with matching normal DNA.[82] In the context of endometrial cancers, MSI status is a component of the molecular classification, a theragnostic marker, and a predictor of clinical outcome.[83]

MSI/MMR testing can be performed by PCR-based methods or immunohistochemistry. PCR-based methods directly compare the length of microsatellite repeats to normal control in 5 or 7 representative DNA regions.[81,84] MSI status is classified into high (MSI-H), low (MSI-L), and microsatellite stable (MSS) when there is > 1, one only, and no abnormalities in the DNA regions, respectively.[81,84] Testing by immunostains requires antibodies to 4 common MMR proteins (MLH1, MSH2, MSH6, and PMS2). Loss of staining in any individual or combination of these 4 proteins indicates MMR deficiency (MMR-D)[85] (Fig. 3A, B). In turn, intact nuclear staining in tumor cells is considered a normal result (ie, MMR-proficient, MMR-P).[86,87] Immunohistochemistry is robust in detecting truncating mutations of MMR genes,[85] but in nontruncating missense mutations, there is residual production of functionally impaired MMR

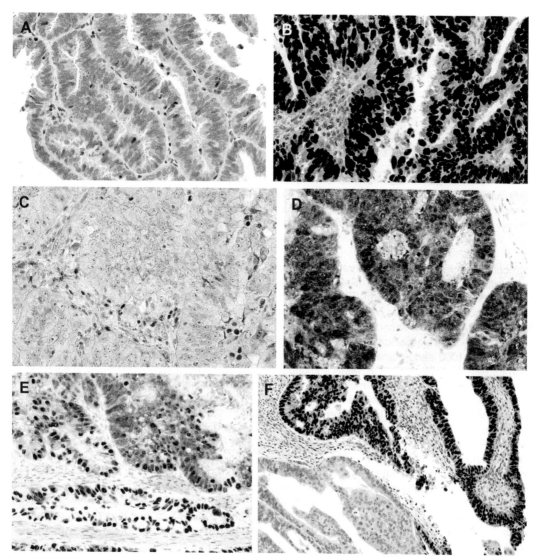

Fig. 2. p53 immunostaining in endometrial cancers. (*A*) Nuclear staining of mixed intensity indicates normal (wild-type) p53 protein, 40x magnification; (*B*) *TP53* missense mutation more commonly leads to nuclear accumulation of nonfunctional p53 protein, resulting in overexpression of p53, 40x magnification; (*C*) complete negative staining in *TP53* null mutations, note the preserved staining in stromal cells and lymphocytes, 40x magnification; (*D*) cyto-plasmic pattern is the rarest pattern of abnormal p53 staining, 20x magnification; (*E*) variable nuclear staining can be observed in the cytoplasmic p53 pattern, 20x magnification; (*F*) intratumoral subclones with different patterns of p53 expression, 40x magni-fication.

proteins that retain immunoreactivity.[88] Fortunately, these potentially false-negative cases are uncommon, and immunoexpression for MMR proteins are largely concordant with MSI status by PCR analysis.[89,90] Defects in MSH2, MSH6, and PMS2 are more likely to be associated with an underlying germline mutation in these genes, whereas MLH1 defects are frequently a result of sporadic *MLH1* promoter methylation.[91] *MLH1* methylation assays can be performed to distinguish sporadic somatic mutations from hereditary germline mutations in endometrial cancers.[83,91]

MSI-H endometrial carcinomas are histologically heterogeneous. They represent a majority of tumors classified as undifferentiated carcinoma (52.9%). Lower proportions of endometrioid (31.0%), serous (16.7%), and clear cell carcinomas (15.6%) are MSI-H.[29,42,90] The histologic features described in association with MMR-D are highly variable, and include nonpapillary and cribriform patterns, mucinous differentiation, and presence of peritumoral and TILs.[85] Even though MSI hypermutated/MMR-D tumors have intermediate prognosis when compared with other

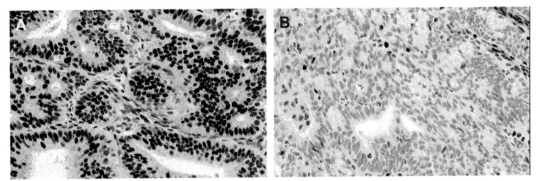

Fig. 3. Mismatch repair protein immunostaining (MMR) for endometrial cancers. (*A*) Retained nuclear expression of MMR indicates MMR proficiency, MLH1, 40x magnification; (*B*) MMR deficient tumors showing complete absence of MMR expression, expression in stromal and inflammatory cells are retained, MLH1, 40x magnification.

molecular subgroups of endometrial cancer, the prognostic value of MSI status alone seems to be limited to early, low-grade and/or endometrioid carcinomas.[2,10,47] It has also been suggested that MSI-H/MMR-D status is associated with a shorter survival.[92–94] In a large-scale study involving greater than 1000 endometrial cancers in which microsatellite status by MSI PCR, MMR immunostains, and *MLH1* promoter hypermethylation were comprehensively evaluated, MSI-H/MMR-D status was not shown to be an independent predictive factor on multivariable analysis.[95] Despite this, MMR-D cancers have high mutational burdens which serve as the basis for treatment with checkpoint inhibitors.[96] Greater benefit from pembrolizumab, a PD-1 inhibitor, has been first reported in patients with metastatic MMR-D colorectal cancers compared with MMR-P cases.[96] The KEYNOTE-158 study also demonstrated clinical benefit of pembrolizumab in MSI-H/MMR-D noncolorectal cancers, including endometrial cancers.[97] Other more recently developed PD-1/PD-L1 inhibitors have also shown superior efficacy in MSI-H/MMR-D tumors[98] that can be independent of PD-L1 status.[99]

DNA POLYMERASE EPSILON

DNA polymerase epsilon (Pol ε) is an enzyme involved in DNA replication and repair.[100] It is a heterotetramer formed by subunits p261, p59, p17, and p12.[101] The *POLE* gene encodes p261, which contains $3' \rightarrow 5'$ exonuclease subdomains[102] that act as the catalytic subunit, and are responsible for the replication fidelity of Pol ε.[103] Defects in the proofreading function of Pol ε are at the core of the tumorigenesis of ultramutated tumors, for which the mutation frequency is typically greater than 100 per megabase.[104] *POLE* mutations are observed in 7% to 10%

endometrial cancers and less frequently in other cancers.[104]

POLE mutated endometrial cancers are almost exclusively of endometrioid histology (96%). They are often high-grade (60%), and rich in tumor-infiltrating and/or peritumoral lymphocytes (84%)[28,105,106] (**Fig. 4**A–D). These tumors are usually seen in younger patients and at earlier stages compared with other molecular groups.[28,107,108]

Molecular classification of *POLE* mutated endometrial cancers has several challenges. As there are no immunohistochemical surrogate markers, DNA sequencing is necessary. The *POLE* subgroup of tumors in the TransPORTEC and ProMisE systems are defined by mutations detected by the sequencing of *POLE* exons 9, 13, and 14, and 9 to 14, respectively.[4,47] The vast majority (96%) of pathogenic *POLE* mutations are exonuclease domain mutations (EDM),[109] and exons 9 to 13 contain greater than 90% *POLE* EDMs.[47] Targeted sequencing assays of these hotspots, for example, the single-gene POLE SNaPshot assay,[110] have been used with success for the streamlining molecular subtyping of endometrial cancers. It is important to classify pathogenic *POLE* mutations because these have prognostic and therapeutic implications. The pathogenic variants are now better delineated (**Fig. 5**). When novel mutations are found, the recently proposed *POLE* genomic alteration score (POLE-score) may be used to determine their pathogenicity. The POLE-score stratifies *POLE* mutations into pathogenic, nonpathogenic, and variants of unknown significance by evaluating single-nucleotide substitutions, insertion–deletion mutations, tumor mutational burden, and variant recurrence.[109]

POLE mutated endometrial cancers have the best prognosis among all 4 molecular subtypes,[2] and consideration of omitting adjuvant therapy in

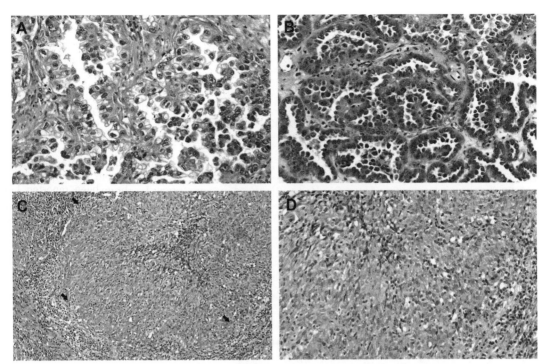

Fig. 4. *POLE* mu-tated endometrial cancers. (*A*) Endometrial carcinoma with *POLE* hotspot mutation involving exon 13 (V411 L). The tumor cells are arranged in papillae lined by clear cells. They are nonimmunoreactive for Napsin A or HNF1B, 40x magnification; (*B*) Endometrial carcinoma with *POLE* hotspot mutation involving exon 13 (V411 L). The tumor cells are arranged in papillae resembling serous carcinoma. The p53 immunostain is wild type, in this case, 40x magnification; (*C*) Endometrial carcinoma with *POLE* hotspot mutation involving exon 9 (P286 R). The tumor cells are arranged in solid sheets with prominent tumor-infiltrating lymphocytes (*arrows*), 20x magnification; (*D*) Endometrial carcinoma with *POLE* hotspot mutation involving exon 9 (P286 R). Solid sheets of cells without gland formation, 40x magnification.

stage I to II *POLE* mutated endometrial cancers is recommended in the 2020 ESGO/ESTRO/ESP guidelines.[11] Similar to MSI hypermutated tumors, *POLE* ultramutated tumors have a high mutational burden,[111] which is positively correlated with response to PD-1 inhibition.[112] Isolated cases of *POLE* mutated endometrial cancers with response to Pembrolizumab have been reported,[111,113] but supporting data from large scale trials are lacking.

It is important to note that targeted *POLE* sequencing may not cover rare mutations and may misinterpret nonpathogenic mutations.[109] Any inconsistencies between clinical impression, histologic appearance, and molecular features should prompt further workup and review.

MARKERS OF DNA DAMAGE RESPONSE (H2AX, DNA-PK, AND FANCD2)

The 2 major pathways of DNA double-strand break (DSB) repair are homologous (requiring a complementary DNA template) and nonhomologous (in the absence of template DNA).[114,115] γ-H2AX status was proposed to further prognostically stratify endometrial carcinomas within the NSMP (ie, copy-number low) and p53-abnormal (ie, copy-number high) groups. H2AX is a variant of histone protein H2A and is involved in both homologous and nonhomologous repair.[116] It responds to DNA DSBs by phosphorylation, forming γ-H2AX at DNA breakage sites.[117,118] γ-H2AX can be detected by immunohistochemistry, and serves as an indicator of DSBs which reflects the level of DNA damage.[119] In the refinement of the Trans-PORTEC system, the cutoff adopted for γ-H2AX positivity was an H-score of $\geq$10/300 [3]. Patients whose tumors that were p53 abnormal/γ-H2AX + or NSMP/γ-H2AX+ were shown to have a shorter disease-free survival than their γ-H2AX-negative counterparts.[3] NSMP tumors also demonstrated a high frequency of *ARID1A* mutations in the same cohort, thus γ-H2AX + status may select more aggressive tumors suited for PARP (poly(ADP-ribose) polymerase) and Ataxia telangiectasia and Rad3-related inhibitors.[3,120] DNA-pk is a key component and positive regulator of nonhomologous end-joining (NHEJ),[3,115] whereas FANCD2 is a negative regulator that

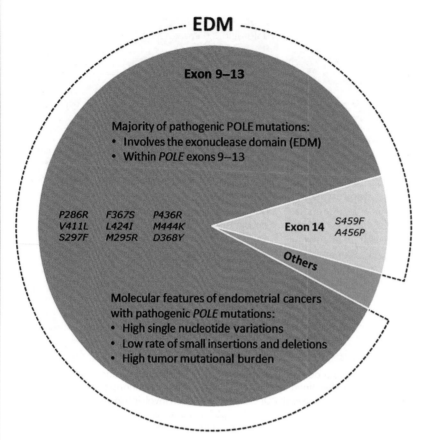

Fig. 5. Pathogenic *POLE* mutations. *Pathogenic *POLE* mutations are mainly found in exonuclease domain mutations (EDM) in exon 9 to 13 (*red*). Other uncommon pathogenic *POLE* mutations in endometrial cancers include exon 14 (*yellow*) mutations. Other possible pathogenic mutations in exon 19 (*grey*) have been reported but their clinical significance is not confirmed. **Established pathogenic *POLE* mutations are displayed in italics.

blocks NHEJ.[121] An immunoprofile of DNA-pk+/FANCD2− indicates NHEJ-proficiency which is responsible for error-prone nonhomologous repair. In the TransPORTEC p53 abnormal group (ie, copy-number high), NHEJ-proficiency stratified a subgroup within p53 abnormal tumors with worse disease-free survival,[3] which may reflect the accumulation of erroneous DSB repairs. The cutoff for the immunostaining interpretation of NHEJ regulator (DNA-pk, FANCD2) was identical to γ-H2AX.[3] These p53 abnormal/NHEJ-proficient tumors also highly expressed PARP-1 immunohistochemically, suggesting sensitivity to PARP inhibitors.[3] Trials involving DNA damage response targeting agents are in progress,[122,123] and the clinical relevance of using these techniques remains to be seen.

TUMORS WITH NO SPECIFIC MOLECULAR PROFILE

Copy-number low tumors do not harbor *POLE* hotspots mutations, *TP53* mutations, or MMR-deficiency.[10,47] Although histologically, NSMP tumors are most commonly low-grade endometrioid carcinomas with squamous differentiation and have low TILs,[26,124] the lack of defining biomarkers is problematic because NSMP tumors constitute approximately to half of all endometrial cancers.[3,9,10]

Recently L1CAM and *CTNNB1*/beta-catenin were explored as such potential markers.[124,125] L1CAM expression by immunohistochemistry predicts worse clinical outcome in p53 wild-type tumors.[125] Likewise, some studies have shown that *CTNNB1* exon 3 mutations are associated with worse outcomes in patients with low-grade endometrioid carcinomas.[126,127] However, other studies have found the opposite: NSMP tumors showing *CTNNB1* mutation and abnormal (nuclear) beta-catenin expression had excellent recurrence-free outcome.[124] Nuclear expression of beta-catenin can be focal (5%–10%) in endometrial cancers,[128] but by adopting a cutoff of less than 10% or ≥10% tumor nuclear expression, studies have achieved good correlation between nuclear beta-catenin and *CTNNB1* mutation.[128,129] *CTNNB1* sequencing may be required when beta-catenin is difficult to interpret or inconclusive.[128]

TUMORS WITH MULTIPLE CLASSIFYING ALTERATIONS

Tumors may be deemed unclassifiable under the TransPORTEC and ProMisE if components are missing or in the TransPORTEC system when multiple classifying alterations are present. These tumors constitute approximately 3% of cases in both the ProMisE confirmation (molecular-defined) and TransPORTEC early-stage endometrial cancer (immunostain surrogate based) cohorts.[9,46] In the confirmation cohort of ProMisE of 319 cases, one molecular-defined "triple-mutated" (MMR-D, POLE EDM, and TP53 mutated) tumor (0.3%) was identified along with 15 tumors (4.7%) with 2 molecular features.[46] Histologically, these were all high-grade tumors (grade III endometrioid, serous, mixed serous-clear cell and undifferentiated carcinomas) and were of variable stages and with different outcomes.[46] In another series, mixed low-grade endometrioid-clear cell carcinoma with p53 aberrant expression and MMR-D have also been reported.[130] In view of these mixed histologic types with complicated mutational profiles, efforts have been made to address the prognostic implications of these endometrial cancers with multiple classifiers. Most importantly, p53 abnormal tumors with either MMR deficiency or POLE mutation have been shown to have significantly better recurrence-free survival than tumors with abnormal p53 expression only.[75] In these cases, the TP53 alteration is thought to arise after the driver POLE or MMR-D alterations as subclonal or late events. POLE mutated plus MSI/MMR-D tumors have rates of recurrence and survival similar to tumors with only POLE alterations.[109] This finding supports prioritizing POLE sequencing before MMR protein immunohistochemistry (if one follows a sequential testing approach).[32] "Triple-mutated" tumors are rare, and their behavior remains uncertain.[75] (**Fig. 6**).

THERAGNOSTIC MARKERS

MMR/MSI and p53/TP53 are primarily molecular surrogate markers that reflect the biological behavior of endometrial cancers, which in turn is associated with prognosis. Clinical trials also stratify patients by molecular classifiers,[99] encouraging clinicians to factor in the tumor molecular subtype for the selection of therapy. In addition, a number of biomarkers with proven predictive power in other malignancies and anatomic sites have entered the realm of endometrial cancer treatment. These include PD-1/PDL1, HER2, and ER/PR, all targetable cell surface/nuclear receptors with well-established targeted therapies and companion immunohistochemistry available.[131–134] These markers further demonstrate correlation

Fig. 6. Unclassifiable tumors and tumors with multiple classifying molecular features.

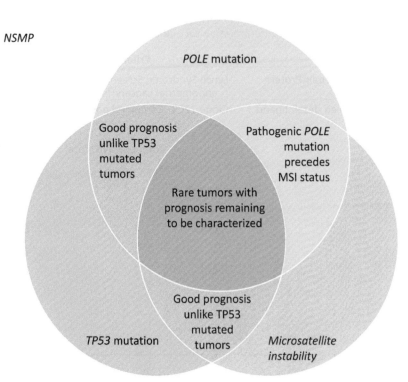

with molecular subtypes, conferring molecular classifiers influence over the selection of these therapies.[2,98,135,136]

PROGRAMMED DEATH-1/PROGRAMMED DEATH-LIGAND 1

PD-1 is a cell surface receptor that regulates T-cell activity. Its ligand PD-L1, which is expressed on tumor and also immune cells, induces inhibitory effects on interaction with PD-1.[137] PD-1/PD-L1 inhibitors restore the activity and antitumor effects of T-cells by blocking PD-1/PD-L1 binding and are approved in many advanced-stage human cancers.[131]

Tumor PD-L1 expression, determined by the combined positive score (CPS), is the highest in endometrial undifferentiated carcinomas (50%–57%), followed by serous (4%–63%) and clear cell carcinomas (15%–75%), and lowest in endometrioid carcinomas (8%–46%).[34,35,41,136,138,139] Increased tumor PD-L1 expression was found in endometrial cancers of higher stage, deeper myometrial invasion, and denser infiltrating lymphocytes.[34,136] PD-L1 expression on immune cells was also associated with higher histologic grade and advanced disease stage.[140] Most PD-L1 high tumors are, from a molecular perspective, POLE mutated or MMR-D.[136,141] The high mutational load in POLE ultramutated and MSI hypermutated tumors leads to formation neoantigens that drives T-cell response.[142] The antibody clones used, assessment methods and cutoffs adopted in these studies,[34,113,140,143] in addition to other scoring methods and PD-L1 antibody clones[144] are listed in **Table 3**.

The standards for the interpretation of PD-L1 immunostain and the associated clinical response have largely been dependent on the clinical settings and reference trials. For example, in KEYNOTE-028, PD-L1 positive locally advanced and metastatic endometrial cancers were found to be responsive to pembrolizumab (a PD-1 inhibitor).[113] Similarly, PD-L1 expression assessed by the Ventana SP142 antibody has demonstrated correlation with response in another trial involving atezolizumab (a PD-L1 inhibitor).[145] In KEYNOTE-158, increased response to pembrolizumab by MMR-D tumors was also observed in endometrial cancers.[97] Others have found MMR-D endometrial cancers respond to another PD-L1 inhibitor, avelumab, but the antitumor activity was independent of PD-L1 status.[99] In view of these findings, before conducting PD-L1 staining, it is advisable to find out the type of drug that would be used, and whether its use needs to be correlated with expression of a companion diagnostic marker.

Table 3
Criteria for biomarker interpretation for endometrial cancers

	Criteria	Interpretation
Mismatch Repair Protein	Lynch Syndrome Screening in endometrial cancers[86,87]	Complete loss of Staining in tumor Cell Nuclei
Programmed death ligand 1	Clone 22C3 Combined positive score[a]	(Number of PD-L1+ tumor and immune cells/Number of tumor cells) × 100
	Total positive score	(Number of PD-L1+ tumor cells/Number of tumor cells) x 100
	Clone 28–8	(Number of PD-L1+ tumor cells/Number of tumor cells) x 100%
	SP142	(Area occupied by PD-L1+ immune cell/Tumor area) x 100%
	SP263	(Number of PD-L1+ tumor cell/Number of tumor cells) x 100%, or (Area occupied by PD-L1+ immune cell/Tumor area occupied by immune cells) x 100%

(continued on next page)

Table 3
(continued)

	Criteria	Interpretation
HER2	Modified from ASCO/CAP breast criteria[154]	0 = Negative: No staining in tumor cells. 1+ = Negative: Faint/barely perceptible, incomplete membrane staining in any proportion, or weak complete staining in <10% of tumor cells. 2+ = Equivocal: intense complete or lateral/basolateral membrane staining in ≤30%, or weak/moderate staining in ≥ 10% tumor cells [b] 3+ = Positive: intense complete or lateral/basolateral membrane staining in > 30% tumor cells
	HER2 testing algorithm specific for p53-abnormal endometrial cancer[162]	0 = Negative: No immunoreactivity or immunoreactivity in <10% of tumor cells. 1+ = Negative: Faint weak and incomplete membranous immunoreactivity in >10% of tumor cells. 2+ = Equivocal: Weak to moderate complete membranous or basolateral immunoreactivity in >10% of tumor cells. [c] 3+ = Positive: Moderate to strong complete membrane or basolateral immunoreactivity in >10% of tumor cells[c]
Estrogen/progesterone receptors	CAP biomarker reporting guidelines	Staining in ≥ 1% tumor cell nuclei[d]

[a] Cutoff of ≥ 1 adopted for KEYNOTE clinical trials.
[b] Confirmation by FISH for HER2 score of 2+ in ASCO/CAP criteria.
[c] Confirmation by DISH for HER2 score of 2+/3+ for p53-abnormal endometrial cancers.
[d] Currently no consensus in cutoff for positivity.

HUMAN EPIDERMAL GROWTH FACTOR RECEPTOR 2

HER2 is encoded by the *ERBB2* gene. HER2 is a cell surface receptor protein and its overexpression is usually a result of gene amplification or less commonly, due to transcriptional deregulation.[146] HER2 overexpression promotes cell proliferation, survival, angiogenesis, and invasion.[146,147] HER2 protein expression may be demonstrated by immunohistochemistry (**Fig. 7**A) while *ERBB2* gene amplification is usually demonstrated by dual-probe fluorescence in situ hybridization (FISH) (**Fig. 7**B) or sequencing. In endometrial cancers, HER2 amplification correlates with histologic grade and stage with amplification rates being highest in serous carcinoma (range 21.4%–29.3%) and clear cell carcinoma (range 22.2%–50.0%), and lowest among grades 1 to 3 endometrioid carcinoma (0.5%, 2.6%, and

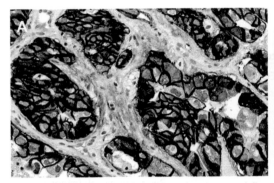 

Fig. 7. HER2 testing by immunohistochemistry and fluorescence in situ hybridization (FISH). (*A*) Complete strong membranous staining in a HER2-overexpressing endometrial cancer, HER2, 40x magnification; (*B*) dual-probe FISH showing increased HER2 (red probe)/CEP17 (green probe) indicating HER2 amplification.

12.7%, respectively).[148–150] In the PORTEC-3 trial, there was a strong correlation between p53 abnormal endometrial cancers with HER2-positive status independent of the tumor histologic type.[135] HER2 amplification is also associated with shorter survival in serous carcinomas.[151]

Patients with advanced or recurrent HER2 overexpressed endometrial serous carcinoma have been shown to benefit from the addition of trastuzumab (a monoclonal anti-HER2 antibody) to conventional chemotherapy.[152,153] The assessment of HER2 immunohistochemistry in endometrial serous carcinoma is, therefore, indicated.

Immunostain evaluation in endometrial cancers is different from breast carcinoma in which complete membranous staining is required. In endometrial serous carcinoma, as apical staining is uncommon, lateral and/or basolateral staining is often observed in the setting of *ERBB2* amplification, and therefore is considered acceptable as positive staining.[154–156] In several studies, the assessment has been based on the Food and Drug Administration (FDA) guidelines,[148,149,151,156,157] while others, including the HER2 analysis from the PORTEC-3 population and therapeutic trials,[135,153] have adopted the American Society of Clinical Oncology/College of American Pathologists (ASCO/CAP) guidelines.[158,159] Both the FDA and all versions of the ASCO/CAP criteria categorizes HER2 staining patterns into scores of 0, 1+, 2+ and 3+, whereby a 3+ score indicates positivity and a 2+ score is recommended for FISH testing, similar to breast cancer.[160] However, some authors considered both 2+ and 3+ as positive,[132,148,156,157,161] which may have resulted in an apparently lowered concordance rate of 59.8% between HER2 immunostain and FISH results.[148] A similar HER2

scoring algorithm developed on p53-abnormal endometrial cancers, assessing the intensity but not the completeness of staining, results in an accuracy of 97% (score 3+) and 100% (score 2+ and 3+) compared against HER2 dual in situ hybridization.[162]

Studies performed on breast cancers suggest that HER2 status predicts response to taxanes, but such findings were not reproducible in endometrial cancers.[148] Although single-agent trastuzumab did not demonstrate treatment efficacy against HER2 overexpressed/amplified endometrial cancers,[132] recent trials of trastuzumab in combination with carboplatin/paclitaxel demonstrated increased progression-free and overall survival in stage III/IV disease endometrial serous carcinoma.[152,153] HER2 overexpression is associated with p53 abnormality and renders anti-HER2 a possible therapeutic option for copy-number high endometrial cancers independent of histologic type.[135] Combination therapy consisting of bevacizumab (a vascular endothelial growth factor A inhibitor) with chemotherapy has recently received renewed interest. A retrospective analysis on the *TP53* mutated subgroup in GOG-86P also revealed improved progression-free and overall survival comparing bevacizumab combination therapy to temsirolimus combination therapy.[163,164] These evidence points to HER2 status as an important factor for the decision of therapy in serous (and other p53 abnormal) endometrial cancers.

ESTROGEN AND PROGESTERONE RECEPTORS

The effect of ER is mediated by nuclear receptor ER,[165] and predominantly through the ER subtype alpha in the endometrium.[166] ER activates cellular signaling pathways and induces the transcription of growth factors and activation in the endometrium.[167,168] ER maintains endometrial proliferation, including the regulation of the menstrual cycle.[169] PR, through PR, inhibits the stimulatory effects of ER in the endometrium.[170] Exposure to PR promotes endometrial epithelial and stromal differentiation, and decreases glandular cellularity, mitosis and atypia.[171] Estrogenic stimulation unopposed by PR increases the risk of developing pathologic hyperplastic and malignant endometrial epithelial neoplasms,[172] in particular ER-positive low-grade endometrioid carcinomas.[167]

ER and PR receptor expression, by immunohistochemistry, is associated with an endometrioid histotype and inversely correlates with histologic grade and stage.[173,174] Compared with other molecular categories, copy-number high endometrial carcinomas have low ER/PR levels.[2]

ER and PR staining are sensitive to tissue ischemia, fixation, and staining protocols,[175] deviation from established parameters can result in loss of staining leading to a false-negative result. For prognostication, cutoffs of 10% and 80% have been proposed to stratify endometrial cancers into high-, intermediate-, and low-risk groups.[176] Clinical trials, however, often use a different cutoff, $\geq 10\%$[177] or scoring systems resembling the Allred score and H-score.[177,178] Systematic reviews and multiple clinical trials have confirmed the efficacy of anti-ERs, in combination with progestins and/or chemotherapy and/or targeted therapy in palliative settings.[133] Tumor ER and PR levels are related to response to single-agent and combination hormonal therapies.[134,179] Nonetheless, further investigation is required to find predictors of response to combinations of newer targeted therapies.[178] In line with breast cancer,[175] the CAP template for biomarker reporting of endometrial carcinoma endorses a cutoff of $\geq 1\%$ for ER/PR positivity, irrespective of intensity,[180] which may be more preferable for practical purposes.

SUMMARY

Classical prognostic pathologic features in endometrial cancer—disease staging and histologic parameters including typing and grading, have long been the core of pathologic assessment. In recent years, molecular methods have proven to be invaluable in providing an additional layer of risk stratification and treatment guidance for patients with endometrial cancer. The molecular classification demonstrates independent predictive power to histologic assessment, correlation with biomarker expression, and treatment response to targeted therapies such as PD1/PD-L1 inhibitors and possibly PARP inhibitors. In the current era of molecular diagnostics, it is essential for practicing pathologists and clinicians to be updated in the molecular classification, as well as the surrogate methods for their application in the diagnosis and treatment of endometrial cancer.

CLINICS CARE POINTS

Pitfalls and recommendations – interpretation of surrogate markers in the molecular classification of endometrial cancers

Pitfalls	Recommendations
• Unrepresentative staining results in inadequate tumor sampling • Presence of undifferentiated/dedifferentiated tumor subclones	Select tumor blocks with adequate tumor volume and representative histology, perform staining on multiple blocks if necessary
• Invalid loss of staining (p53, MMR) interpreted as a genuine aberrant result	Ensure intact staining in internal control, standardize tissue fixation, processing, and staining protocol
• Uninterpretable/unclassifiable staining results (eg, loss of internal control, anomalous staining patterns)	Repeat staining on different blocks, avoid dated archived tissue, review staining procedures

Clinical impact and significance

- Accurate prognostication – the addition of molecular classification to clinical and histologic assessment improves prognostication

- Identifying high-risk groups – p53 mutant low-grade endometrial cancers may require adjuvant therapy

- De-escalation of therapy – omission of adjuvant therapy should be considered in early-stage POLE mutant tumors

- Selection of biomarker – p53 mutant tumors carry a high rate of HER2 overexpression

- Selection of targeted therapy – POLE mutant and MMR deficient tumors show increased response to PD-L1 inhibitors

Challenges in application
• Limited materials for molecular/surrogate testing
○ High correlation between preoperative biopsy and hysterectomy specimen
○ Sequential approach (ProMisE classification system) may reduce tissue requirement
• Limited resources for performing *POLE* sequencing
○ Prioritizing MMR immunostaining reduces cases required for *POLE* sequencing
○ Selecting high-grade, serous-like but heterogenous tumors with prominent TILs
• Distinguishing nonpathogenic *POLE* mutations from pathogenic mutations
○ Targeted sequencing of *POLE* exons 9 to 13/4 or exonuclease domain
• Distinguishing *TP53* passenger mutations from driver mutations
○ Search for multiple p53 subclones by immunostain and histology

REFERENCES

1. Bokhman JV. Two pathogenetic types of endometrial carcinoma. Gynecol Oncol 1983;15(1):10–7.
2. Kandoth C, Schultz N, Cherniack AD, et al. Integrated genomic characterization of endometrial carcinoma. Nature 2013;497(7447):67–73.
3. Auguste A, Genestie C, De Bruyn M, et al. Refinement of high-risk endometrial cancer classification using DNA damage response biomarkers: a Trans-PORTEC initiative. Mod Pathol 2018;31(12):1851–61.
4. Kommoss S, McConechy MK, Kommoss F, et al. Final validation of the ProMisE molecular classifier for endometrial carcinoma in a large population-based case series. Ann Oncol 2018;29(5):1180–8.
5. Matius-Guiu X, Anderson L, Buza N, et al. Endometrial Cancer Histopathology Reporting Guide. Sydney, Australia: International Collaboration on Cancer Reporting, ISBN 978-1-922324-26-9; 2021.
6. Gultekin M, Yildiz F, Ozyigit G, et al. Comparison of FIGO 1988 and 2009 staging systems for endometrial carcinoma. Med Oncol 2012;29(4):2955–62.
7. Kim CH, Soslow RA, Park KJ, et al. Pathologic ultrastaging improves micrometastasis detection in sentinel lymph nodes during endometrial cancer staging. Int J Gynecol Cancer 2013;23(5):964–70.
8. Amin MB, Edge SB, American Joint Committee on C. AJCC cancer staging manual. 2017.
9. Stelloo E, Nout RA, Osse EM, et al. Improved Risk Assessment by Integrating Molecular and Clinicopathological Factors in Early-stage Endometrial Cancer-Combined Analysis of the PORTEC Cohorts. Clin Cancer Res 2016;22(16):4215–24.
10. Talhouk A, McConechy MK, Leung S, et al. A clinically applicable molecular-based classification for endometrial cancers. Br J Cancer 2015;113(2):299–310.
11. Concin N, Matias-Guiu X, Vergote I, et al. ESGO/ESTRO/ESP guidelines for the management of patients with endometrial carcinoma. Int J Gynecol Cancer 2021;31(1):12–39.
12. Idos GE, Kwok J, Bonthala N, et al. The Prognostic Implications of Tumor Infiltrating Lymphocytes in Colorectal Cancer: A Systematic Review and Meta-Analysis. Scientific Rep 2020;10(1):3360.
13. Dieci MV, Radosevic-Robin N, Fineberg S, et al. Update on tumor-infiltrating lymphocytes (TILs) in breast cancer, including recommendations to assess TILs in residual disease after neoadjuvant therapy and in carcinoma in situ: A report of the International Immuno-Oncology Biomarker Working Group on Breast Cancer. Semin Cancer Biol 2018;52:16–25.
14. Lee N, Zakka LR, Mihm MC, et al. Tumour-infiltrating lymphocytes in melanoma prognosis and cancer immunotherapy. Pathology 2016;48(2):177–87.
15. Paijens ST, Vledder A, de Bruyn M, et al. Tumor-infiltrating lymphocytes in the immunotherapy era. Cell Mol Immunol 2021;18(4):842–59.
16. Zhang S, Minaguchi T, Xu C, et al. PD-L1 and CD4 are independent prognostic factors for overall survival in endometrial carcinomas. BMC Cancer 2020;20(1):127.
17. de Jong RA, Leffers N, Boezen HM, et al. Presence of tumor-infiltrating lymphocytes is an independent prognostic factor in type I and II endometrial cancer. Gynecol Oncol 2009;114(1):105–10.
18. Raffone A, Travaglino A, Raimondo D, et al. Tumor-infiltrating lymphocytes and POLE mutation in endometrial carcinoma. Gynecol Oncol 2021 2021;161(2):621–8.
19. Howitt BE, Shukla SA, Sholl LM, et al. Association of Polymerase e–Mutated and Microsatellite-Instable Endometrial Cancers With Neoantigen Load, Number of Tumor-Infiltrating Lymphocytes, and Expression of PD-1 and PD-L1. JAMA Oncol 2015;1(9):1319–23.
20. Peters EEM, León-Castillo A, Smit V, et al. Defining Substantial Lymphovascular Space Invasion in Endometrial Cancer. Int J Gynecol Pathol 2021. https://doi.org/10.1097/PGP.0000000000000806. In press.
21. Bosse T, Peters EE, Creutzberg CL, et al. Substantial lymph-vascular space invasion (LVSI) is a significant risk factor for recurrence in endometrial

cancer–A pooled analysis of PORTEC 1 and 2 trials. Eur J Cancer 2015;51(13):1742–50.

22. Peters EEM, Léon-Castillo A, Hogdall E, et al. Substantial Lymphovascular Space Invasion Is an Adverse Prognostic Factor in High-risk Endometrial Cancer. Int J Gynecol Pathol 2021. https://doi.org/10.1097/PGP.0000000000000805. In press.

23. Peters EEM, Bartosch C, McCluggage WG, et al. Reproducibility of lymphovascular space invasion (LVSI) assessment in endometrial cancer. Histopathology 2019;75(1):128–36.

24. Raffone A, Travaglino A, Mascolo M, et al. TCGA molecular groups of endometrial cancer: Pooled data about prognosis. Gynecol Oncol 2019; 155(2):374–83.

25. Lynch HT, Drescher KM, de la Chapelle A. Immunology and the Lynch syndrome. Gastroenterology 2008;134(4):1246–9.

26. Hussein YR, Soslow RA. Molecular insights into the classification of high-grade endometrial carcinoma. Pathology 2018;50(2):151–61.

27. Hoang LN, McConechy MK, Köbel M, et al. Histotype-genotype correlation in 36 high-grade endometrial carcinomas. Am J Surg Pathol 2013;37(9): 1421–32.

28. Hussein YR, Weigelt B, Levine DA, et al. Clinicopathological analysis of endometrial carcinomas harboring somatic POLE exonuclease domain mutations. Mod Pathol 2015;28(4):505–14.

29. DeLair DF, Burke KA, Selenica P, et al. The genetic landscape of endometrial clear cell carcinomas. J Pathol 2017;243(2):230–41.

30. Travaglino A, Raffone A, Mascolo M, et al. TCGA Molecular Subgroups in Endometrial Undifferentiated/Dedifferentiated Carcinoma. Pathol Oncol Res 2020;26(3):1411–6.

31. Travaglino A, Raffone A, Gencarelli A, et al. TCGA Classification of Endometrial Cancer: the Place of Carcinosarcoma. Pathol Oncol Res 2020;26(4): 2067–73.

32. Kim SR, Cloutier BT, Leung S, et al. Molecular subtypes of clear cell carcinoma of the endometrium: Opportunities for prognostic and predictive stratification. Gynecol Oncol 2020;158(1): 3–11.

33. Baniak N, Fadare O, Köbel M, et al. Targeted Molecular and Immunohistochemical Analyses of Endometrial Clear Cell Carcinoma Show that POLE Mutations and DNA Mismatch Repair Protein Deficiencies Are Uncommon. Am J Surg Pathol 2019;43(4).

34. Jin C, Hacking S, Liang S, et al. PD-L1/PD-1 Expression in Endometrial Clear Cell Carcinoma: A Potential Surrogate Marker for Clinical Trials. Int J Surg Pathol 2020;28(1):31–7.

35. Willis BC, Sloan EA, Atkins KA, et al. Mismatch repair status and PD-L1 expression in clear cell carcinomas of the ovary and endometrium. Mod Pathol 2017;30(11):1622–32.

36. Cagaanan A, Stelter B, Vu N, et al. HER2 Expression in Endometrial Cancers Diagnosed as Clear Cell Carcinoma. Int J Gynecol Pathol 2021;41(2): 132–41.

37. Halle MK, Tangen IL, Berg HF, et al. HER2 expression patterns in paired primary and metastatic endometrial cancer lesions. Br J Cancer 2018; 118(3):378–87.

38. Reid-Nicholson M, Iyengar P, Hummer AJ, et al. Immunophenotypic diversity of endometrial adenocarcinomas: implications for differential diagnosis. Mod Pathol 2006;19(8):1091–100.

39. Rosa-Rosa JM, Leskelä S, Cristóbal-Lana E, et al. Molecular genetic heterogeneity in undifferentiated endometrial carcinomas. Mod Pathol 2016;29(11): 1390–8.

40. Hacking S, Jin C, Komforti M, et al. MMR deficient undifferentiated/dedifferentiated endometrial carcinomas showing significant programmed death ligand-1 expression (sp 142) with potential therapeutic implications. Pathol Res Pract 2019; 215(10):152552.

41. Sloan EA, Ring KL, Willis BC, et al. PD-L1 Expression in Mismatch Repair-deficient Endometrial Carcinomas, Including Lynch Syndrome-associated and MLH1 Promoter Hypermethylated Tumors. Am J Surg Pathol 2017;41(3):326–33.

42. Ramalingam P, Masand RP, Euscher ED, et al. Undifferentiated Carcinoma of the Endometrium: An Expanded Immunohistochemical Analysis Including PAX-8 and Basal-Like Carcinoma Surrogate Markers. Int J Gynecol Pathol 2016;35(5): 410–8.

43. Howitt BE, Dong F, Vivero M, et al. Molecular Characterization of Neuroendocrine Carcinomas of the Endometrium: Representation in All 4 TCGA Groups. Am J Surg Pathol 2020;44(11): 1541–8.

44. Espinosa I, Lee CH, D'Angelo E, et al. Undifferentiated and Dedifferentiated Endometrial Carcinomas With POLE Exonuclease Domain Mutations Have a Favorable Prognosis. Am J Surg Pathol 2017;41(8): 1121–8.

45. Gilks CB, Oliva E, Soslow RA. Poor interobserver reproducibility in the diagnosis of high-grade endometrial carcinoma. Am J Surg Pathol 2013;37(6): 874–81.

46. Talhouk A, McConechy MK, Leung S, et al. Confirmation of ProMisE: A simple, genomics-based clinical classifier for endometrial cancer. Cancer 2017; 123(5):802–13.

47. Stelloo E, Bosse T, Nout RA, et al. Refining prognosis and identifying targetable pathways for high-risk endometrial cancer; a TransPORTEC initiative. Mod Pathol 2015;28(6):836–44.

48. Stelloo E, Nout RA, Naves LC, et al. High concordance of molecular tumor alterations between pre-operative curettage and hysterectomy specimens in patients with endometrial carcinoma. Gynecol Oncol 2014;133(2):197–204.

49. Plotkin A, Kuzeljevic B, De Villa V, et al. Interlaboratory Concordance of ProMisE Molecular Classification of Endometrial Carcinoma Based on Endometrial Biopsy Specimens. Int J Gynecol Pathol 2020;39(6):537–45.

50. Talhouk A, Hoang LN, McConechy MK, et al. Molecular classification of endometrial carcinoma on diagnostic specimens is highly concordant with final hysterectomy: Earlier prognostic information to guide treatment. Gynecol Oncol 2016;143(1):46–53.

51. Bosse T, Nout RA, McAlpine JN, et al. Molecular Classification of Grade 3 Endometrioid Endometrial Cancers Identifies Distinct Prognostic Subgroups. Am J Surg Pathol 2018;42(5):561–8.

52. León-Castillo A, de Boer SM, Powell ME, et al. Molecular Classification of the PORTEC-3 Trial for High-Risk Endometrial Cancer: Impact on Prognosis and Benefit From Adjuvant Therapy. J Clin Oncol 2020;38(29):3388–97.

53. Talhouk A, McAlpine JN. New classification of endometrial cancers: the development and potential applications of genomic-based classification in research and clinical care. Gynecol Oncol Res Pract 2016;3:14.

54. McAlpine J, Leon-Castillo A, Bosse T. The rise of a novel classification system for endometrial carcinoma; integration of molecular subclasses. J Pathol 2018;244(5):538–49.

55. Olivier M, Hollstein M, Hainaut P. TP53 mutations in human cancers: origins, consequences, and clinical use. Cold Spring Harb Perspect Biol 2010; 2(1):a001008.

56. Schultheis AM, Martelotto LG, De Filippo MR, et al. TP53 Mutational Spectrum in Endometrioid and Serous Endometrial Cancers. Int J Gynecol Pathol 2016;35(4):289–300.

57. Bae HS, Kim H, Young Kwon S, et al. Should endometrial clear cell carcinoma be classified as Type II endometrial carcinoma? Int J Gynecol Pathol 2015; 34(1):74–84.

58. Fadare O, Gwin K, Desouki MM, et al. The clinicopathologic significance of p53 and BAF-250a (ARID1A) expression in clear cell carcinoma of the endometrium. Mod Pathol 2013;26(8):1101–10.

59. Yano M, Ito K, Yabuno A, et al. Impact of TP53 immunohistochemistry on the histological grading system for endometrial endometrioid carcinoma. Mod Pathol 2019;32(7):1023–31.

60. Brett MA, Atenafu EG, Singh N, et al. Equivalent Survival of p53 Mutated Endometrial Endometrioid Carcinoma Grade 3 and Endometrial Serous Carcinoma. Int J Gynecol Pathol 2021;40(2):116–23.

61. Raffone A, Travaglino A, Cerbone M, et al. Diagnostic accuracy of p53 immunohistochemistry as surrogate of TP53 sequencing in endometrial cancer. Pathol Res Pract 2020;216(8):153025.

62. Soussi T, Leroy B, Taschner PEM. Recommendations for Analyzing and Reporting TP53 Gene Variants in the High-Throughput Sequencing Era. Hum Mutat 2014;35(6):766–78.

63. Lukashchuk N, Vousden KH. Ubiquitination and degradation of mutant p53. Mol Cell Biol 2007; 27(23):8284–95.

64. Kobel M, Ronnett BM, Singh N, et al. Interpretation of P53 Immunohistochemistry in Endometrial Carcinomas: Toward Increased Reproducibility. Int J Gynecol Pathol 2019; 38(Suppl 1):S123–31.

65. Köbel M, Piskorz AM, Lee S, et al. Optimized p53 immunohistochemistry is an accurate predictor of TP53 mutation in ovarian carcinoma. J Pathol Clin Res 2016;2(4):247–58.

66. Alsner J, Jensen V, Kyndi M, et al. A comparison between p53 accumulation determined by immunohistochemistry and TP53 mutations as prognostic variables in tumours from breast cancer patients. Acta Oncol 2008;47(4):600–7.

67. Alkushi A, Lim P, Coldman A, et al. Interpretation of p53 immunoreactivity in endometrial carcinoma: establishing a clinically relevant cut-off level. Int J Gynecol Pathol 2004;23(2): 129–37.

68. Cho KR, Cooper K, Croce S, et al. International Society of Gynecological Pathologists (ISGyP) Endometrial Cancer Project: Guidelines From the Special Techniques and Ancillary Studies Group. Int J Gynecol Pathol 2019;38.

69. Singh N, Piskorz AM, Bosse T, et al. p53 immunohistochemistry is an accurate surrogate for TP53 mutational analysis in endometrial carcinoma biopsies. J Pathol 2020;250(3):336–45.

70. Coronado PJ, Vidart JA, Lopez-asenjo JA, et al. P53 overexpression predicts endometrial carcinoma recurrence better than HER-2/neu overexpression. Eur J Obstet Gynecol Reprod Biol 2001; 98(1):103–8.

71. McCluggage WG, Soslow RA, Gilks CB. Patterns of p53 immunoreactivity in endometrial carcinomas: 'all or nothing' staining is of importance. Histopathology 2011;59(4):786–8.

72. van Esterik M, Van Gool IC, de Kroon CD, et al. Limited impact of intratumour heterogeneity on molecular risk assignment in endometrial cancer. Oncotarget 2017;8(15):25542–51.

73. Agrawal L, Engel KB, Greytak SR, et al. Understanding preanalytical variables and their effects on clinical biomarkers of oncology and immunotherapy. Semin Cancer Biol 2018;52(Pt 2):26–38.

74. Chen W, Frankel WL. A practical guide to biomarkers for the evaluation of colorectal cancer. Mod Pathol 2019;32(1):1–15.

75. Leon-Castillo A, Gilvazquez E, Nout R, et al. Clinicopathological and molecular characterisation of 'multiple-classifier' endometrial carcinomas. J Pathol 2020;250(3):312–22.

76. Garrido-Ramos MA. Satellite DNA: An Evolving Topic. Genes (Basel) 2017;8(9).

77. Dieringer D, Schlötterer C. Two distinct modes of microsatellite mutation processes: evidence from the complete genomic sequences of nine species. Genome Res 2003;13(10): 2242–51.

78. Li G-M. Mechanisms and functions of DNA mismatch repair. Cell Res 2008;18(1):85–98.

79. Modrich P, Lahue R. Mismatch repair in replication fidelity, genetic recombination, and cancer biology. Annu Rev Biochem 1996;65:101–33.

80. Lynch HT, de la Chapelle A. Genetic susceptibility to non-polyposis colorectal cancer. J Med Genet 1999;36(11):801–18.

81. Umar A, Boland CR, Terdiman JP, et al. Revised Bethesda Guidelines for hereditary nonpolyposis colorectal cancer (Lynch syndrome) and microsatellite instability. J Natl Cancer Inst 2004;96(4): 261–8.

82. Dietmaier W, Wallinger S, Bocker T, et al. Diagnostic Microsatellite Instability: Definition and Correlation with Mismatch Repair Protein Expression. Cancer Res 1997;57(21):4749–56.

83. Kurnit KC, Westin SN, Coleman RL. Microsatellite instability in endometrial cancer: New purpose for an old test. Cancer 2019;125(13):2154–63.

84. Boland CR, Thibodeau SN, Hamilton SR, et al. A National Cancer Institute Workshop on Microsatellite Instability for cancer detection and familial predisposition: development of international criteria for the determination of microsatellite instability in colorectal cancer. Cancer Res 1998;58(22): 5248–57.

85. Karamurzin Y, Rutgers JKL. DNA Mismatch Repair Deficiency in Endometrial Carcinoma. Int J Gynecol Pathol 2009;28(3):239–55.

86. Hampel H, Frankel W, Panescu J, et al. Screening for Lynch Syndrome (Hereditary Nonpolyposis Colorectal Cancer) among Endometrial Cancer Patients. Cancer Res 2006;66(15):7810–7.

87. Wong S, Hui P, Buza N. Frequent loss of mutation-specific mismatch repair protein expression in nonneoplastic endometrium of Lynch syndrome patients. Mod Pathol 2020; 33(6):1172–81.

88. Raevaara TE, Korhonen MK, Lohi H, et al. Functional significance and clinical phenotype of nontruncating mismatch repair variants of MLH1. Gastroenterology 2005;129(2):537–49.

89. Stelloo E, Jansen AML, Osse EM, et al. Practical guidance for mismatch repair-deficiency testing in endometrial cancer. Ann Oncol 2017;28(1): 96–102.

90. McConechy MK, Talhouk A, Li-Chang HH, et al. Detection of DNA mismatch repair (MMR) deficiencies by immunohistochemistry can effectively diagnose the microsatellite instability (MSI) phenotype in endometrial carcinomas. Gynecol Oncol 2015;137(2):306–10.

91. Bruegl AS, Djordjevic B, Urbauer DL, et al. Utility of MLH1 methylation analysis in the clinical evaluation of Lynch Syndrome in women with endometrial cancer. Curr Pharm Des 2014;20(11): 1655–63.

92. Cosgrove CM, Cohn DE, Hampel H, et al. Epigenetic silencing of MLH1 in endometrial cancers is associated with larger tumor volume, increased rate of lymph node positivity and reduced recurrence-free survival. Gynecol Oncol 2017; 146(3):588–95.

93. Mackay HJ, Gallinger S, Tsao MS, et al. Prognostic value of microsatellite instability (MSI) and PTEN expression in women with endometrial cancer: results from studies of the NCIC Clinical Trials Group (NCIC CTG). Eur J Cancer 2010;46(8):1365–73.

94. Ruz-Caracuel I, Ramón-Patino JL, López-Janeiro Á, et al. Myoinvasive Pattern as a Prognostic Marker in Low-Grade, Early-Stage Endometrioid Endometrial Carcinoma. Cancers (Basel) 2019;11(12).

95. McMeekin DS, Tritchler DL, Cohn DE, et al. Clinicopathologic Significance of Mismatch Repair Defects in Endometrial Cancer: An NRG Oncology/ Gynecologic Oncology Group Study. J Clin Oncol 2016;34(25):3062–8.

96. Le DT, Uram JN, Wang H, et al. PD-1 Blockade in Tumors with Mismatch-Repair Deficiency. N Engl J Med 2015;372(26):2509–20.

97. Marabelle A, Le DT, Ascierto PA, et al. Efficacy of Pembrolizumab in Patients With Noncolorectal High Microsatellite Instability/Mismatch Repair-Deficient Cancer: Results From the Phase II KEYNOTE-158 Study. J Clin Oncol 2020;38(1): 1–10.

98. Green AK, Feinberg J, Makker V. A Review of Immune Checkpoint Blockade Therapy in Endometrial Cancer. Am Soc Clin Oncol Educ Book 2020;(40):238–44.

99. Konstantinopoulos PA, Luo W, Liu JF, et al. Phase II Study of Avelumab in Patients With Mismatch Repair Deficient and Mismatch Repair Proficient Recurrent/Persistent Endometrial Cancer. J Clin Oncol 2019;37(30):2786–94.

100. Park VS, Pursell ZF. POLE proofreading defects: Contributions to mutagenesis and cancer. DNA Repair 2019;76:50–9.

101. Bermudez VP, Farina A, Raghavan V, et al. Studies on human DNA polymerase epsilon and GINS complex and their role in DNA replication. J Biol Chem 2011;286(33):28963–77.

102. Kesti T, Flick K, Keränen S, et al. DNA Polymerase ε Catalytic Domains Are Dispensable for DNA Replication, DNA Repair, and Cell Viability. Mol Cell 1999;3(5):679–85.

103. Korona DA, Lecompte KG, Pursell ZF. The high fidelity and unique error signature of human DNA polymerase epsilon. Nucleic Acids Res 2011; 39(5):1763–73.

104. Rayner E, van Gool IC, Palles C, et al. A panoply of errors: polymerase proofreading domain mutations in cancer. Nat Rev Cancer 2016;16(2):71–81.

105. López-Reig R, Fernández-Serra A, Romero I, et al. Prognostic classification of endometrial cancer using a molecular approach based on a twelve-gene NGS panel. Scientific Rep 2019; 9(1):18093.

106. McConechy MK, Talhouk A, Leung S, et al. Endometrial Carcinomas with POLE Exonuclease Domain Mutations Have a Favorable Prognosis. Clin Cancer Res 2016;22(12):2865–73.

107. Raffone A, Travaglino A, Gabrielli O, et al. Clinical features of ProMisE groups identify different phenotypes of patients with endometrial cancer. Arch Gynecol Obstet 2021;303(6):1393–400.

108. Imboden S, Nastic D, Ghaderi M, et al. Phenotype of POLE-mutated endometrial cancer. PLoS One 2019;14(3):e0214318.

109. León-Castillo A, Britton H, McConechy MK, et al. Interpretation of somatic POLE mutations in endometrial carcinoma. J Pathol 2020;250(3): 323–35.

110. Devereaux KA, Weiel JJ, Pors J, et al. Prospective molecular classification of endometrial carcinomas: institutional implementation, practice, and clinical experience. Mod Pathol 2021. https://doi.org/10.1038/s41379-021-00963-y. In press.

111. Mehnert JM, Panda A, Zhong H, et al. Immune activation and response to pembrolizumab in POLE-mutant endometrial cancer. J Clin Invest 2016; 126(6):2334–40.

112. Yarchoan M, Hopkins A, Jaffee EM. Tumor Mutational Burden and Response Rate to PD-1 Inhibition. N Engl J Med 2017;377(25):2500–1.

113. Ott PA, Bang YJ, Berton-Rigaud D, et al. Safety and Antitumor Activity of Pembrolizumab in Advanced Programmed Death Ligand 1-Positive Endometrial Cancer: Results From the KEYNOTE-028 Study. J Clin Oncol 2017;35(22):2535–41.

114. Scully R, Xie A. Double strand break repair functions of histone H2AX. Mutat Res 2013;750(1–2): 5–14.

115. Lieber MR. The mechanism of double-strand DNA break repair by the nonhomologous DNA end-joining pathway. Annu Rev Biochem 2010;79: 181–211.

116. Collins PL, Purman C, Porter SI, et al. DNA double-strand breaks induce H2Ax phosphorylation domains in a contact-dependent manner. Nat Commun 2020;11(1):3158.

117. DeMicco A, Bassing CH. Deciphering the DNA damage histone code. Cell Cycle 2010;9(19): 3842–7.

118. Bonner WM, Redon CE, Dickey JS, et al. Gamma-H2AX and cancer. Nat Rev Cancer 2008;8(12): 957–67.

119. Matthaios D, Foukas PG, Kefala M, et al. γ-H2AX expression detected by immunohistochemistry correlates with prognosis in early operable non-small cell lung cancer. Onco Targets Ther 2012;5: 309–14.

120. Shen J, Peng Y, Wei L, et al. ARID1A Deficiency Impairs the DNA Damage Checkpoint and Sensitizes Cells to PARP Inhibitors. Cancer Discov 2015;5(7): 752–67.

121. Adamo A, Collis SJ, Adelman CA, et al. Preventing nonhomologous end joining suppresses DNA repair defects of Fanconi anemia. Mol Cell 2010; 39(1):25–35.

122. Jamieson A, Bosse T, McAlpine JN. The emerging role of molecular pathology in directing the systemic treatment of endometrial cancer. Ther Adv Med Oncol 2021;13, 17588359211035959.

123. van den Heerik ASVM, Horeweg N, de Boer SM, et al. Adjuvant therapy for endometrial cancer in the era of molecular classification: radiotherapy, chemoradiation and novel targets for therapy. Int J Gynecol Cancer 2021;31(4):594–604.

124. De Leo A, de Biase D, Lenzi J, et al. ARID1A and CTNNB1/β-Catenin Molecular Status Affects the Clinicopathologic Features and Prognosis of Endometrial Carcinoma: Implications for an Improved Surrogate Molecular Classification. Cancers 2021; 13(5):950.

125. Kommoss FKF, Karnezis AN, Kommoss F, et al. L1CAM further stratifies endometrial carcinoma patients with no specific molecular risk profile. Br J Cancer 2018;119(4):480–6.

126. Kurnit KC, Kim GN, Fellman BM, et al. CTNNB1 (beta-catenin) mutation identifies low grade, early stage endometrial cancer patients at increased risk of recurrence. Mod Pathol 2017;30(7): 1032–41.

127. Liu Y, Patel L, Mills GB, et al. Clinical significance of CTNNB1 mutation and Wnt pathway activation in endometrioid endometrial carcinoma. J Natl Cancer Inst 2014;106(9).

128. Kim G, Kurnit KC, Djordjevic B, et al. Nuclear β-catenin localization and mutation of the CTNNB1 gene: a context-dependent association. Mod Pathol 2018;31(10):1553–9.

129. Costigan DC, Dong F, Nucci MR, et al. Clinicopathologic and Immunohistochemical Correlates of CTNNB1 Mutated Endometrial Endometrioid Carcinoma. Int J Gynecol Pathol 2020;39(2):119–27.

130. Ida N, Nakamura K, Saijo M, et al. DNA mismatch repair deficiency and p53 abnormality are age-related events in mixed endometrial carcinoma with a clear cell component. Pathol - Res Pract 2021;220:153383.

131. Alsaab HO, Sau S, Alzhrani R, et al. PD-1 and PD-L1 Checkpoint Signaling Inhibition for Cancer Immunotherapy: Mechanism, Combinations, and Clinical Outcome. Front Pharmacol 2017;8:561.

132. Fleming GF, Sill MW, Darcy KM, et al. Phase II trial of trastuzumab in women with advanced or recurrent, HER2-positive endometrial carcinoma: a Gynecologic Oncology Group study. Gynecol Oncol 2010;116(1):15–20.

133. van Weelden WJ, Massuger L, Pijnenborg JMA, et al. Anti-estrogen Treatment in Endometrial Cancer: A Systematic Review. Front Oncol 2019;9:359.

134. Thigpen JT, Brady MF, Alvarez RD, et al. Oral Medroxyprogesterone Acetate in the Treatment of Advanced or Recurrent Endometrial Carcinoma: A Dose-Response Study by the Gynecologic Oncology Group. J Clin Oncol 1999;17(6):1736.

135. Vermij L, Horeweg N, Leon-Castillo A, et al. HER2 Status in High-Risk Endometrial Cancers (PORTEC-3): Relationship with Histotype, Molecular Classification, and Clinical Outcomes. Cancers 2021;13(1):44.

136. Pasanen A, Ahvenainen T, Pellinen T, et al. PD-L1 Expression in Endometrial Carcinoma Cells and Intratumoral Immune Cells: Differences Across Histologic and TCGA-based Molecular Subgroups. Am J Surg Pathol 2020;44(2):174–81.

137. Freeman GJ, Long AJ, Iwai Y, et al. Engagement of the PD-1 immunoinhibitory receptor by a novel B7 family member leads to negative regulation of lymphocyte activation. J Exp Med 2000;192(7):1027–34.

138. Engerud H, Berg HF, Myrvold M, et al. High degree of heterogeneity of PD-L1 and PD-1 from primary to metastatic endometrial cancer. Gynecol Oncol 2020;157(1):260–7.

139. Kir G, Soylemez T, Olgun ZC, et al. Correlation of PD-L1 expression with immunohistochemically determined molecular profile in endometrial carcinomas. Virchows Arch 2020;477(6):845–56.

140. Sungu N, Yildirim M, Desdicioglu R, et al. Expression of Immunomodulatory Molecules PD-1, PD-L1, and PD-L2, and their Relationship With Clinicopathologic Characteristics in Endometrial Cancer. Int J Gynecol Pathol 2019;38(5):404–13.

141. Li Z, Joehlin-Price AS, Rhoades J, et al. Programmed Death Ligand 1 Expression Among 700 Consecutive Endometrial Cancers: Strong Association With Mismatch Repair Protein Deficiency. Int J Gynecol Cancer 2018;28(1):59–68.

142. Schumacher TN, Schreiber RD. Neoantigens in cancer immunotherapy. Science 2015;348(6230):69–74.

143. Makker V, Taylor MH, Aghajanian C, et al. Lenvatinib Plus Pembrolizumab in Patients With Advanced Endometrial Cancer. J Clin Oncol 2020;38(26):2981–92.

144. Huang T-H, Cheng W, Wang Y-H. Interpretation According to Clone-Specific PD-L1 Cutoffs Reveals Better Concordance in Muscle-Invasive Urothelial Carcinoma. Diagnostics 2021;11(3):448.

145. Fleming GF, Emens LA, Eder JP, et al. Clinical activity, safety and biomarker results from a phase Ia study of atezolizumab (atezo) in advanced/recurrent endometrial cancer (rEC). J Clin Oncol 2017;35(15_suppl):5585.

146. Moasser MM. The oncogene HER2: its signaling and transforming functions and its role in human cancer pathogenesis. Oncogene 2007;26(45):6469–87.

147. Diver EJ, Foster R, Rueda BR, et al. The Therapeutic Challenge of Targeting HER2 in Endometrial Cancer. Oncologist 2015;20(9):1058–68.

148. Grushko TA, Filiaci VL, Mundt AJ, et al. An exploratory analysis of HER-2 amplification and overexpression in advanced endometrial carcinoma: a Gynecologic Oncology Group study. Gynecol Oncol 2008;108(1):3–9.

149. Morrison C, Zanagnolo V, Ramirez N, et al. HER-2 is an independent prognostic factor in endometrial cancer: association with outcome in a large cohort of surgically staged patients. J Clin Oncol 2006;24(15):2376–85.

150. Peiró G, Mayr D, Hillemanns P, et al. Analysis of HER-2/neu amplification in endometrial carcinoma by chromogenic in situ hybridization. Correlation with fluorescence in situ hybridization, HER-2/neu, p53 and Ki-67 protein expression, and outcome. Mod Pathol 2004;17(3):277–87.

151. Santin AD, Bellone S, Van Stedum S, et al. Amplification of c-erbB2 oncogene: a major prognostic indicator in uterine serous papillary carcinoma. Cancer 2005;104(7):1391–7.

152. Fader AN, Roque DM, Siegel E, et al. Randomized Phase II Trial of Carboplatin-Paclitaxel Versus Carboplatin-Paclitaxel-Trastuzumab in Uterine Serous Carcinomas That Overexpress Human Epidermal Growth Factor Receptor 2/neu. J Clin Oncol 2018;36(20):2044–51.

153. Fader AN, Roque DM, Siegel E, et al. Randomized Phase II Trial of Carboplatin-Paclitaxel Compared with Carboplatin-Paclitaxel-Trastuzumab in Advanced (Stage III-IV) or Recurrent Uterine Serous Carcinomas that Overexpress Her2/Neu (NCT01367002): Updated Overall Survival Analysis. Clin Cancer Res 2020;26(15):3928–35.

154. Buza N. HER2 Testing in Endometrial Serous Carcinoma: Time for Standardized Pathology Practice to Meet the Clinical Demand. Arch Pathol Lab Med 2020;145(6):687–91.

155. Buza N, English DP, Santin AD, et al. Toward standard HER2 testing of endometrial serous carcinoma: 4-year experience at a large academic center and recommendations for clinical practice. Mod Pathol 2013;26(12):1605–12.

156. Buza N, Roque DM, Santin AD. HER2/neu in Endometrial Cancer: A Promising Therapeutic Target With Diagnostic Challenges. Arch Pathol Lab Med 2014;138(3):343–50.

157. Slomovitz BM, Broaddus RR, Burke TW, et al. Her-2/neu overexpression and amplification in uterine papillary serous carcinoma. J Clin Oncol 2004; 22(15):3126–32.

158. Wolff AC, Hammond MEH, Allison KH, et al. Human Epidermal Growth Factor Receptor 2 Testing in Breast Cancer: American Society of Clinical Oncology/College of American Pathologists Clinical Practice Guideline Focused Update. J Clin Oncol 2018;36(20):2105–22.

159. Wolff AC, Hammond ME, Schwartz JN, et al. American Society of Clinical Oncology/College of American Pathologists guideline recommendations for human epidermal growth factor receptor 2 testing in breast cancer. J Clin Oncol 2007; 25(1):118–45.

160. Wolff AC, Hammond MEH, Allison KH, et al. Human Epidermal Growth Factor Receptor 2 Testing in Breast Cancer: American Society of Clinical Oncology/College of American Pathologists Clinical Practice Guideline Focused Update. Arch Pathol Lab Med 2018;142(11):1364–82.

161. Togami S, Sasajima Y, Oi T, et al. Clinicopathological and prognostic impact of human epidermal growth factor receptor type 2 (HER2) and hormone receptor expression in uterine papillary serous carcinoma. Cancer Sci 2012;103(5):926–32.

162. Vermij L, Singh N, Leon-Castillo A, et al. Performance of a HER2 testing algorithm specific for p53-abnormal endometrial cancer. Histopathology 2021;79(4):533–43.

163. Leslie KK, Filiaci VL, Mallen AR, et al. Mutated p53 portends improvement in outcomes when bevacizumab is combined with chemotherapy in advanced/recurrent endometrial cancer: An NRG Oncology study. Gynecol Oncol 2021;161(1):113–21.

164. Aghajanian C, Filiaci V, Dizon DS, et al. A phase II study of frontline paclitaxel/carboplatin/bevacizumab, paclitaxel/carboplatin/temsirolimus, or ixabepilone/carboplatin/bevacizumab in advanced/recurrent endometrial cancer. Gynecol Oncol 2018;150(2):274–81.

165. Paterni I, Granchi C, Katzenellenbogen JA, et al. Estrogen receptors alpha (ERα) and beta (ERβ): subtype-selective ligands and clinical potential. Steroids 2014;90:13–29.

166. Leslie KK, Thiel KW, Reyes HD, et al. The Estrogen Receptor Joins Other Cancer Biomarkers as a Predictor of Outcome. Obstet Gynecol Int 2013;2013: 479541.

167. Rodriguez AC, Blanchard Z, Maurer KA, et al. Estrogen Signaling in Endometrial Cancer: a Key Oncogenic Pathway with Several Open Questions. Horm Cancer 2019;10(2–3):51–63.

168. Lösel R, Wehling M. Nongenomic actions of steroid hormones. Nat Rev Mol Cell Biol 2003;4(1):46–55.

169. Groothuis PG, Dassen HH, Romano A, et al. Estrogen and the endometrium: lessons learned from gene expression profiling in rodents and human. Hum Reprod Update 2007;13(4):405–17.

170. Kim JJ, Kurita T, Bulun SE. Progesterone action in endometrial cancer, endometriosis, uterine fibroids, and breast cancer. Endocr Rev 2013;34(1):130–62.

171. Wheeler DT, Bristow RE, Kurman RJ. Histologic alterations in endometrial hyperplasia and well-differentiated carcinoma treated with progestins. Am J Surg Pathol 2007;31(7):988–98.

172. Brinton LA, Felix AS. Menopausal hormone therapy and risk of endometrial cancer. J Steroid Biochem Mol Biol 2014;142:83–9.

173. Carcangiu ML, Chambers JT, Voynick IM, et al. Immunohistochemical evaluation of estrogen and progesterone receptor content in 183 patients with endometrial carcinoma. Part I: Clinical and histologic correlations. Am J Clin Pathol 1990;94(3): 247–54.

174. Obeidat BR, Matalka II, Mohtaseb AA, et al. Selected immuno-histochemical markers in curettage specimens and their correlation with final pathologic findings in endometrial cancer patients. Pathol Oncol Res 2013;19(2):229–35.

175. Hammond ME, Hayes DF, Dowsett M, et al. American Society of Clinical Oncology/College of American Pathologists guideline recommendations for immunohistochemical testing of estrogen and progesterone receptors in breast cancer (unabridged version). Arch Pathol Lab Med 2010;134(7):e48–72.

176. van Weelden WJ, Reijnen C, Küsters-Vandevelde HVN, et al. The cutoff for estrogen and progesterone receptor expression in endometrial cancer revisited: a European Network for Individualized Treatment of Endometrial Cancer collaboration study. Hum Pathol 2021;109:80–91.

177. Covens AL, Filiaci V, Gersell D, et al. Phase II study of fulvestrant in recurrent/metastatic endometrial carcinoma: A Gynecologic Oncology Group Study. Gynecol Oncol 2011;120(2):185–8.

178. Slomovitz BM, Jiang Y, Yates MS, et al. Phase II Study of Everolimus and Letrozole in Patients With Recurrent Endometrial Carcinoma. J Clin Oncol 2015;33(8):930–6.

179. Singh M, Zaino RJ, Filiaci VJ, et al. Relationship of estrogen and progesterone receptors to clinical outcome in metastatic endometrial carcinoma: a Gynecologic Oncology Group Study. Gynecol Oncol 2007;106(2):325–33.

180. Longacre TA, Broaddus R, Chuang LT, et al. Template for Reporting Results of Biomarker Testing of Specimens From Patients With Carcinoma of the Endometrium. Arch Pathol Lab Med 2017; 141(11):1508–12.

181. Alexa M, Hasenburg A, Battista MJ. The TCGA Molecular Classification of Endometrial Cancer and Its Possible Impact on Adjuvant Treatment Decisions. Cancers (Basel) 2021;13(6).

182. Ramalingam P, Croce S, McCluggage WG. Loss of expression of SMARCA4 (BRG1), SMARCA2 (BRM) and SMARCB1 (INI1) in undifferentiated carcinoma of the endometrium is not uncommon and is not always associated with rhabdoid morphology. Histopathology 2017;70(3):359–66.

183. Koo Y-J, Kim D-Y, Kim K-R, et al. Small cell neuroendocrine carcinoma of the endometrium: A clinicopathologic study of six cases. Taiwanese J Obstet Gynecol 2014;53(3):355–9.

Uncommon and Difficult High-Grade Endometrial Carcinomas

Jelena Mirkovic, MD, PhD[a,b,*]

KEYWORDS

- Dedifferentiated endometrial carcinoma • Undifferentiated endometrial carcinoma
- Mesonephric-like carcinoma of the endometrium • Gastric-type endometrial carcinoma
- Endometrial carcinoma with germ cell or trophoblastic-like components

Key points

- Distinct types of high-grade endometrial carcinoma have been described and included in the current World Health Organization classification.
- Undifferentiated/dedifferentiated carcinoma is not limited to arising in association with low-grade endometrioid carcinoma but can be seen in association with various types of high-grade carcinoma.
- Mesonephric-like carcinoma of the endometrium (and the ovary) is a tumor exhibiting the classic morphologic and immunohistochemical features of mesonephric carcinomas without association with mesonephric remnants/hyperplasia.
- Gastric-type endometrial carcinoma is currently defined by gastric-type morphology, with at least focal immunohistochemical expression of one or more gastrointestinal markers (HIK1083, MUC6, CK20, and CDX2), absent or minimal (arbitrarily defined as <5%) expression of ER, absence of cervical involvement on the histologic examination of the entire cervix, and absence of any component of typical endometrioid morphology.
- Mullerian endometrial (and ovarian) carcinomas with germ cell/trophoblastic-like components are rare aggressive tumors typically affecting postmenopausal patients with poor response to chemotherapy and early recurrence. They are now recognized to have a somatic origin and are characterized by genomic instability.

ABSTRACT

This article presents features of uncommon high-grade endometrial carcinomas that often pose a significant diagnostic challenge. An update on undifferentiated and dedifferentiated endometrial carcinoma is first provided, followed by discussions on more recently defined entities such as mesonephric-like carcinoma of the endometrium and gastric-type endometrial carcinomas. Finally, endometrial carcinoma with germ cell or trophoblastic-like components is discussed.

UNDIFFERENTIATED AND DEDIFFERENTIATED ENDOMETRIAL CARCINOMA

INTRODUCTION

Undifferentiated endometrial carcinoma, an aggressive pathologic subtype of endometrial cancer, defined in 2005 as a malignant epithelial neoplasm characterized by a total absence of glandular differentiation and a patternless solid growth of tumor cells, with absent or minimal

[a] Division of Laboratory Medicine and Molecular Diagnostics, Anatomic Pathology, Sunnybrook Health Sciences Centre, 2075 Bayview Avenue, Room E401, Toronto, Ontario M4N 3M5, Canada; [b] Department of Laboratory Medicine and Pathobiology, University of Toronto, Toronto, Ontario, Canada
* Division of Laboratory Medicine and Molecular Diagnostics, Anatomic Pathology, Sunnybrook Health Sciences Centre, 2075 Bayview Avenue, Room E401, Toronto, Ontario M4N 3M5, Canada.
E-mail address: Jelena.mirkovic@sunnybrook.ca

Surgical Pathology 15 (2022) 301–314
https://doi.org/10.1016/j.path.2022.02.007
1875-9181/22/© 2022 Elsevier Inc. All rights reserved.

neuroendocrine differentiation.[1] It was next recognized that undifferentiated carcinoma can be associated with low-grade endometrioid carcinoma, in which case the term "dedifferentiated carcinoma" applies.[2] Before the 2020 WHO classification of female genital tract tumors, dedifferentiated carcinoma was strictly defined as composed of undifferentiated carcinoma and a low-grade endometrioid carcinoma (FIGO grade 1 or 2) components.[1–4] It is now recognized that dedifferentiated carcinoma can also arise in the background of high-grade endometrial carcinoma.

MICROSCOPIC FEATURES

Undifferentiated endometrial carcinoma, either pure or as a component of dedifferentiated carcinoma, is characterized by a diffuse population of noncohesive epithelioid cells with a monotonous appearance (Fig. 1A). It often exhibits extensive geographic necrosis, lymphovascular invasion, and prominent tumor-infiltrating lymphocytes. Rhabdoid morphology and/or a prominent myxoid stroma can be encountered. Tumors may show focal areas of abrupt keratinization, marked nuclear pleomorphism, and multinucleation. Focal alveolar, nested, vaguely corded, or trabecular growth pattern and focal spindling, may be present.[5] Prototypical dedifferentiated carcinoma is characterized by an abrupt transition between undifferentiated carcinoma and low-grade endometrioid carcinoma (Fig. 1B). Undifferentiated carcinoma can also arise in the background of high-grade endometrial carcinoma (Fig. 1C), including endometrioid,[6–8] clear cell,[7,9] serous,[10] high-grade tumors with ambiguous morphology, as well as various types of mixed carcinomas.[7,11] In this setting, the undifferentiated component has been described as intermixed with the differentiated components.

IMMUNOHISTOCHEMISTRY

Pankeratin (Fig. 1D), cytokeratin (CK)8/18, and epithelial membrane antigen (EMA), are usually focally but strongly positive.[1,2] E-cadherin is usually entirely negative (Fig. 1E) or focal.[7] Estrogen receptor (ER, Fig. 1F) and progesterone receptor (PR) are usually not expressed.[7] Likewise, PAX8 is usually negative (~80–90% of cases). Diffuse expression of one or more of these markers, although infrequent, does not necessarily exclude the diagnosis of UC. Claudin-4 is frequently negative.[12]

SMARCA4 expression is lost in ~30% of cases, while INI1 expression is lost in ~5–10% cases.[13,14] In dedifferentiated endometrial carcinoma, loss of SMARCA4 expression is frequently limited to undifferentiated component.[13] Rhabdoid morphology is not correlated with loss of SMARCA4/INI1 expression.[14] Loss of claudin-4, PAX8, ER, and PR staining are more common in SMARCA4/INI1 deficient tumors.[8,12]

Mismatch repair protein loss of expression, most commonly concurrent MLH1 (Fig. 1G) and PMS2 loss, is seen in 45% to 70% of the cases.[6,7,13,15] In dedifferentiated endometrial carcinoma, the abnormality is most commonly seen across the entire tumor (including both the undifferentiated and differentiated carcinoma components).

Aberrant p53 expression is reported in ~15 to 30% of undifferentiated/dedifferentiated endometrial carcinomas, while most cases exhibit wild type p53 staining (Fig. 1H).[6,7] Frequency of p53 abnormal expression depends on the SMARCA4/INI1 mutational status. While approximately 50% of SMARCA4/INI1-intact cases exhibited abnormal p53 expression, only 5% of the SMARCA4/INI1-deficient cases exhibited abnormal p53 expression in one study.[8]

CyclinD1 was diffusely and strongly positive in 50% of the cases in one study.[16] CD34 was positive in 30% of the cases, with diffuse expression in 6%.[17] P16 was diffusely positive in 34% of the cases.[7] Synaptophysin and chromogranin are usually negative or focal. According to the recent recommendations on high-grade endometrial carcinomas by the International Society of Gynecologic Pathologists, immunohistochemical expression of neuroendocrine markers should be restricted to less than 10% of tumor cells in undifferentiated carcinoma.[5]

MOLECULAR FEATURES

Undifferentiated and dedifferentiated endometrial carcinomas exhibit genetic heterogeneity with the representation of all 4 groups of the Cancer Genome Atlas classification.[6,18] Most commonly they are hypermutated and microsatellite unstable tumors.[6,19] They have relatively frequent mutations in genes commonly altered in endometrial carcinomas such as PTEN, PIK3CA, CTNNB1, TP53, and POLE exonuclease domain.[6,13,19–21] In addition, they exhibit the frequent inactivation of core SWI/SNF complex proteins. In dedifferentiated endometrial carcinomas, mutually exclusive inactivating SMARCA4 (~35%) or SMARCB1 (~10%) mutations, as well as concurrent inactivating mutations involving ARID1A/ARID1B (~25%) are described.[15,22] Similar findings are seen in UCs.[19]

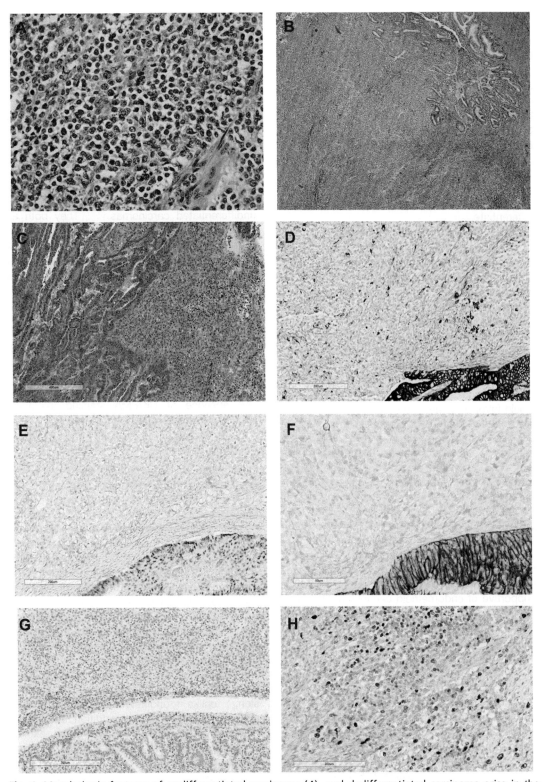

Fig. 1. Morphologic features of undifferentiated carcinoma (*A*), and dedifferentiated carcinoma arise in the background of low-grade endometrioid carcinoma (*B*) and high-grade (serous) carcinoma (*C*). Undifferentiated carcinoma is characterized by focal pan-cytokeratin expression (*D*), loss of ER (*E*), loss of e-cadherin (*F*), loss of MMR nuclear expression (MLH1 in this example) (*G*), and p53 wild type staining (*H*).

DIFFERENTIAL DIAGNOSIS

The most important differential diagnoses of dedifferentiated carcinoma are endometrioid carcinoma and carcinosarcoma. Pure undifferentiated carcinoma has a long list of entities in a differential, including high-grade endometrioid carcinoma, SMARCA4 deficient uterine sarcoma, and high-grade endometrial stromal sarcoma (HG ESS) among others. Some of these, such as melanoma, lymphoid malignancies, and high-grade neuroendocrine carcinoma are easily distinguishable by a limited panel of immunohistochemistry stains, and others can be more challenging to differentiate.

Endometrioid Carcinoma

Recognizing dedifferentiated/undifferentiated endometrial carcinoma as a distinct entity is important, as it confers a worse prognosis compared with FIGO3 endometrioid carcinoma.[1] Endometrioid carcinoma, particularly with solid growth and/or poor fixation, may seem noncohesive and therefore mimic UC. The assessment is best performed in well-preserved areas of the tumor, in which cell cohesion (nesting, defined grouping) and at least focal glandular formation would favor endometrioid carcinoma. In contrast, the undifferentiated carcinoma component of dedifferentiated carcinoma is characterized by the lack of cellular cohesion and glandular formation. Focal rhabdoid morphology is also helpful. In the appropriate morphologic setting, immunohistochemistry stains can be helpful. In general, absent or focal CK/EMA, negative PAX8/ER/E-cadherin, along with loss of INI1 or SMARCA4 would favor undifferentiated carcinoma component over endometrioid carcinoma. Conversely, diffuse retained expression of keratins, E-cadherin, PAX8, and hormone receptors would be supportive of endometrioid carcinoma. However, it is important to note that expression of PAX8 and ER can be significant in a minority of undifferentiated carcinomas[7] and lost in some high-grade endometrioid carcinomas.

SMARCA4 Deficient Uterine Sarcoma

SMARCA4 deficient uterine sarcoma, a recently described aggressive sarcoma, has overlapping features with UC, including epithelioid cells, rhabdoid morphology, noncohesive cell growth, necrosis, prominent lymphovascular invasion, and SMARCA4 loss.[23–25] Undifferentiated sarcoma affects young patients, in contrast to UC which predominantly affects peri or postmenopausal women. Phyllodiform-like growth mimicking adenosarcoma, if present, favors SMARCA4-deficient uterine sarcoma, while overt nuclear pleomorphism, if present, favors undifferentiated endometrial carcinoma. Unlike ~ 30% of UCs, sarcomas are p53 wild type, and unlike up to 60% of UCs, they exhibit normal MMR immunohistochemistry expression. Sarcomas are also usually entirely negative for CKs, EMA, and claudin-4. Unlike UC, they have a low mutation burden. In a minority of cases, molecular testing may be required to classify the tumor.

High-Grade Endometrial Stromal Sarcoma

Among the HG ESSs, those with YWHAE-NUTM2 fusion are the most challenging to distinguish from undifferentiated carcinomas.[26,27] They both are characterized by monomorphic epithelioid cells with brisk mitoses, but the nested pattern can be seen in YWHAE-NUTM2 HG ESS, and this is unusual of undifferentiated endometrial carcinoma. They are both typically negative for ER and PR. In addition, diffuse and strong Cyclin D1, which is characteristic of this type of HG ESS, is also present in 50% of undifferentiated endometrial carcinoma.[16] In cases whereby there is no associated component of low-grade endometrial stromal sarcoma or differentiated carcinoma, respectively, and tumor shows diffuse and strong CyclinD1 and absence of CK/EMA staining, molecular studies may be necessary for diagnosis.

Carcinosarcoma

Dedifferentiated carcinomas and carcinosarcomas both show a low-power biphasic appearance and may exhibit myxoid stroma. However, carcinosarcoma is characterized by a malignant mesenchymal component that is usually diffusely atypical, pleomorphic, and mitotically active. Spindle cell morphology, as well as heterologous differentiation, are also in keeping with a true mesenchymal component. Dedifferentiated carcinoma can contain areas of spindled cells, but this should be a focal finding. Likewise, dedifferentiated carcinoma can have areas of prominent myxoid matrix deposition, which by itself is not diagnostic of sarcomatous transformation. The vast majority of carcinosarcomas exhibit p53 mutation/abnormal immunohistochemistry expression, unlike undifferentiated/dedifferentiated endometrial carcinomas. In addition, undifferentiated carcinoma, unlike carcinosarcoma, exhibits frequent microsatellite instability and MMR immunohistochemistry loss.[28,29]

It is important to note that undifferentiated carcinoma can rarely be seen as a component in a carcinosarcoma, most frequently in those that are MMR-deficient (41% of MMR-deficient carcinosarcomas in a recent study).[30] Also, sarcomatous transformation in undifferentiated/dedifferentiated endometrial carcinomas was described recently in 3 cases, one of which exhibited true heterologous differentiation.[31]

UNDIFFERENTIATED CARCINOMAPATHOLOGIC: KEY FEATURES

- Diffuse population of noncohesive epithelioid cells with uniform round nuclei and scant cytoplasm

- Geographic necrosis, lymphovascular invasion, and prominent tumor-infiltrating lymphocytes

- Occasionally rhabdoid morphology, often in a myxoid stroma

- Focal alveolar, nested, vaguely corded, or trabecular growth pattern and focal spindling may be present

- By immunohistochemistry, loss or diminished expression of e-cadherin, PAX8, ER, PR, and claudin-4 and focal CK expression is typical

- SMARCA4/INI1 loss and p53 abnormalities seen in a subset of cases

- Microsatellite unstable tumors with frequent

- MMR loss

- Genetically heterogeneous, belonging to all 4 groups of TCGA classification (predominance of hypermutated/microsatellite unstable tumors)

DEDIFFERENTIATED CARCINOMAPATHOLOGIC: KEY FEATURES

- Abrupt transition between undifferentiated carcinoma and low-grade endometrioid carcinoma is prototypical

- Can also arise in the background of highgrade endometrial carcinoma

---

MESONEPHRIC-LIKE CARCINOMA OF THE ENDOMETRIUM

DEFINITION

Mesonephric-like carcinoma of the endometrium can be defined as a tumor exhibiting the classic morphologic and immunohistochemistry features of mesonephric carcinoma, occurring outside of the cervix and without association with mesonephric remnants/hyperplasia.

INTRODUCTION

Mesonephric carcinomas, which most frequently arise in the uterine cervix, are rare gynecologic malignant tumors characterized by variable histologic patterns, and because of their frequent association with mesonephric remnant/hyperplasia are thought to be mesonephric in origin. In 2016, a study by McFarland et al.[32] described a series of 12 adenocarcinomas of the uterine corpus and ovary characterized by striking morphologic and immunophenotypic similarities to mesonephric carcinoma, but with features unusual for tumors that would be derived from mesonephric remnants.[32] None of these cases had any associated mesonephric remnants. Uterine tumors were centered in the endometrium with subsequent myometrial invasion and most of the ovarian tumors were associated with endometriosis. They were named mesonephric-like adenocarcinomas because it was debated whether they represent mesonephric adenocarcinomas that arise in the endometrium/ovary or Müllerian adenocarcinomas mimicking mesonephric adenocarcinoma. Growing body of evidence supports a Müllerian origin of these tumors.[33]

MICROSCOPIC FEATURES

Mesonephric-like carcinomas of the endometrium, just like mesonephric carcinomas, are typically heterogeneous and exhibit an admixture of architectural patterns which may include tubular, ductal/glandular, solid, papillary, sex cord-like, retiform, glomeruloid, and spindle cell patterns (**Fig. 2**). In most cases, the tubular and/or ductal growth patterns are conspicuous or predominant. The tubules often contain luminal eosinophilic colloid-like material, with variable prominence. No squamous or mucinous elements are present. Some cases may exhibit heterologous mesenchymal differentiation, such as cartilage.[34] The nuclear features of mesonephric-like carcinomas are often reminiscent of those in papillary thyroid carcinomas with nuclear overlapping, grooves, open to vesicular chromatin and pseudoinclusions.[32,35,36] Although typically absent, one study reported cases with hobnail-type cells or cytoplasmic clearing.[35] Mitotic index and degree of nuclear atypia are variable. Coagulative tumor necrosis may be present. Unlike cervical mesonephric carcinomas, mesonephric remnants/hyperplasia have not been identified in any of the endometrial mesonephric-like carcinomas reported in the literature.

In addition, several variants have been reported. A case report of corded and hyalinized

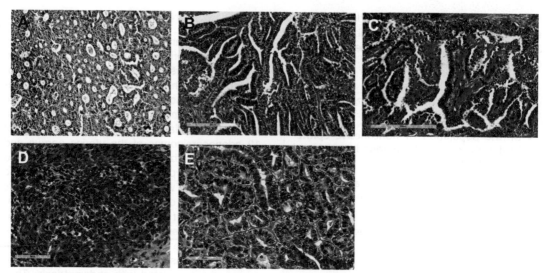

Fig. 2. Morphologic features of endometrial mesonephric-like carcinoma. Tumors exhibit the admixture of architectural patterns such as tubular (*A*), ductal/retiform (*B*), papillary (*C*), and solid (*D*). This tumor frequently shows nuclear features reminiscent of thyroid papillary carcinoma (*E*).

mesonephric-like adenocarcinoma of the endometrium that mimicked corded and hyalinized endometrioid carcinoma has been described.[37] A dedifferentiated endometrial mesonephric-like adenocarcinoma with a *KRAS* mutation present in both components was also recently reported.[38] Moreover, we have anecdotally seen mesonephric-like endometrial and ovarian carcinomas with sarcomatous differentiation, a phenomenon that can rarely occur in cervical mesonephric carcinomas (so-called "mesonephric carcinosarcoma"). Finally, just like in the ovary, endometrial mesonephric-like carcinomas may exist in association with, and sharing identical mutations with, other histologic components such as low-grade endometrioid carcinoma,[39] further supporting a Müllerian origin of these tumors.

In cytology specimens, mesonephric-like adenocarcinomas exhibit a monotonous population of small cells with scant to moderate cytoplasm and abundant nuclear grooves arranged in tight, overlapping, 3-dimensional clusters. Occasionally, papillary or tubular architecture, as well as extracellular hyaline globules, may be seen.[40]

IMMUNOHISTOCHEMISTRY

The immunohistochemical profile of endometrial mesonephric-like carcinoma is akin to that of mesonephric carcinomas (**Fig. 3**). As these are rare neoplasms, it is important to note that the following data are based on a limited number of cases available up to date (**Table 1**). Most tumors are positive for TTF1 (69%–100%) with distribution

ranging from focal to diffuse.[32,35,41] GATA3 is also frequently positive (14%–100%) with distribution ranging from only focal to diffuse.[32,34,35,41] An inverse relationship between GATA3 and TTF1 expression was noted in a subset of cases, with areas that were positive for GATA3 being completely negative for TTF1, and vice versa.[36,41] These tumors are also positive for PAX8 (100% in 2 studies).[32,41]

ER and PR are typically entirely negative, with only a minority of cases exhibiting focal staining (ER 0%–50%, PR 0%–7%).[32,34,35,41] P53 is wild type.[32,34,35] P16 is typically patchy positive.[32,34] Luminal CD10 expression is often present (80%–100%).[32,34,35,41] These tumors may be focally positive for calretinin in a subset of cases (0%–50%).[32,34,35,41] Napsin-A and HNF1B are negative in all of the cases reported in the literature.[32,35] In a very limited number of cases tested, thyroglobulin, WT1, and inhibin are negative (expression reported in 0/5, 0/5, and 0/3 cases, respectively).[32]

MOLECULAR FEATURES

Mesonephric-like adenocarcinomas exhibit strikingly similar molecular aberrations to cervical mesonephric adenocarcinomas including the canonical activation of *KRAS* and gain of 1q. Nonetheless, and unlike most cervical mesonephric carcinomas, mesonephric-like adenocarcinomas harbor genetic alterations frequently reported in Müllerian tumors such as *PIK3CA*, *PTEN*, and *CTNNB1*.[35,36,42] These findings support the concept that mesonephric-like carcinomas are

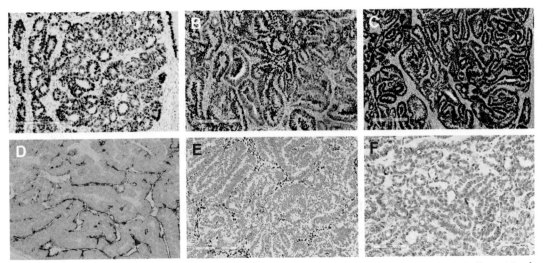

Fig. 3. Immunohistochemistry features of endometrial mesonephric-like carcinoma. Tumors are typically positive for (*A*) PAX8, (*B*) GATA3, (*C*) TTF-1, (*D*) luminal CD10, negative for (*E*) ER, and are (*F*) p53 wild type.

Müllerian in origin, in contrast to cervical mesonephric carcinomas which arise from preexisting Wolffian remnants.

DIFFERENTIAL DIAGNOSIS

Mesonephric Carcinoma

Mesonephric-like carcinomas exhibit strikingly similar morphologic and immunohistochemical features to mesonephric carcinoma. While mesonephric carcinomas are typically associated with mesonephric remnants/hyperplasia and most commonly arise in the cervix, mesonephric-like carcinomas arise in the endometrium (and ovary) and have no association with mesonephric remnants/hyperplasia. Molecular analysis may be of value, as pathogenic variants frequently seen in Müllerian carcinomas such as *PIK3CA*, *PTEN*, and *CTNNB1* would favor mesonephric-like carcinoma over true mesonephric carcinoma.

Endometrioid Carcinoma

Mesonephric-like carcinomas of the endometrium are most likely to be mistaken as endometrioid carcinomas. Absence of squamous and mucinous differentiation, admixture of different architectural patterns, presence of tubules with dense eosinophilic secretions, cytologic features akin to that of papillary thyroid carcinoma, combined with the absence of ER/PR staining, positivity for TTF1 and/or GATA3, and luminal CD10 expression would favor mesonephric-like carcinoma over endometrioid carcinoma.

Serous Carcinoma

Mesonephric-like carcinoma can show papillary architecture and relatively high-grade nuclear atypia and may be mistaken for serous carcinoma. Wild type p53 staining and patchy p16 expression, in addition to classic morphologic and immunohistochemistry, would support mesonephric-like carcinoma over endometrial serous carcinoma.[33]

Clear Cell Carcinoma

Both mesonephric-like carcinoma of the endometrium and clear cell carcinoma are characterized by the admixture of architectural patterns such as tubules and cysts with intraluminal eosinophilic secretions, and both are typically ER/PR negative, p16 patchy, and with infrequent p53 abnormalities. Hobnailing and cytoplasmic clearing, although described in a few cases in the literature, are not a classic feature of mesonephric-like carcinoma. The absence of HNF1β and Napsin-A expression in the limited number of mesonephric-like carcinomas of the endometrium tested highlights a potential role for these markers in differentiating these tumors from clear cell carcinomas, particularly in cases with overlapping morphology.

PROGNOSIS

The cumulative body of evidence shows that mesonephric-like carcinomas are aggressive neoplasms, which often present at the advanced stage and have frequent distant recurrences.[34,35,43,44]

A multi-institutional study of 44 mesonephric-like carcinomas of the uterine corpus and 25 mesonephric-like carcinomas of the ovary highlights the aggressive nature of these tumors.[45] In

Table 1
Immunohistochemistry staining pattern in mesonephric-like carcinoma of the endometrium

IHC Stain	Typical Staining Pattern	Overall % Positive and (Range of Positive Cases per Study)	# Positive Cases per Study and References
PAX8	+	100% (100%)	7/7[32] 4/4[41]
GATA3	+ variable distribution	69% (14%–100%)	1/7[32] 11/11[34] 15/16[35] 4/4[41]
TTF1	+ variable distribution	78% (69%–100%)	6/7[32] 11/16[35] 4/4[41]
ER	-(infrequently focal)	15% (0%–50%)	0/7[32] 0/11[34] 6/21[35] 2/4[41]
PR	-(infrequently focal)	3% (0%–7%)	0/6[32] 0/11[34] 1/15[35]
Luminal CD10	+ variable distribution	94% (80%–100%)	5/6[32] 11/11[34] 10/10[35] 3/4[41]
calretinin	+/-usually focal	28% (0%–50%)	1/2[32] 3/11[34] 5/15[35] 0/4[41]
P53	wild type	all wild type	0/4[32] 0/11[34] 0/7[35]
P16	Patchy +	all patchy +	0/5[32] 0/11[34]
Napsin A	-	0	0/7[32] 0/5[35]
HNF1beta	-	0	0/6[32] 0/2[35]
WT1	-	0	0/5[32]

this study, 58% of patients with mesonephric-like carcinoma of the endometrium presented at an advanced stage, 32% presented with lymph node metastases, and 59% were associated with recurrence. The 5-year progression-free survival was 27.5% and the 5-year overall survival/disease-specific survival was 72%. The majority (64%) of the uterine corpus tumors recurred in the lungs, a finding also previously reported in other studies.[34,35,43,44] This contrasts to the relatively infrequent rate of lung metastasis in mesonephric-like carcinomas of the ovary (25%) and nonmesonephric endometrial carcinomas (<5%).[46,47] Furthermore, in this study, overall and disease-specific survival of patients with this tumor type was better than for carcinosarcoma, but significantly worse compared with low-grade endometrioid carcinomas. The behavior was most similar to high-grade endometrioid carcinoma, suggesting that these tumors should be regarded as high-grade tumors.

ENDOMETRIAL GASTRIC-TYPE CARCINOMA

INTRODUCTION

Gastric-type glandular lesions of the lower female genital tract, especially of the uterine cervix, have

ENDOMETRIAL MESONEPHRIC-LIKE CARCINOMA - PATHOLOGIC KEY FEATURES

- Morphologic, immunohistochemical, and molecular similarity to mesonephric carcinoma

- Heterogeneous architecture with the admixture of patterns

- No squamous or mucinous differentiation

- Tubules with luminal dense eosinophilic secretions with variable prominence

- Nuclear features akin to papillary thyroid carcinoma (overlapping, grooves, open to vesicular chromatin, pseudoinclusions)

- Absence of associated mesonephric remnants/hyperplasia

- Typical immunohistochemistry profile includes expression of PAX8, GATA3, TTF1, and luminal CD10, absence of ER and PR, and wild type p53

- Microsatellite stable

- Canonical activating KRAS mutations and gain of 1q in most cases, similar to mesonephric carcinoma

- A subset harbor genetic alterations frequently reported in Müllerian tumors, such as PIK3CA, PTEN, and CTNNB1

- Aggressive neoplasms, often presenting at an advanced stage with frequent distant recurrences most commonly to the lungs

received attention in the gynecologic pathology literature in recent years. Unlike cervical gastric-type adenocarcinoma which is now a well-defined entity, endometrial carcinoma with gastric and/or intestinal differentiation has been reported in literature predominantly as rarely isolated case reports.[48–50] Recently, a concept of and diagnostic criteria for diagnosis of gastric (gastrointestinal)-type mucinous carcinoma of the endometrium was proposed[51] and the entity was recognized by the current WHO classification.[52]

MICROSCOPIC FEATURES

Although defining features of this entity are still evolving, according to the current proposal in Wong and colleagues,[51] these tumors should be characterized using the same gastric-type morphologic features defined by Kojima and colleagues for cervical gastric-type adenocarcinoma,[53] namely voluminous, pale eosinophilic or clear cytoplasm with distinct cell borders and/or intestinal-type morphologic features (goblet cells) (Fig. 4).

In the very limited studies, the immunoprofile of these tumors is similar to the cervical counterpart.[51] At least focal immunohistochemical expression of one or more of the gastrointestinal markers HIK1083, MUC6, CK20, and CDX2, along with absent or minimal (arbitrarily defined as <5%) expression of ER and PR, is preferable for the diagnosis of endometrial gastric-type adenocarcinoma. In addition, abnormal (mutant) p53 staining can be observed in this tumor type, and such a result would be supportive of the diagnosis (see **Fig. 4**). However, none of these results should be the sole criterion for demonstrating gastric/gastrointestinal differentiation because none of these are specific markers.

Importantly, the tumor should be centered in the uterine corpus, and cervical glandular or stromal involvement following the histologic examination of the entire cervix should be absent. It is suggested that any component of typical endometrioid morphology should also be absent as well. However, it is important to note that a case report of endometrial carcinoma with striking morphologic heterogeneity, including endometrioid, serous, clear cell, conventional mucinous, and gastric-like areas arising in association with gastric-type metaplasia of the endometrium has been described.[54]

DIFFERENTIAL DIAGNOSIS

Gastric-type adenocarcinoma of the uterine cervix is the major differential diagnostic consideration, which can be excluded by assuring that cervical glandular or stromal involvement following the histologic examination of the entire cervix is absent.

Endometrioid carcinoma with mucinous differentiation is another major differential diagnostic consideration. Mucinous differentiation in an endometrioid carcinoma can be extensive, but there are usually areas with conventional endometrioid morphology, as well as other types of metaplasia (squamous, secretory, tubal). In addition, the mucinous appearance in this setting tends to resemble endocervical-type epithelium rather than the clear to eosinophilic, granular to the foamy appearance of gastric-type mucinous epithelium. Substantial ER expression (>5% as suggested in Wong and colleagues[51]) would also argue against gastric-type endometrial carcinoma.

Clear cell carcinoma may be entertained in the differential because of the abundant clear cytoplasm, feature shared with gastric-type adenocarcinoma. However, the absence of mixed architectural patterns of clear cell carcinoma and absence of

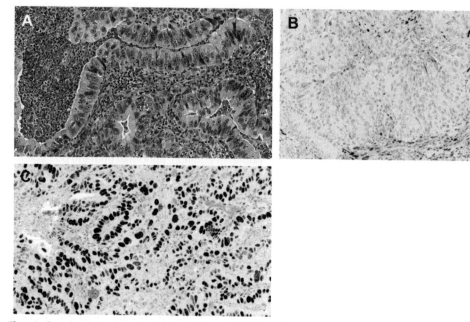

Fig. 4. Gastric-type adenocarcinoma. Microscopically, the neoplasm has mucinous morphology; nuclei are enlarged and markedly atypical, and cytoplasm has a foamy/frothy appearance (*A*). Carcinomas with gastric-type differentiation are typically negative for progesterone receptor (*B*) and often show abnormal p53 staining (*C*), (overexpression in this example).

Napsin-A expression by immunohistochemistry would favor gastric-type adenocarcinoma.

Metastasis to the endometrium, from a gastrointestinal or pancreaticobiliary adenocarcinoma, should be excluded before confidently assigning a diagnosis of primary endometrial gastric-type adenocarcinoma, particularly in biopsy material. Clinical history and radiologic findings may be of substantial help. Immunohistochemistry is generally of limited value, unless tumor is PAX8 positive, which would support gynecologic origin.

PROGNOSIS

Case reports and small series of endometrial gastric type carcinomas[49,51,54,55] suggest that these tumors exhibit clinically aggressive behavior. Larger studies are needed.

ENDOMETRIAL CARCINOMA WITH TROPHOBLASTIC/GERM CELL-LIKE COMPONENTS

INTRODUCTION

Endometrial (and ovarian) carcinomas with Müllerian and germ cell/trophoblastic-like components are rare tumors typically affecting postmenopausal patients. Although rare cases of pure germ cell tumor and nongestational pure choriocarcinoma have been described in this age group,

---

ENDOMETRIAL GASTRIC-TYPE ADENOCARCINOMA - PATHOLOGIC KEY FEATURES

- Evolving concept, but currently defined as a carcinoma with voluminous, pale eosinophilic or clear cytoplasm with distinct cell borders and/or intestinal-type morphologic features (goblet cells).

- At least focal immunohistochemical expression of one or more of the gastrointestinal markers HIK1083, MUC6, CK20, and CDX2

- Absent or minimal (arbitrarily defined as <5%) expression of ER.

- Absence of cervical involvement on the histologic examination of the entire cervix

- Difficult High-Grade Endometrial Carcinomas 309

- Absence of any component of typical endometrioid morphology

---

most present in combination with a Müllerian component.[56,57] Thus, they are now recognized to have a somatic origin and are characterized by genomic instability.[56,58,59] Unlike germ cell tumors, they are often characterized by and aggressive clinical course with poor response to chemotherapy and early recurrence.

MICROSCOPIC FEATURES

Endometrial (and ovarian) carcinomas with Müllerian and germ cell or trophoblastic components exhibit a wide morphologic spectrum (**Fig. 5**). The type and amount of both Müllerian and germ cell/trophoblastic-like components can vary significantly. For example, the Müllerian component has been reported as high-grade serous carcinoma, endometrioid carcinoma, clear cell carcinoma, large cell neuroendocrine carcinoma, and carcinosarcoma, among others.[56,58,59] The germ cell-like component most frequently exhibits features of the yolk sac tumor, while the trophoblastic-like component is most commonly a choriocarcinoma.[57] There may be significant overlap in morphologic and immunohistochemistry features between the Müllerian and germ cell-like components.[59,60] For example, the yolk-sac tumor component can exhibit prominent glandular morphology and positivity with EMA, BerEP4 and CK7, besides yolk-sac tumor markers.[59]

MOLECULAR FEATURES

In a study of tumors with mixed germ cell and epithelial features, Skala and colleagues[56] identified two distinct groups: (1) tumors with background endometriosis and endometrioid carcinoma-like mutations (*PTEN, PIK3CA, FGFR2,* and *CTNNB1*) and (2) tumors with high-grade morphology and *TP53* and *PIK3CA* mutations. In a study by Acosta and colleagues,[58] next-generation sequencing of paired samples demonstrated that the mutational profile of the Müllerian and germ cell-like components of the tumor is typically almost identical, with driver mutations being those expected in the specific subtype of the Müllerian component present. In contrast, mutations characteristic of germ cell tumors and gestational trophoblastic tumors were absent, and FISH for i(12p) was negative.[58] In a study including mixed tumors with Müllerian and choriocarcinomatous components, the Müllerian component showed lineage-characteristic alterations, while the choriocarcinomatous component shared some of these as well as demonstrating novel alterations.[61] These studies support the notion that the germ cell tumor/trophoblastic-like component of these tumors is somatically derived.

PROGNOSIS AND IMPLICATIONS

Unlike pure germ cell tumors, tumors with mixed Müllerian and germ cell components are often characterized by an aggressive clinical course with poor response to chemotherapy and early recurrence. However, it is not yet clear whether the presence

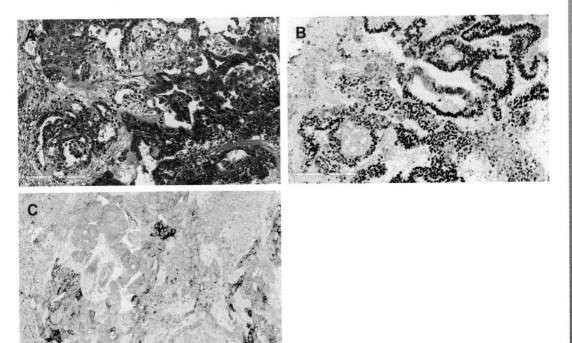

Fig. 5. Mullerian carcinoma with yolk sac differentiation. The yolk sac component shows primitive cells poorly forming glands and papillary structures resembling **Schiller**–Duval bodies (*A*). Expression of SALL4 (*B*) and glypican-3 (*C*) supports germ cell differentiation.

of germ cell and trophoblastic-like somatic components are independent predictors of unfavorable
outcomes. Given the somatic origin of germ cell/
trophoblastic components in these tumors, the patient may be best managed with treatments established for the Müllerian components. However,
whether additional therapeutic options might be
helpful should be explored further. For example,
high-level PD-L1 expression was identified in the
choriocarcinoma component, but not a carcinomatous component, of a series of mixed tumors suggesting a potential role for immunotherapy in this
setting.[61] Further study is necessary regarding the
best therapeutic option for these tumors.

**ENDOMETRIAL CARCINOMA WITH
TROPHOBLASTIC/GERM CELL-LIKE
COMPONENTS - PATHOLOGIC KEY FEATURES**

- Endometrial (and ovarian) carcinomas with
  Müllerian and germ cell or trophoblastic-
  like components exhibit a wide morphologic
  spectrum.

- Careful morphologic evaluation is needed for
  this diagnosis. Immunohistochemistry can
  help, but there can be immunohistochemical
  overlap between the Müllerian and germ
  cell-like components

- When arising in postmenopausal patients,
  these tumors have a somatic origin and are
  characterized by genomic instability

- Unlike pure germ cell tumors, they are often
  characterized by an aggressive clinical course
  with poor response to chemotherapy and
  early recurrence.

- Presence of apparently pure yolk-sac tumor
  or trophoblastic tumor in a postmenopausal
  woman should prompt a search for an un-
  sampled Müllerian carcinoma component.

DISCLOSURE

The author has nothing to disclose.

REFERENCES

1. Altrabulsi B, Malpica A, Deavers MT, et al. Undifferentiated carcinoma of the endometrium. Am J Surg
   Pathol 2005;29:1316–21.
2. Silva EG, Deavers MT, Bodurka DC, et al. Association of low-grade endometrioid carcinoma of the
   uterus and ovary with undifferentiated carcinoma: a
   new type of dedifferentiated carcinoma? Int J Gynecol Pathol 2006;25:52–8.
3. Kurman R. International Agency for Research on
   Cancer, WHO classification of tumours of female
   reproductive organs. 4th edition. International
   Agency for Research on Cancer; 2014.
4. Silva EG, Deavers MT, Malpica A. Undifferentiated
   carcinoma of the endometrium: a review. Pathology
   2007;39:134–8.
5. Murali R, Davidson B, Fadare O, et al. High-grade
   Endometrial Carcinomas: Morphologic and Immunohistochemical Features, Diagnostic Challenges and
   Recommendations. Int J Gynecol Pathol 2019;
   38(Suppl 1):S40–63.
6. Rosa-Rosa JM, Leskela S, Cristobal-Lana E, et al.
   Molecular genetic heterogeneity in undifferentiated
   endometrial carcinomas. Mod Pathol 2016;29:
   1390–8.
7. Ramalingam P, Masand RP, Euscher ED, et al. Undifferentiated Carcinoma of the Endometrium: An
   Expanded Immunohistochemical Analysis Including
   PAX-8 and Basal-Like Carcinoma Surrogate
   Markers. Int J Gynecol Pathol 2016;35:410–8.
8. Hoang LN, Lee YS, Karnezis AN, et al. Immunophenotypic features of dedifferentiated endometrial carcinoma - insights from BRG1/INI1-deficient tumours.
   Histopathology 2016;69:560–9.
9. Lee SE, Park HY, Shim SH, et al. Dedifferentiated
   carcinoma with clear cell carcinoma of the endometrium: A case report. Pathol Int 2017;67:472–6.
10. Al-Hussaini M, Lataifeh I, Jaradat I, et al. Undifferen-
    tiated Endometrial Carcinoma, an Immunohisto-
    chemical Study Including PD-L1 Testing of a Series
    of Cases From a Single Cancer Center. Int J Gynecol
    Pathol 2018;37:564–74.
11. Tafe LJ, Garg K, Chew I, et al. Endometrial and
    ovarian carcinomas with undifferentiated compo-
    nents: clinically aggressive and frequently underre-
    cognized neoplasms. Mod Pathol 2010;23:781–9.
12. Tessier-Cloutier B, Soslow RA, Stewart CJR, et al.
    Frequent loss of claudin-4 expression in dedifferen-
    tiated and undifferentiated endometrial carcinomas.
    Histopathology 2018;73:299–305.
13. Karnezis AN, Hoang LN, Coatham M, et al. Loss of
    switch/sucrose non-fermenting complex protein
    expression is associated with dedifferentiation in endo-
    metrial carcinomas. Mod Pathol 2016;29:302–14.
14. Ramalingam P, Croce S, McCluggage WG. Loss of
    expression of SMARCA4 (BRG1), SMARCA2
    (BRM) and SMARCB1 (INI1) in undifferentiated car-
    cinoma of the endometrium is not uncommon and is
    not always associated with rhabdoid morphology.
    Histopathology 2017;70:359–66.
15. Stewart CJ, Crook ML. SWI/SNF complex deficiency
    and mismatch repair protein expression in undiffer-
    entiated and dedifferentiated endometrial carci-
    noma. Pathology 2015;47:439–45.
16. Shah VI, McCluggage WG. Cyclin D1 does not
    distinguish YWHAE-NUTM2 high-grade endometrial
    stromal sarcoma from undifferentiated endometrial
    carcinoma. Am J Surg Pathol 2015;39:722–4.

17. Shah VI, Ramalingam P, McCluggage WG. CD34 expression in undifferentiated endometrial carcinoma. Histopathology 2016;69:894–7.

18. Travaglino A, Raffone A, Mascolo M, et al. TCGA Molecular Subgroups in Endometrial Undifferentiated/Dedifferentiated Carcinoma. Pathol Oncol Res 2020;26:1411–6.

19. Kobel M, Hoang LN, Tessier-Cloutier B, et al. Undifferentiated Endometrial Carcinomas Show Frequent Loss of Core Switch/Sucrose Nonfermentable Complex Proteins. Am J Surg Pathol 2018;42:76–83.

20. Espinosa I, Lee CH, D'Angelo E, et al. Undifferentiated and Dedifferentiated Endometrial Carcinomas With POLE Exonuclease Domain Mutations Have a Favorable Prognosis. Am J Surg Pathol 2017;41:1121–8.

21. Kuhn E, Ayhan A, Bahadirli-Talbott A, et al. Molecular characterization of undifferentiated carcinoma associated with endometrioid carcinoma. Am J Surg Pathol 2014;38:660–5.

22. Coatham M, Li X, Karnezis AN, et al. Concurrent ARID1A and ARID1B inactivation in endometrial and ovarian dedifferentiated carcinomas. Mod Pathol 2016;29:1586–93.

23. Kolin DL, Dong F, Baltay M, et al. SMARCA4-deficient undifferentiated uterine sarcoma (malignant rhabdoid tumor of the uterus): a clinicopathologic entity distinct from undifferentiated carcinoma. Mod Pathol 2018;31:1442–56.

24. Kolin DL, Quick CM, Dong F, et al. SMARCA4-deficient Uterine Sarcoma and Undifferentiated Endometrial Carcinoma Are Distinct Clinicopathologic Entities. Am J Surg Pathol 2020;44:263–70.

25. Lin DI, Allen JM, Hecht JL, et al. SMARCA4 inactivation defines a subset of undifferentiated uterine sarcomas with rhabdoid and small cell features and germline mutation association. Mod Pathol 2019;32:1675–87.

26. Lee CH, Ali RH, Rouzbahman M, et al. Cyclin D1 as a diagnostic immunomarker for endometrial stromal sarcoma with YWHAE-FAM22 rearrangement. Am J Surg Pathol 2012;36:1562–70.

27. Lee CH, Marino-Enriquez A, Ou W, et al. The clinicopathologic features of YWHAE-FAM22 endometrial stromal sarcomas: a histologically high-grade and clinically aggressive tumor. Am J Surg Pathol 2012;36:641–53.

28. Hoang LN, Ali RH, Lau S, et al. Immunohistochemical survey of mismatch repair protein expression in uterine sarcomas and carcinosarcomas. Int J Gynecol Pathol 2014;33:483–91.

29. Jenkins TM, Hanley KZ, Schwartz LE, et al. Mismatch Repair Deficiency in Uterine Carcinosarcoma: A Multi-institution Retrospective Review. Am J Surg Pathol 2020;44:782–92.

30. Segura SE, Pedra Nobre S, Hussein YR, et al. DNA Mismatch Repair-deficient Endometrial Carcinosarcomas Portend Distinct Clinical, Morphologic, and Molecular Features Compared With Traditional Carcinosarcomas. Am J Surg Pathol 2020;44:1573–9.

31. Vroobel KM, Attygalle AD. Sarcomatous Transformation in Undifferentiated/Dedifferentiated Endometrial Carcinoma: An Underrecognized Phenomenon and Diagnostic Pitfall. Int J Gynecol Pathol 2020;39:485–92.

32. McFarland M, Quick CM, McCluggage WG. Hormone receptor-negative, thyroid transcription factor 1-positive uterine and ovarian adenocarcinomas: report of a series of mesonephric-like adenocarcinomas. Histopathology 2016;68:1013–20.

33. da Silva EM, Fix DJ, Sebastiao APM, et al. Mesonephric and mesonephric-like carcinomas of the female genital tract: molecular characterization including cases with mixed histology and matched metastases. Mod Pathol 2021;34:1570–87.

34. Na K, Kim HS. Clinicopathologic and Molecular Characteristics of Mesonephric Adenocarcinoma Arising From the Uterine Body. Am J Surg Pathol 2019;43:12–25.

35. Euscher ED, Bassett R, Duose DY, et al. Mesonephric-like Carcinoma of the Endometrium: A Subset of Endometrial Carcinoma With an Aggressive Behavior. Am J Surg Pathol 2020;44:429–43.

36. Lin DI, Shah N, Tse JY, et al. Molecular profiling of mesonephric and mesonephric-like carcinomas of cervical, endometrial and ovarian origin. Gynecol Oncol Rep 2020;34:100652.

37. Patel V, Kipp B, Schoolmeester JK. Corded and hyalinized mesonephric-like adenocarcinoma of the uterine corpus: report of a case mimicking endometrioid carcinoma. Hum Pathol 2019;86:243–8.

38. Choi S, Na K, Kim SW, et al. Dedifferentiated Mesonephric-like Adenocarcinoma of the Uterine Corpus. Anticancer Res 2021;41:2719–26.

39. Yano M, Shintani D, Katoh T, et al. Coexistence of endometrial mesonephric-like adenocarcinoma and endometrioid carcinoma suggests a Mullerian duct lineage: a case report. Diagn Pathol 2019;14:54.

40. Kezlarian B, Muller S, Werneck Krauss Silva V, et al. Cytologic features of upper gynecologic tract adenocarcinomas exhibiting mesonephric-like differentiation. Cancer Cytopathol 2019;127:521–8.

41. Pors J, Cheng A, Leo JM, et al. A Comparison of GATA3, TTF1, CD10, and Calretinin in Identifying Mesonephric and Mesonephric-like Carcinomas of the Gynecologic Tract. Am J Surg Pathol 2018;42:1596–606.

42. Mirkovic J, McFarland M, Garcia E, et al. Targeted Genomic Profiling Reveals Recurrent KRAS Mutations in Mesonephric-like Adenocarcinomas of the Female Genital Tract. Am J Surg Pathol 2018;42:227–33.

43. Horn LC, Hohn AK, Krucken I, et al. Mesonephric-like adenocarcinomas of the uterine corpus: report of a case series and review of the literature

indicating poor prognosis for this subtype of endometrial adenocarcinoma. J Cancer Res Clin Oncol 2020;146:971–83.

44. Kolin DL, Costigan DC, Dong F, et al. A Combined Morphologic and Molecular Approach to Retrospectively Identify KRAS-Mutated Mesonephric-like Adenocarcinomas of the Endometrium. Am J Surg Pathol 2019;43:389–98.

45. Pors J, Segura S, Chiu DS, et al. Clinicopathologic Characteristics of Mesonephric Adenocarcinomas and Mesonephric-like Adenocarcinomas in the Gynecologic Tract: A Multi-institutional Study. Am J Surg Pathol 2021;45:498–506.

46. Paik ES, Yoon A, Lee YY, et al. Pulmonary metastasectomy in uterine malignancy: outcomes and prognostic factors. J Gynecol Oncol 2015;26:270–6.

47. Labi FL, Evangelista S, Di Miscia A, et al. FIGO Stage I endometrial carcinoma: evaluation of lung metastases and follow-up. Eur J Gynaecol Oncol 2008;29:65–6.

48. Abiko K, Baba T, Ogawa M, et al. Minimal deviation mucinous adenocarcinoma ('adenoma malignum') of the uterine corpus. Pathol Int 2010;60:42–7.

49. Hino M, Yamaguchi K, Abiko K, et al. Magnetic resonance imaging findings and prognosis of gastric-type mucinous adenocarcinoma (minimal deviation adenocarcinoma or adenoma malignum) of the uterine corpus: Two case reports. Mol Clin Oncol 2016; 4:699–704.

50. McCarthy WA, Makhijani R, Miller K, et al. Gastric-Type Endometrial Adenocarcinoma: Report of Two Cases in Patients From the United States. Int J Surg Pathol 2018;26:377–81.

51. Wong RW, Ralte A, Grondin K, et al. Endometrial Gastric (Gastrointestinal)-type Mucinous Lesions: Report of a Series Illustrating the Spectrum of Benign and Malignant Lesions. Am J Surg Pathol 2020;44: 406–19.

52. Lokuhetty D, White VA, Watanabe R. Female genital tumours. 5th edition. Internal Agency for Research on Cancer (IARC); 2020.

53. Kojima A, Mikami Y, Sudo T, et al. Gastric morphology and immunophenotype predict poor outcome in mucinous adenocarcinoma of the uterine cervix. Am J Surg Pathol 2007;31:664–72.

54. Travaglino A, Raffone A, Gencarelli A, et al. Endometrial Gastric-type Carcinoma: An Aggressive and Morphologically Heterogenous New Histotype Arising From Gastric Metaplasia of the Endometrium. Am J Surg Pathol 2020;44:1002–4.

55. Wong RW, Talia KL, McCluggage WG. Endometrial Gastric-type Carcinoma: An Aggressive and Morphologically Heterogenous New Histotype Arising From Gastric Metaplasia of the Endometrium. Am J Surg Pathol 2020;44:1736–7.

56. Skala SL, Liu CJ, Udager AM, et al. Molecular characterization of uterine and ovarian tumors with mixed epithelial and germ cell features confirms frequent somatic derivation. Mod Pathol 2020;33:1989–2000.

57. Rawish KR, Buza N, Zheng W, et al. Endometrial Carcinoma With Trophoblastic Components: Clinicopathologic Analysis of a Rare Entity. Int J Gynecol Pathol 2018;37:174–90.

58. Acosta AM, Sholl LM, Cin PD, et al. Malignant tumours of the uterus and ovaries with Mullerian and germ cell or trophoblastic components have a somatic origin and are characterised by genomic instability. Histopathology 2020;77:788–97.

59. McNamee T, Damato S, McCluggage WG. Yolk sac tumours of the female genital tract in older adults derive commonly from somatic epithelial neoplasms: somatically derived yolk sac tumours. Histopathology 2016;69:739–51.

60. Roma AA, Przybycin CG. Yolk sac tumor in postmenopausal patients: pure or associated with adenocarcinoma, a rare phenomenon. Int J Gynecol Pathol 2014;33:477–82.

61. Xing D, Zheng G, Pallavajjala A, et al. Lineage-Specific Alterations in Gynecologic Neoplasms with Choriocarcinomatous Differentiation: Implications for Origin and Therapeutics. Clin Cancer Res 2019;25:4516–29.

Update on Uterine Mesenchymal Neoplasms

Elizabeth C. Kertowidjojo, MD, MPH, PhD, Jennifer A. Bennett, MD*

KEYWORDS

- Uterus • PEComa • UTROSCT • Leiomyosarcoma • High-grade endometrial stromal sarcoma
- Inflammatory myofibroblastic tumor • Molecular

Key points

- There is considerable morphologic and immunohistochemical overlap among uterine mesenchymal neoplasms.
- Classification of uterine mesenchymal neoplasms is continuously evolving as molecular testing identifies novel alterations in these tumors.
- Molecular testing is not only diagnostic, but can also provide important therapeutic (ie, actionable targets) and prognostic information.

ABSTRACT

This review focuses on recent advances in epithelioid and myxoid uterine mesenchymal neoplasms, a category of tumors whereby diagnostic criteria have been rapidly evolving due to advances in molecular testing. Pertinent clinicopathological and molecular features are highlighted for perivascular epithelioid cell tumors, uterine tumors resembling ovarian sex cord tumors, BCOR/BCORL1-altered high-grade endometrial stromal sarcomas, and inflammatory myofibroblastic tumors. Novel developments in epithelioid and myxoid leiomyosarcomas are briefly discussed, and differential diagnoses with key diagnostic criteria are provided for morphologic mimickers.

OVERVIEW

Molecular pathology is rapidly becoming the cornerstone for diagnosing uterine mesenchymal neoplasms as many tumors show striking morphologic and immunohistochemical overlap. Such techniques have reshaped the classification of these tumors and hence, resulted in improved characterization of their clinicopathological and prognostic features. Furthermore, the potential for targeted therapy in many of these neoplasms emphasizes the importance of ancillary molecular testing, allowing for proper diagnosis and treatment. In this review, we focus specifically on epithelioid and myxoid neoplasms, highlighting 2 entities within each section, followed by a brief overview of recent advances in variant (epithelioid and myxoid) leiomyosarcomas.

EPITHELIOID MESENCHYMAL NEOPLASMS

PERIVASCULAR EPITHELIOID CELL TUMOR (PEComa)

Clinical Features

In the gynecologic tract, the uterine corpus is the most common site; however, PEComas have also been reported in the cervix,[1–4] vagina,[5–7] broad ligament,[6,8–10] ovary,[5,11–13] and vulva.[14,15] Patients are typically in their fifth to sixth decades, though a broad age range (6–79 years) has been reported.[5,7,16,17] Presenting symptoms are nonspecific, frequently consisting of abnormal uterine bleeding, abdominopelvic pain, or a mass on physical examination or imaging.[16] Most PEComas are sporadic; however,

Department of Pathology, University of Chicago Medicine, 5837 South Maryland Avenue, MC 6101, Chicago, IL 60637, USA
* Corresponding author.
E-mail address: jabennett@bsd.uchicago.edu

Surgical Pathology 15 (2022) 315–340
https://doi.org/10.1016/j.path.2022.02.008
1875-9181/22/© 2022 Elsevier Inc. All rights reserved.

approximately 10% are associated with tuberous sclerosis.[5,16,18]

Gross Features

Grossly, PEComas are often solitary, ranging in size from 0.2 to 25 (mean: 6.5) cm.[5,6,16] They are well-circumscribed or infiltrative myometrial masses, with a pink, tan-brown, or white cut surface. Occasionally, they may be polypoid/pedunculated with protrusion into the endometrial cavity, and a subset may show hemorrhage or necrosis. Rarely, widespread variably-sized nodules (PEComatosis) are present, a phenomenon most commonly associated with tuberous sclerosis.[19,20]

Microscopic Features

On low-power, tumors can display a well-circumscribed pushing border or show frank invasion, with destructive or permeative growth.[5,16] A variety of architectural patterns may be seen, with the most common being sheets or nests surrounded by delicate vasculature (**Fig. 1**).[16] Most

PEComas are epithelioid, but occasionally a spindled component is present.[5,16,21] Epithelioid cells typically have clear-to-eosinophilic and granular cytoplasm, though a subset shows more densely eosinophilic cytoplasm, imparting a rhabdoid appearance.[16,22] A range of cytologic atypia and mitotic activity can be seen. Tumor cell necrosis or lymphovascular invasion may be present. Stromal hyalinization is often noted, and when extensive, the tumor may be termed sclerosing PEComa.[23] Other features occasionally observed include a radial/perivascular distribution of tumor cells, intranuclear pseudoinclusions, multinucleated cells, and melanin pigment.[6,16,22]

PEComas with *TFE3* fusions (discussed below) are often comprised of epithelioid cells with abundant clear cytoplasm arranged in a nested to alveolar patterns (**Fig. 2**).[24] Rare PEComas with lymphangioleiomyomatosis (LAM)-like morphology have also been reported, typically in the setting of tuberous sclerosis and/or pulmonary LAM.[16,25]

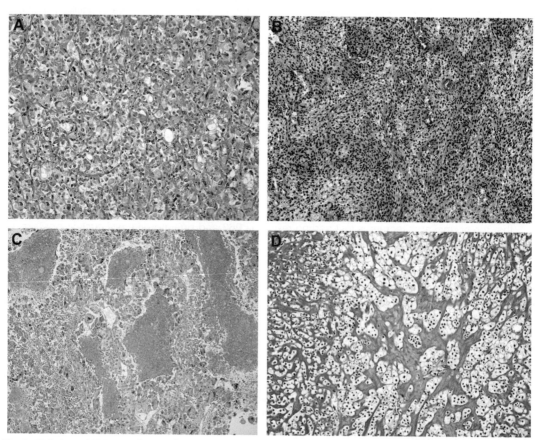

Fig. 1. *TSC*-altered PEComa. Sheets of epithelioid cells with clear to eosinophilic and granular cytoplasm (*A*). Spindle cell component (*B*). Malignant PEComa with tumor cell necrosis, severe atypia, and brisk mitoses (*C*). Sclerosing PEComa (*D*).

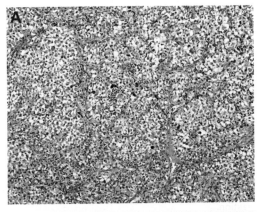

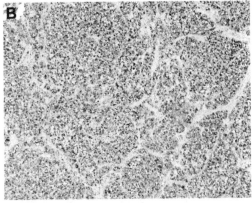

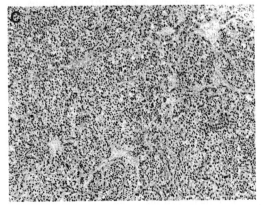

Fig. 2. *TFE3*-translocation associated PEComa. Nests of epithelioid cells with clear cytoplasm surrounded by delicate vasculature. Melanin pigment is present (*A*). Cells are diffusely positive for HMB-45 (*B*) and TFE3 (*C*).

Immunohistochemistry

PEComas coexpress melanocytic and smooth muscle markers. Large studies have shown HMB-45 to be the most sensitive melanocytic marker, though the extent and intensity of staining are highly variable.[5,16,26,27] Other melanocytic markers, such as melan-A, MiTF, and PNL2 are variably expressed.[16,26,28,29] Previously, melanocytic markers were considered to be predominantly expressed in epithelioid cells while spindle cells were more often positive for myogenic markers (desmin, SMA, and caldesmon).[6,27] However, more recent studies have shown strong and diffuse desmin and caldesmon expression regardless of cell morphology.[5,16] Cathepsin K, a protease regulated by microphthalmia transcription factor , is often strong and diffuse.[16,30] Although not specific, strong and diffuse nuclear expression of TFE3 is common in *TFE3* translocation-associated PEComas.[24] However, TFE3 staining does not unequivocally indicate a rearrangement as TFE3 is expressed at low levels in many cell types[31]; thus, weak staining should be interpreted with caution. *TFE3* translocation-associated PEComas are also strongly HMB-45 positive, with focal or absent expression of melan-A, MiTF, and smooth muscle markers.[16,21,27,31]

Molecular

Several recurrent molecular alterations have been identified, with the most common involving inactivation of *TSC1* or *TSC2*. This may occur in the setting of tuberous sclerosis, but is more commonly sporadic.[21,32] TSC1 and TSC2 interact with TBC1D7 to form the heterotrimeric tuberous sclerosis complex, which ultimately inhibits the mammalian target of rapamycin (mTOR).[33,34] Hence, inactivation of TSC1/TSC2 leads to constitutive activation of mTOR, resulting in cell growth and proliferation. Consequently, therapy with mTOR inhibitors has been proposed in these tumors with varying success.[35–37] Currently, the AMPECT phase II trial, the first prospective study evaluating mTOR inhibitors in malignant PEComas, is underway.[38,39]

A recent study by Bennett and colleagues[27] found that 83% (5/6) of *TSC*-altered PEComas classified as malignant based on the modified gynecologic-specific criteria (discussed below) harbored concurrent alterations in *TP53*, *ATRX*, or *RB1*. These alterations were absent in PEComas classified as uncertain malignant potential. Two other studies also reported similar findings in malignant PEComas.[21,40] Microsatellite instability has been detected in 2 PEComas, one showing MLH1/PMS2 loss without any genomic alterations in mismatch repair genes and the other with MSH2/MSH6 loss and 2 copy deletion of *MSH2*.[27,41]

The second molecular subgroup harbors *TFE3* rearrangements. Transcription factor E3 (TFE3) is a member of the MiTF family and is involved in autophagy and lysosome biogenesis.[42] *SFPQ/PSF-TFE3* is the most prevalent fusion, though several

Table 1
PEComa risk prediction algorithms

Tumor Classification	General (Folpe 2005)[6]	Gynecologic-Specific (Schoolmeester 2014)[5]	Modified Gynecologic-Specific (Bennett 2018 and WHO 2020)[16,48]
Benign	No atypical features	<4 features	N/A
Uncertain malignant potential	Nuclear pleomorphism/ multi-nucleated giant cells, or size >5 cm	<4 features	<3 features
Malignant	≥2 features	≥4 features	≥3 features

Atypical Features: Size > 5 cm, high-grade atypia, > 1 mitosis/12 mm² (equivalent to 50 HPF), necrosis, lymphovascular invasion.
Abbreviations: N/A, not applicable; WHO, world health organization.

other partners have been reported.[21,43] *TFE3* translocation-associated PEComas lack concurrent *TSC1/TSC2* mutations, suggesting a distinct tumorigenesis pathway.[21,44,45] Hence, this variant may not be responsive to mTOR inhibitors. The efficacy of different immunotherapies, such as crizotinib and tivantinib, is currently being explored in other *TFE3*-rearranged neoplasms.[46,47]

Finally, *RAD51B* fusions have been identified in a small subset of PEComas, partnering with *RRAGB* or *OPHN1*.[16,21] In 2 tumors with *RAD51B* fusions, concurrent *TSC2* mutations were detected, proposing that the 2 are not mutually exclusive.[21] While no distinct morphology was associated with these tumors, all had brisk mitoses (>10 per 10 high power fields [HPF]) and showed aggressive behavior, suggesting that this fusion may be associated with poor prognosis.[16,21]

Prognosis

Risk prediction for malignant behavior in PEComas is based on the evaluation of size, atypia, mitoses, tumor cell necrosis, and lymphovascular invasion, and 3 main algorithms incorporating these features have previously been proposed (**Table 1**). The study by Bennett and colleagues[16] included 32 uterine PEComas and showed that the prior algorithms resulted in misclassification of up to 36% of aggressive PEComas as benign. Hence, the study proposed a modified gynecologic-specific algorithm whereby ≥ 3 atypical features are required to diagnose malignancy. Furthermore, as histologically benign PEComas rarely displayed aggressive behavior, they also proposed the elimination of the term benign, classifying all gynecologic PEComas as either malignant or of uncertain malignant potential. This approach has since been endorsed by the 2020 World Health Organization Classification of Female Genital Tumors.[48]

Key Features
Perivascular Epithelioid Cell Tumor

- Nests and sheets of epithelioid (+/− spindle) cells surrounded by delicate vasculature.

- Coexpression of melanocytic and myogenic markers.

- Two distinct molecular subgroups:

  ○ *TSC1/TSC2*-altered: Most commonly sporadic but may occur in the setting of tuberous sclerosis. Concurrent alterations in *TP53*, *ATRX*, and *RB1* may portend aggressive behavior.

  ○ *TFE3*-translocation associated: Predominantly epithelioid cells with nested to alveolar growth and clear to eosinophilic cytoplasm; HMB-45 and TFE3 often strong and diffuse but Melan-A, MiTF, and myogenic markers are typically focal or negative.

- Modified gynecologic-specific criteria for risk prediction categorize PEComas as malignant if ≥ 3 worrisome features (**Table 1**) are present, with the remainder classified as uncertain malignant potential.

UTERINE TUMOR RESEMBLING OVARIAN SEX CORD TUMOR (UTROSCT)

Clinical Features

UTROSCTs may present with nonspecific symptoms, including abnormal uterine bleeding, postmenopausal bleeding, pelvic discomfort, or infertility, while a subset is incidental.[49–52] A potential association with tamoxifen therapy has also been proposed.[53] They typically affect women in their fifties (range: 12–86 years),[54,55] with those harboring *GREB1*-fusions presenting at a later age than those with *ESR1*-rearrangements (median: 65 vs 47 years).[52] Most tumors are confined to the uterus at diagnosis; however, serosal rupture or metastases occasionally occur.[54–57]

Gross Features

Tumors are variable in size, ranging from 0.4 to 22 (mean: 5.1–6.6) cm,[54,55,58] and may be submucosal and polypoid, intramural, or subserosal; rare tumors arise in or involve the cervix.[54,58–60] Most are well-circumscribed, tan-white-yellow, solid, soft and fleshy nodules, but occasionally may be ill-defined, solid and cystic, or entirely cystic. Hemorrhage and necrosis are uncommon.

Microscopic Features

UTROSCTs are generally well-circumscribed and while they may abut the adjacent endometrium, its involvement is exceedingly rare.[49,52] Irregular borders with focal myometrial invasion or incorporation of adjacent myometrium may occur, but overt invasion is uncommon (**Fig. 3**). As their name implies, UTROSCTs are composed of structures resembling ovarian sex cord tumors, including trabeculae, cords, small nests, solid or hollow tubules, and retiform patterns, the latter of which can be extensive.[49,61] Cells are typically small, round to ovoid, with minimal atypia, inconspicuous to occasionally prominent nucleoli, scant to moderately abundant eosinophilic or vacuolated cytoplasm, and infrequent mitoses (<5/10 HPF).[49,55,58] Stromal hyalinization, myxoid change, Leydig-like cells, foam cells, rhabdoid cells, and nuclear grooves may be present (**Fig. 4**).[50,55,62,63] A delicate capillary network is observed in most tumors, while lymphovascular invasion and necrosis are uncommon.[54,55]

The recent identification of 2 molecular subgroups (discussed below) has revealed several morphologic differences. Those with *ESR1*-fusions are primarily composed of sex cord-like elements, while those with *GREB1*-rearrangements may show a fascicular component. While some reports document no definitive sex cord-like elements in the latter,[52] others have described at least focal sex cord-like differentiation,[55,57,64,65] suggesting that these tumors are part of the UTROSCT family. A small series detected recurring *ESR1-NCOA2* fusions in UTROSCTs with a prominent component (≥ 50%) of rhabdoid cells.[63]

Immunohistochemistry

UTROSCTs are polyphenotypic, with variable expression of sex cord (inhibin, calretinin, SF1, FOXL2, WT1, CD99, CD56, melan-A), myogenic (SMA, desmin, caldesmon), epithelial (cytokeratins, EMA), and hormonal (ER, PR, AR) markers (**Fig. 5**).[50,51,55,59,62,66] In one study, 92% and 50% of tumors were positive for at least one myogenic or sex cord marker, respectively, with co-expression of sex cord, epithelial, and myogenic markers occurring in 33%.[51] In another series, 70% of UTROSCTs were inhibin positive, while most of the remaining tumors were positive for another sex cord marker.[55] CD10 is positive in about 50% of tumors,[50,51,55,61,62] while INI-1 and BRG-1 are retained.[52,57,63]

Molecular

Until recently, the pathogenesis of UTROSCTs was enigmatic as they lacked fusions characteristic of low-grade endometrial stromal tumors (*JAZF1-SUZ12*, *PHF1*)[58,67] and mutations typically seen in ovarian sex cord neoplasms (*FOXL2*, *DICER1*).[59,66] Dickson et al. and Croce et al.[57,64] were the first to detect fusions in UTROSCTs, which included *ESR1-NCOA3*, *ESR1-NCOA2*, *GREB1-NCOA2*, and *GREB1-CTNNB1*. However, on retrospective review, a previously described "undifferentiated uterine sarcoma" with a *GREB1-NCOA2* fusion and morphologic and immunohistochemical features suggestive of UTROSCT is now considered to be the first report of a recurring rearrangement in these tumors.[56] ESR1 (estrogen receptor 1) is a ligand-dependent transcription factor that binds estrogen, NCOA1-3 (nuclear receptor coactivator 1–3) is a family of p160 steroid receptor coactivators that stimulate transcription in a hormone-dependent manner, and GREB1 (growth regulation by estrogen in breast cancer) is involved in the canonical estrogen-estrogen receptor signaling pathway.[52,55,63,64]

Lee and colleagues[52] subsequently described 4 uterine sarcomas harboring *GREB1*-fusions (partnered with *NCOA2*, *NR4A3*, *SS18*, *NCOA1*), but with variable amounts of sex cord differentiation and infrequent expression of more specific sex cord markers (calretinin, inhibin), raising the question as to whether these represent a "poorly differentiated" UTROSCT versus a novel entity. The largest UTROSCT molecular study reported to date detected *NCOA*-fusions (paired with *ESR1* or *GREB1*) in 82% (18/22) of tumors[55]. The remaining 4 were negative for fusions by molecular testing. Recently, a UTROSCT harboring a *GTF2A1-NCOA2* rearrangement was described.[68]

Rare genomic events described in UTROSCTs include *FOXL2* gain, single copy-number loss of

DICER1, chromosome 11 loss, chromosome 1q gain, and isolated mutations in homologous recombination repair genes (ARID1A, ATR, FANCE).[55,69] Dickson et al.[64] reported the upregulation of ESR1, WT1, AR, HOXA10, HOXA11, and PBX1 mRNA levels, but no significant increase in NCOA2 or NCOA3. They also showed that ESR1-and GREB1-rearranged UTROSCTs grouped closely with low-grade endometrial stromal sarcomas harboring JAZF1-SUZ12 or JAZF1-PHF1 fusions by unsupervised hierarchical clustering of RNA-sequencing data. However, UTROSCTs formed a cluster distinct from endometrial stromal tumors using unsupervised hierarchical clustering of genome-wide DNA methylation data.[70]

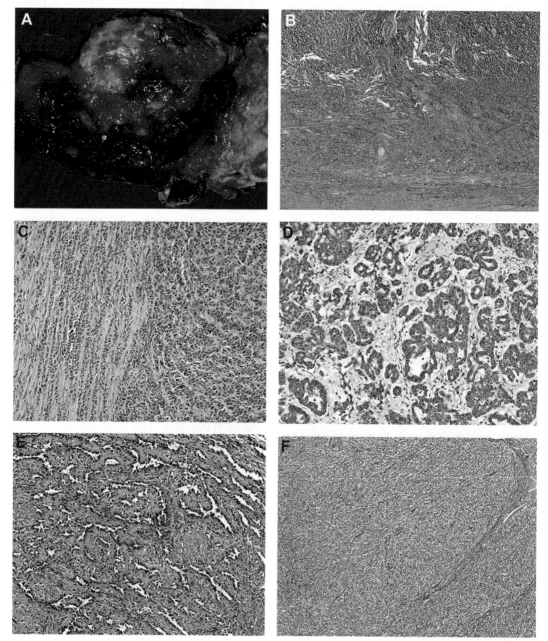

Fig. 3. Uterine tumor resembling ovarian sex cord tumor. Yellow-tan polypoid mass (A). Irregular borders with focal myometrial invasion (B). Corded, trabecular (C), tubular (D), and retiform (E) growth patterns. GREB1-NCOA2 tumor with conspicuous fascicular growth (F).

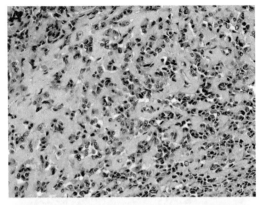

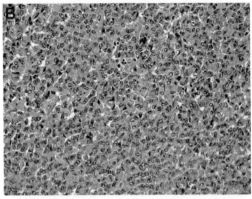

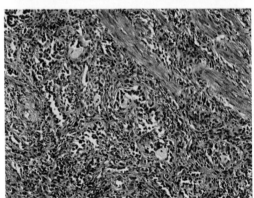

Fig. 4. Uterine tumor resembling ovarian sex cord tumor. Small ovoid cells with scant cytoplasm percolating throughout a hyalinized stroma (A). Cells with prominent rhabdoid morphology (B). Scattered foam cells (C).

Prognosis

In the largest series of UTROSCTs with follow-up data (range: 6–135 months), recurrences (local and distant) occurred in 24% (8/34) of patients.[54] These tumors were more likely to present in older patients and were larger with necrosis, significant nuclear atypia, increased mitoses (≥2/10 HPF), lymphovascular invasion, and cervical extension; however, only necrosis and increased mitoses

were statistically significant. Although follow-up for UTROSCTs with molecular data is limited, it seems that those with *GREB1* and *GTF2A1* fusions portend a more aggressive course.[55–57,68,71,72] In addition, 3 of the 5 UTROSCTs with *ESR1-NCOA2* fusions recurred (with a time to recurrence ranging from 7 to 32 years; no follow-up available for the others), all of which had a prominent component (≥50%) of rhabdoid cells.[55,63] This emphasizes how these tumors may have prolonged disease-free intervals, recognizing the importance of classifying them as uncertain malignant potential.

Key Features
Uterine Tumor Resembling Ovarian Sex Cord Tumor

- Tumor of uncertain malignant potential, with late recurrences and extended disease-free intervals.

- Sex cord-like morphology including cords, trabeculae, small nests, tubules, and retiform structures.

- Polyphenotypic with coexpression of sex cord, myogenic, epithelial, and hormonal markers.

- Two primary molecular subgroups:

  ○ *ESR1*-fusions: Often premenopausal, conspicuous sex cord-like differentiation, more likely to be positive for sex cord markers, suggested to have a more favorable outcome unless a prominent rhabdoid component (≥ 50%) and *ESR1-NCOA2* fusion are present.

  ○ *GREB1*-fusions: Often postmenopausal, fascicular component, sex cord-like elements may be focal or absent, sex cord markers may be negative, favored to portend a more aggressive clinical course.

EPITHELIOID LEIOMYOSARCOMA (LMS)

According to the 2020 World Health Organization Classification of Female Genital Tumors, the epithelioid variant of LMS is diagnosed when greater than 50% of the tumor is comprised of nests, cords, nodules, or sheets of round/polygonal cells with eosinophilic or clear cytoplasm, and meets at least one of the following criteria: moderate to severe cytologic atypia, tumor cell necrosis, or ≥4 mitoses/2.4 mm² (equivalent to 10 HPFs whereby each field is 0.55 mm in diameter

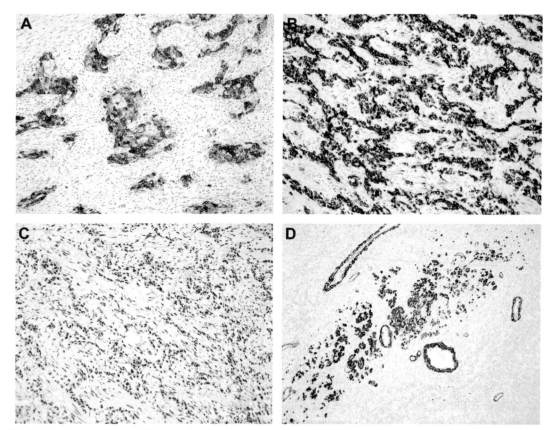

Fig. 5. Uterine tumor resembling ovarian sex cord tumor. Tumors may express sex cord (*A*, inhibin), epithelial (*B*, CAM5.2), hormonal (*C*, ER), and myogenic (*D*, caldesmon) markers.

and 0.24 mm^2 in area) **(Fig. 6)**.[48] However, Chapel et al.[73] recently analyzed the largest series of epithelioid LMS (n = 81) and proposed a revised classification system. In this system, each epithelioid smooth muscle tumor should be assessed for the presence of ≥ 2+ nuclear atypia (defined as nuclei >2-fold larger than normal myocyte nucleus), ≥ 4 mitoses/2.4 mm^2, and tumor cell necrosis. The presence of at least 2 features is compatible with LMS, while a diagnosis of smooth muscle tumor of uncertain malignant potential (STUMP) should be rendered if only one feature is present. If all features are absent, the tumor should be assessed for an infiltrative border, atypical mitoses, size (≥ 5 cm), and lymphovascular invasion. The presence of at least one feature is diagnostic of STUMP, whereas the absence of all features is compatible with leiomyoma. Using this system, all their epithelioid LMS had at least 2 worrisome features, and 78% of patients were alive with disease or dead of disease. In contrast, 3 tumors were classified as epithelioid STUMP, and in the 2 patients with follow-up, both were alive without disease. No tumors met the criteria for epithelioid leiomyoma, suggesting that this is an exceedingly rare diagnosis that should be made with caution.

As the 2 main studies on epithelioid smooth muscle tumors preceding the study by Chapel et al. were limited due to small sample size and lack of ancillary testing, little was known about their immunoprofile, pathogenesis, and behavior compared with conventional LMS.[74,75] The recent series by Chapel et al.[73] demonstrated that most epithelioid LMS were positive, usually strongly but with variable extent for smooth muscle markers (SMA, desmin, caldesmon), and typically negative for melanocytic markers (HMB-45, Melan-A, PNL2, MiTF). Most tumors (73%; 19/26) showed focal cathepsin K expression of variable intensity, while ER and PR were positive in greater than 50%, and fumarate hydratase, BRG-1, and INI-1 were retained. Based on limited data (n = 9), the molecular profiles of epithelioid LMS seem similar to conventional LMS, with alterations detected in *ATRX,*

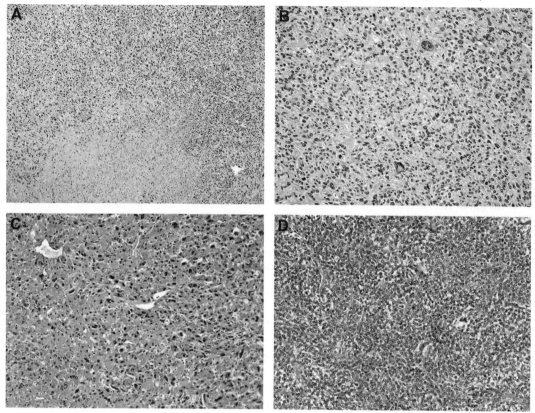

Fig. 6. Epithelioid leiomyosarcoma. Tumor cell necrosis (*A*), mitoses, and atypia (*B*). Pleomorphic tumor with densely eosinophilic cytoplasm (*C*). Uniform atypia characteristic of tumors with *PGR* fusions (*D*).

TP53, *PTEN*, and *CDKN2A*.[73] While one tumor harbored a *TSC2* variant of uncertain significance, the morphology and immunoprofile were incompatible with PEComa. Although the immunohistochemical and molecular profiles are comparable between epithelioid and conventional LMS, disease-specific survival was significantly decreased for the former, with a 5-year survival of 35% versus 46%.[73]

Recently, Chiang et al.[76] described a subset of epithelioid LMS with *PGR* fusions (35%; 6/17), most commonly partnering with *NR4A3*. This fusion was not detected in other morphologic mimickers including endometrial stromal tumors with epithelioid change and PEComas. All tumors with *PGR* fusions were FIGO stage I or II, and 3 were centered in the cervix. The epithelioid component was uniformly atypical but lacked overt pleomorphism. Five showed an admixed spindle cell component, that was of low- or intermediate-grade. All 6 were positive for desmin, ER, and PR, but negative for CD10 (n = 5) and HMB-45 (n = 4); caldesmon was positive in one. Two patients were alive with disease at 75 and 180 months, 3 were alive and well at 1,

9, and 96 months, and the sixth was lost to follow-up.

Key Features
Epithelioid Leiomyosarcoma

- The current WHO classification requires only one worrisome feature for the diagnosis of epithelioid leiomyosarcoma (moderate to severe atypia, $\geq$ 4 mitoses/2.4 mm^2, tumor cell necrosis). However, recent evidence shows that epithelioid leiomyosarcoma consistently shows 2 or more of these features and that tumors with only one feature are rare and are best classifed as STUMP.

- Shares similar immunohistochemical and molecular profiles with conventional leiomyosarcoma.

- Significantly decreased 5-year survival rate in contrast to conventional leiomyosarcoma.

- Subset harbor *PGR* fusions and lack overt nuclear pleomorphism; the clinical significance of this cohort remains to be determined.

Differential Diagnosis Epithelioid Mesenchymal Neoplasms

- Entities detailed in the text are summarized in **Table 2**
- Epithelioid leiomyoma
  - Exceedingly rare and should be treated as a diagnosis of exclusion
  - Well-circumscribed nodule lacking an infiltrative border
  - ≤ 5 cm
  - No tumor cell necrosis
  - At most mild atypia
  - ≤ 4 mitoses/2.4 mm^2
- Low-grade endometrial stromal sarcoma with sex cord-like elements:
  - < 50% sex cord differentiation
  - Classic low-grade component present
  - Tongue-like/permeative growth
  - CD10+, ER+, PR+
  - *JAZF1, PHF1* fusions; no *ESR1, NCOA* fusions
- High-grade endometrial stromal sarcoma:
  - +/− spindle cell component and myxoid stroma
  - Cyclin D1+, CD10+, BCOR+/-
  - *YWHAE, BCOR, BCORL1* alterations
- *SMARCA4*-deficient uterine sarcoma:
  - Young age (mean: 36 years)
  - Sheets of monomorphic large epithelioid cells, +/− rhabdoid cells, +/− adenosarcoma-like features
  - Cytokeratins, EMA, claudin-4, PAX8 usually negative
  - Mismatch repair protein proficient, BRG-1 (rarely INI-1) deficient
  - *SMARCA4* (rarely *SMARCB1)* mutations; no *PIK3CA* and *PTEN* mutations
- Undifferentiated/dedifferentiated carcinoma:
  - +/− differentiated carcinoma
  - Cytokeratins, EMA, claudin-4, PAX8 +/− (usually focal if positive)
  - Mismatch repair protein deficiency (~50%), SWI/SNF protein deficiency common
  - Concurrent endometrial carcinoma mutations (*PTEN, PIK3CA, CTNNB1, TP53*)
- Undifferentiated uterine sarcoma:
  - Diagnosis of exclusion
  - Lacks morphologic, immunohistochemical, and molecular features characteristic of recognized entities

Table 2
Key morphologic, immunohistochemical, and molecular findings of epithelioid mesenchymal neoplasms

Feature	PEComa	Epithelioid Leiomyosarcoma	UTROSCT
Age, range	6–79 y	26–81 y	12–86 y
Morphology	• Epithelioid cells with clear to eosinophilic and granular cytoplasm • +/− spindle cells • Delicate vasculature • Variable atypia and mitoses	• >50% epithelioid cells • Clear cell change uncommon • Moderate to severe atypia • Frequent tumor cell necrosis and brisk mitoses	• Sex cord-like elements • Occasionally fascicular growth (*GREB1*-rearranged tumors) • Small round cells with minimal atypia and infrequent mitoses
Immunohistochemistry			Polyphenotypic with variable coexpression of epithelial, sex cord, myogenic, and hormonal markers
Melanocytic markers	• HMB-45 usually strong/diffuse (>50%) • Melan-A, MiTF, PNL2 variable	Usually negative (at most focally positive)	
Myogenic markers	Variable, often strong/diffuse	Strong staining, variable distribution	
Cathepsin K	Strong/diffuse	Focal, variable staining intensity	
Molecular	• *TSC1/TSC2* alterations • Subset with *TFE3* fusions • Concurrent *ATRX*, *TP53*, *RB1* alterations may be seen in malignant PEComas	• *ATRX*, *TP53*, *PTEN*, *CDKN2A* alterations • Subset with *PGR* fusions	• *ESR1* fusions • *GREB1* fusions

MYXOID MESENCHYMAL NEOPLASMS

HIGH-GRADE ENDOMETRIAL STROMAL SARCOMA (HGESS) WITH *BCOR* ALTERATIONS

Clinical Features

BCOR-altered HGESS present with nonspecific symptoms including dysmenorrhea and abdominopelvic pain. They occur over a wide age range, with those harboring *BCOR* internal tandem duplication (ITD) presenting at an earlier age (range: 14–62, median: 44 years)[77–82] compared with those with *BCOR* fusions (range: 23–79, median: 54 years).[81,83] No significant age difference is evident between patients with *ZC3H7B-BCOR* tumors versus those with other partner genes.[81] While all stages have been reported, advanced-stage disease at presentation is more common for both *BCOR*-fusion and ITD tumors.[80,81]

Gross Features

Tumors are often large and bulky (range: 1.5–14.5, median: 9.7 cm)[80,83] and may be polypoid, myometrial-based, or both. Serosal involvement/ulceration, as well as extrauterine disease may be present. Tumors are tan-pink-yellow to gray-white, soft and fleshy, occasionally with areas of hemorrhage, necrosis, or a gelatinous appearance.[83–85]

Microscopic Features

Overall, the morphology of *ZC3H7B-BCOR* tumors differs from those harboring *BCOR* ITD; however, some overlap occurs. The number of reported HGESS partnering with genes other than *ZC3H7B* is limited, but evidence thus far supports a morphology more analogous to ITD tumors.[81,86] Low-power examination of all subtypes is similar, characterized by a broad pushing border often with irregular borders and/or tongue-like invasion.[78,80,81,83]

ZC3H7B-BCOR HGESS is comprised of haphazard fascicles of mildly to moderately atypical, but uniform spindle cells with intermediate-sized, round to ovoid and elongated nuclei with irregular contours, inconspicuous nucleoli, and evenly dispersed chromatin (**Fig. 7**). Infrequently, a focal epithelioid component or marked pleomorphism is observed.[83–85,87,88] Scant to moderate eosinophilic cytoplasm is often noted, but occasionally may be blue-gray and abundant or vacuolated, the latter imparting a signet ring-like appearance.[83,85,87] Mitoses range from 1 to 50 (median: 14.5) per 10 HPFs, with most tumors having at least 10/10 HPF.[83] Variable amounts of myxoid stroma, which may form microcysts or lakes, are present in most, while a subset show focal stromal collagenization or collagen plaques.[81,83,85,87,89] Small arterioles lacking perivascular whorling is common, but hemangiopericytoma-like and thick-walled vessels are infrequent.[83,85] Necrosis, often infarct-type, is present in over half of reported tumors and lymphovascular invasion in nearly two-thirds.[83] Rarely, osseous metaplasia, benign endometrial glands, or round "ball-like" proliferations of spindle cells are noted.[83,85,89] Unlike HGESS with *YWHAE-*

NUTM2A/B fusions[90] or *BCOR* ITD, a conventional or fibromyxoid low-grade ESS is not appreciated.

In contrast, HGESS with *BCOR* ITD often consists of 3 components: high-grade spindle cells (resembling those in *ZC3H7B-BCOR* tumors), high-grade round cells, and low-grade spindle cells (**Fig. 8**). Sheets of intermediate-sized epithelioid cells with round to ovoid nuclei, coarse chromatin, small nucleoli, and scant cytoplasm characterize the round cell component, while the low-grade component consists of fascicles of bland cells resembling low-grade fibrous/fibromyxoid ESS.[77–80] Mitoses are brisk in the high-grade components but rare in the low-grade component. Myxoid and/or collagenous stroma is appreciated, at least focally in most tumors, and tumor cell necrosis and lymphovascular invasion are common.[78–80] Small vessels with prominent walls have been reported in one case series,[78] but otherwise, the vasculature is not well described.

Immunohistochemistry

All *ZC3H7B-BCOR* HGESS are CD10 positive, with most (85%; 11/13) having strong and diffuse cyclin D1 expression.[83,85,87,89,91] BCOR is diffusely

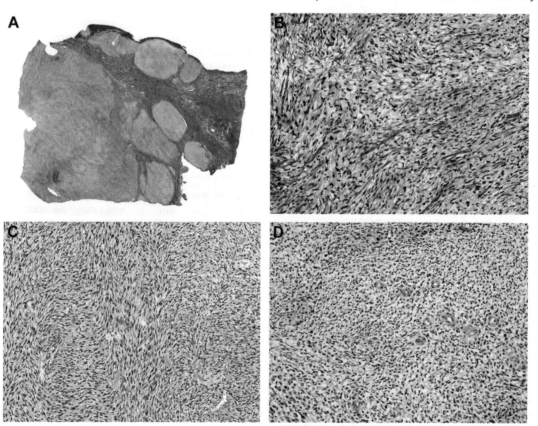

Fig. 7. High-grade endometrial stromal sarcoma with *ZC3H7B-BCOR* fusion. Tongue-like/permeative growth (*A*). Fascicles of atypical spindle cells in a myxoid stroma (*B*). Scattered hyaline plaques (*C*). Small arterioles without perivascular cuffing (*D*).

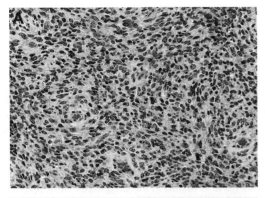

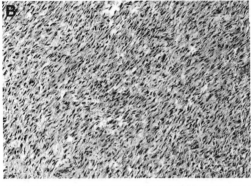

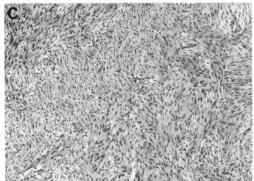

Fig. 8. High-grade endometrial stromal sarcoma with *BCOR* internal tandem duplication. High-grade round cell component with brisk mitoses (*A*). High-grade spindle cell component (*B*). Low-grade spindle cell component (*C*).

positive in 50% (10/20) and usually strong in intensity; however, one tumor showed weak staining.[79,83,85,87,89,91] Smooth muscle markers are generally negative, but focal SMA expression may be seen in up to 30% (6/20).[83,85,87,89,91] ER and PR are positive in about 25%,[83,85,87,89,91] while panTRK is usually expressed.[92] Although only tested in a small number of tumors, ALK,[85,89] CD117,[85,91] CD34,[85,91] and WT1[85,89] are negative, and p53 shows wild-type expression.[85,93]

The high-grade components of HGESS with *BCOR* ITD are strongly and diffusely cyclin D1

and BCOR positive, with most (83%; 5/6) focally expressing CD10.[77–79] Desmin is focally positive in 60% (3/5), ER in 50% (3/6), and PR in 25% (1/4), while SMA and caldesmon are negative.[77–79,82] PanTRK is positive[92] and p53 shows wild-type expression.[93] The low-grade spindle cell component stains like a low-grade ESS, with strong and diffuse BCOR expression reported in 2 tumors.[79]

Molecular

Historically, *BCOR*-altered HGESS were often diagnosed as either myxoid LMS or undifferentiated uterine sarcoma.[79,84] However, identification of *BCOR* alterations in these tumors, along with features typical of other ESS (endometrial involvement, tongue-like myometrial invasion, lymphovascular invasion, CD10 positivity) led to their recognition by most as a distinct subtype of HGESS.[83,84] BCL-6 corepressor (BCOR) is one of the core proteins of the noncanonical polycomb repressive complex 1.1 (PRC1.1), which is involved in transcriptional repression via histone modification.[94,95] *BCOR* alterations in HGESS include fusions, ITD, inversions, and mutations. *ZC3H7B-BCOR* is the most common rearrangement described, with most fusions occurring between exon 10 of *ZC3H7B* and exon 7 of *BCOR*; however, fusions involving *ZC3H7B* exons 11 or 12 and *BCOR* exons 8 or 9 have been reported.[81,82,84,87,89,91,96,97] In addition, a subset of *ZC3H7B-BCOR* HGESS also harbor the reciprocal fusion (*BCOR-ZC3H7B*), but its role in tumorigenesis and/or progression remains to be elucidated.[81,87,96–98] Recently, novel *BCOR* gene partners have been detected including *L3MBTL2*, *EP300*, *NUTM2G*, *MAP7D2*, *RALGPS1*, *RGAG1*, *CREBBP*, *ING3*, *NUGGC*, *KMT2D*, and *LPP*.[81,88] An *EPC1-BCOR* fusion has also been described in a tumor morphologically compatible with HGESS arising in a background of pelvic endometriosis.[86] A distinct subset of *BCOR*-altered HGESS harbor ITD of *BCOR* exon 15, located near the C-terminus, with most duplications involving 29 to 33 amino acids.[77–81] Other rare genomic *BCOR* alterations include chromosome X inversion or truncating mutations, the latter coexisting with either *ZC3H7B-BCOR* or *YWHAE-NUTM2E* fusions.[81,82]

Activation of the cyclin D1-CDK4 kinase, either though *CDK4* or *CCND2* amplification, or *CDKN2A/2B* loss has been reported in 65% of *BCOR*-rearranged HGESS.[81] *MDM2* amplifications have been described in 45% to 100%, usually in those with *ZC3H7B* fusions; however, it was also detected in one tumor harboring a *BCOR-LPP* rearrangement.[81,88] *FRS2* amplification, *HMGA2* rearrangements, and *TP53* mutations occur in 40%, 15%, and 10% of tumors, respectively. Infrequent genomic aberrations include *PDGFRA, KDR, ERBB3,* and *KIT* amplifications, *NF1, NF2,* and *PTCH1* inactivating truncating mutations, and *NCOR2, FGF6,* and *CREBBP* alterations. In contrast, *CDK4* or *MDM2* amplifications have not been detected in *BCOR* ITD tumors, although 20% harbor *CDKN2A/2B* homozygous deletions. Rare alterations in *ARID1A, TP53, CTNNB1, PASK,* and *STAG2* have also been described in this group.

By targeted RNA expression analysis, *BCOR*-altered HGESS show high expression of *NTRK3, FGFR3, RET, BCOR, GLI1,* and *PTCH1,* and low *ESR1* expression, with more striking upregulation in ITD tumors.[92] These tumors also show the upregulation of cell cycle/proliferation pathways, morphogenesis/development, translation, and spliceosome genes, and downregulation of those involved in immunity.[82] Recently, DNA methylation analysis recognized distinct signatures between *YWHAE-* and *BCOR*-rearranged HGESS.[70]

Prognosis

As this is an emerging entity and the number of reported cases is low, follow-up data are limited. Nonetheless, it seems that recurrences (local and distant) are common in *ZC3H7B-BCOR* HGESS, mostly occurring within 3 years of diagnosis, and many patients succumb to disease (range: 19–80 months).[82–85,91] Even less information is available for ITD tumors; however, one patient is alive and free of disease after 22 years, while a second patient recurred 7 years after diagnosis, and died from her disease the following year.[78]

HIGH-GRADE ENDOMETRIAL STROMAL SARCOMA (HGESS) WITH BCOR ALTERATIONS

BCORL1 is interchangeable with BCOR in PRC1.1, binding with CTBP1 instead of BCL-6 for transcriptional repression.[95] Lin et al.[99] recently published a series of 12 HGESS with *BCORL1* alterations. Two molecular subgroups were evident, one characterized by *BCORL1* fusions (most commonly with *JAZF1*), ITD, or homozygous deletions, and the second with *BCORL1* truncating mutations, half of which also harbored a fusion typical of low-grade ESS. Spindle and epithelioid cells with at least moderate cytologic atypia and brisk mitoses (mean: 12.3 per 10 HPF) were seen in the first group, while the second showed uniform nuclei, with an epithelioid component in 40% and a lower mitotic index (mean: 5.6 per 10 HPF). Myxoid stroma (86% vs 80%), fibrosis/collagen plaques (57% vs 40%), and tumor cell necrosis (57% vs 20%) were present in both cohorts.

All tested tumors were CD10 positive, most showed ER, PR, desmin, and SMA, expression. Cyclin D1 was rarely positive and BCOR was not performed. Concurrent alterations included *CDKN2A/2B* homozygous deletions (33%), *NF1* or *NF2* alterations (33% and 25%, respectively), and *CDK4/MDM2* amplification (17%). Follow-up was available in 10 patients, and aggressive behavior occurred in 9. Despite the low numbers, *BCORL1*-altered HGESS overlap morphologically and share a similar disease course with *BCOR*-altered HGESS; thus, it is important to ensure this gene is tested in the diagnostic work-up.

Key Features
HIGH-GRADE Endometrial Stromal Sarcoma with *BCOR/BCORL1* Alterations

- *BCOR* alterations include fusions (most commonly with *ZC3H7B*), internal tandem duplication, inversions, and mutations.

  - *ZC3H7B-BCOR*: Haphazard fascicles of atypical uniform spindle cells often in a myxoid stroma, usually CD10 and cyclin D1 positive, 50% BCOR positive, may show concurrent activation of cyclin D1-CDK4 kinase and/or *MDM2* amplification.

  - *BCOR* internal tandem duplication: High-grade round cells, high-grade spindle cells, and low-grade spindle cells in a myxoid stroma, cyclin D1 and BCOR positive, usually CD10 positive, lack concurrent *MDM2/CDK4* amplifications.

- *BCORL1*-alterated tumors:

  - *BCORL1* fusions (most commonly with *JAZF1*), internal tandem duplication, or homozygous deletions: Spindle and epithelioid cells with at least moderate atypia.

  - *BCORL1* truncating mutations: Spindle cells with uniform atypia, 40% with epithelioid component, 50% with concurrent fusion typical of low-grade ESS.

INFLAMMATORY MYOFIBROBLASTIC TUMOR (IMT)

Clinical Features

IMTs typically arise in the uterine corpus and, much less commonly, the cervix.[100,101] A subset is associated with pregnancy, involving the placental disc or membranes, or may be expelled with delivery or shortly thereafter.[102–108] Presenting symptoms include abnormal bleeding or symptoms related to mass effect. Occasionally, the tumor is an incidental finding at Cesarean section or surgery.[100] Patients are often premenopausal (mean: 39–44 years), though a broad age range (6–78 years) has been reported.[100,101,109,110] Malignant IMTs, however, tend to occur in older women (mean: 50 years).[111]

Gross Features

Grossly, most IMTs are intramural, though polypoid intracavitary growth can occur.[100] Tumors can measure up to 20 cm; however, most are less than 10 (mean: 7.5) cm.[100,101,112] They can be firm or soft with a tan-white, whorled cut

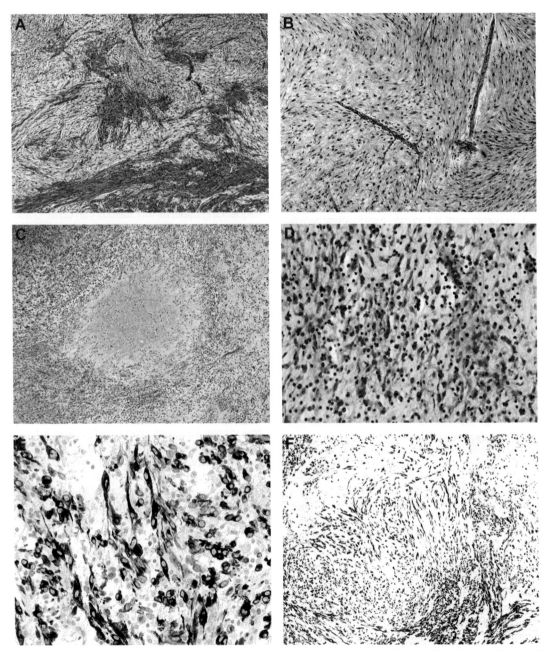

Fig. 9. Inflammatory myofibroblastic tumor. Mixture of compact/fascicular and myxoid patterns (*A*). Myxoid pattern with elongated, thin-walled vessels (*B*). Small focus of the hyalinized pattern surrounded by a brisk inflammatory infiltrate (*C*). Lymphoplasmacytic inflammation (*D*). Granular cytoplasmic ALK staining (*E*). Myxoid pattern with strong and diffuse desmin expression (*F*).

surface that is often myxoid or gelatinous. Margins can be irregular, and hemorrhage and necrosis may be observed.[100,112]

Microscopic Features

On low power, IMTs may be well-circumscribed, have irregular margins, or be frankly infiltrative.[100] Architecturally, they display 3 patterns, which may be admixed: 1) myxoid pattern with hypocellular areas and dispersed tumor cells in a myxoid background, 2) compact/fascicular pattern with cellular areas of intersecting fascicles or storiform growth, and 3) hyalinized pattern with a dense collagenous matrix and inconspicuous cells (**Fig. 9**).[100,101,109] Myofibroblastic cells are often spindled or stellate, with pale eosinophilic cytoplasm, and can appear decidualized if pregnancy-associated; rarely epithelioid cells are present.[111] Nuclei are granular or vesicular and may show prominent nucleoli. Atypia is usually minimal but occasionally moderate or severe, while mitoses are variable. Ganglion-like and Touton giant cells are infrequently present. The inflammatory component is typically lymphoplasmacytic but may be mixed and of variable intensity and distribution. Thin-walled elongated/ectatic vessels are often conspicuous.

Epithelioid inflammatory myofibroblastic sarcoma (EIMS), an aggressive variant of IMT, most commonly occurs in the peritoneum but has recently been described in the gynecologic tract (ovary and uterus).[111,113-115] This subtype is composed of sheets of epithelioid cells with large vesicular nuclei and prominent nucleoli, as well as a minor spindle cell component (<5%) with similar nuclear features to the epithelioid cells, all percolating throughout a myxoid to occasionally collagenous stroma. It is often neutrophil-rich and can lack plasma cells.

Immunohistochemistry

Granular cytoplasmic staining for ALK is highly sensitive and specific; however, extent and intensity are variable.[100,109,116,117] Perinuclear accentuation may also be present in IMTs, while EIMS usually show distinct nuclear membrane staining.[111,113] In one study, ALK D5F3 clone demonstrated greater sensitivity, staining intensity, and correlation with ALK rearrangements compared with the traditional ALK1 clone.[118] However, a recent pooled analysis of different ALK clones showed that ALK1, 5A4, and D5F3 are comparable in terms of sensitivity and specificity.[119]

In 2 series, Bennett and colleagues[100,110] reported frequent expression of smooth muscle markers (SMA, desmin, caldesmon, transgelin)

and endometrial stromal markers (CD10, IFITM1), with focal weak BCOR staining noted in 40% of tumors. All were p53 wildtype, while p16 was aberrantly expressed in 35%, with 5 tumors being completely negative, and 3 strongly and diffusely positive. This contrasts with a previous series whereby all IMTs studied (n = 12) were p53 wildtype but consistently showed patchy p16 expression.[120] In pregnancy-associated tumors, PR is strong and diffuse, while ER is variably expressed.[102,106,117]

Molecular

Approximately 75% of uterine IMTs harbor ALK gene rearrangements detected by FISH, with those reported as negative often showing complex genetic rearrangements.[100,109,117,121,122] RNA sequencing increases detection sensitivity to 80%-90%, as it allows for the identification of intrachromosomal rearrangements, including those involving FN1 and IGFBP5.[100,109] However, it is important to ensure the entire ALK gene is covered by the sequencing panel as IMT fusions can occur outside of exons 17 to 20 (the region involved by most ALK-rearranged non-small cell lung cancers).[106] Various partner genes have been identified including TIMP3, THBS1, IGFBP5, DES, FN1, DCTN1, SEC31, TPM3, PPP1CB, TNS1, and SYN3.[100,109,121-123] Pregnancy-associated IMTs are enriched in TIMP3-ALK and THBS1-ALK fusions, both of which are involved in endometrial remodeling during implantation and pregnancy,[100,105-107,109] and short-tandem repeat genotyping has confirmed these tumors are maternally derived.[104] Rare IMTs with non-ALK fusions have been reported, including ETV6-NTRK,[124] TIMP3-RET,[105] TIMP3-ROS1,[108] and FN1-ROS1.[125] The sole uterine EIMS harbored a RANBP2-ALK fusion, as has been described in other sites.[111,113,115]

The presence of ALK fusions raises the possibility for targeted therapy. Crizotinib is an ATP-competitive inhibitor that inhibits ALK kinase and fusion proteins with proven efficacy in the treatment of ALK-rearranged non-small cell lung cancer.[126] While there is mounting evidence in its utility in extrauterine ALK-rearranged IMTs, experience in the gynecologic tract is limited.[127-129] Recently, Kyi et al.[130] described durable responses (at least 12 months) to ALK inhibitors in 4 patients with uterine IMT, 3 of whom derived further benefit from a second-generation ALK inhibitor after disease progression or crizotinib intolerance.

Other molecular alterations in IMTs have not been well-documented. Bennett et al.[110] detected CDKN2A alterations in 2 malignant IMTs, which showed complete absence of p16 staining, while in another study, one malignant IMT harbored a concurrent *MTOR* mutation and *CDKN2A/B* loss.[111]

Prognosis

Although originally described as indolent,[112] extrauterine disease at diagnosis and recurrence have been reported in a subset of IMTs; thus, it is best regarded as a neoplasm of low malignant potential.[100,101] Features suggestive of aggressive behavior include infiltrative borders, size $\geq$ 7 cm, moderate to severe atypia, brisk mitoses ($\geq$ 10/10 HPF),[131] and tumor cell necrosis; however, histologically bland tumors have recurred.[100] Recently, Collins et al.[111] described 9 malignant IMTs and while all demonstrated at least one of the above features, 2 only showed one atypical feature (infiltrative growth or atypia ranging from mild to severe), but both of the latter also presented with extrauterine disease. In all reported pregnancy-associated IMTs, aside from one with peritoneal disease at diagnosis,[111] recurrences have not been documented.[100,102,103,105–107,109]

Key Features
Inflammatory Myofibroblastic Tumor

- Neoplasm of low malignant potential, as recurrences and extrauterine spread have been reported.

- Morphologically composed of at least one of the 3 patterns—myxoid, compact/fascicular, and hyalinized.

- ALK immunohistochemistry is highly sensitive and specific for *ALK* fusions regardless of the clone used.

- Confirmation of *ALK* rearrangement has both diagnostic and therapeutic implications, as ALK inhibitors may be of use in managing patients with recurrent or refractory disease.

MYXOID LEIOMYOSARCOMA

According to the 2020 World Health Organization Classification of Female Genital Tumors, if any one of the following criteria is fulfilled, a diagnosis of myxoid LMS can be made: irregular margins/infiltrative borders, moderate to severe atypia, tumor cell necrosis, or > 1 mitosis/2.4 mm² (**Fig. 10**).[48] Myxoid LMS can be deceptively bland and lack brisk proliferation, which explains why morphologic criteria are different than for conventional leiomyosarcoma. Studies suggest that myxoid LMS is more aggressive than its conventional counterpart, with a reported 5-year survival of 11%.[132–134]

In the largest series of myxoid LMS by Parra-Herran et al.[134] (n = 25), all tumors were positive for at least one smooth muscle marker. SMA was the most sensitive, with 9 expressing all 3 markers. In a subsequent study of 9 myxoid smooth muscle tumors, all showed expression (usually strong and diffuse) for at least 2 myogenic markers.[135] Aberrant p53 and p16 staining has been described in 50% of tumors,[120] while CD10 is positive in 67%–75%[134,135] and ER in 75%.[135] BCOR is expressed in a subset, but is typically weak and focal, and ALK is negative.[135,136] Approximately 50% of myxoid LMS are positive for PLAG1, including all tumors with a *PLAG1*-rearrangement (discussed below), as well as a subset lacking *PLAG1* fusions.[135,136]

The molecular phenotype of myxoid LMS is largely unknown due to its rarity. Whole-exome sequencing has shown a low total mutational burden but relatively high burden of copy-number variations.[135] Genes most likely to be implicated included those involved in epigenetic regulation, chromatin remodeling, and RNA metabolism. *TP53* mutations and *CDKN2A* deletions appear are uncommon.[120,135] Recently, rearrangements involving *PLAG1* were detected in five myxoid LMS.[136,137] *PLAG1* (pleomorphic adenoma gene 1) is part of the PLAG family encoding zinc finger transcription factors involved in cell proliferation and survival.[138–140] Translocation results in the activation of PLAG1 by the promoter of the fusion partner.[141,142] Partner genes include *TRPS1*, *RAD51B*, and *TRIM13*.

Key Features
Myxoid Leiomyosarcoma

- Only one worrisome feature (infiltrative borders/irregular margins, moderate to severe atypia, > 1 mitosis/2.4 mm², tumor cell necrosis) is needed to diagnose myxoid leiomyosarcoma.

- More aggressive than conventional leiomyosarcoma.

- Express at least one smooth muscle marker and approximately 50% are PLAG1 positive.

- Have a low total mutational burden but relatively high burden of copy-number variations, with *PLAG1* fusions described in a small subset.

Differential Diagnosis Myxoid Mesenchymal Neoplasms

- Entities detailed in the text are summarized in **Table 3**
- Leiomyoma with hydropic change
  - Classic areas of leiomyoma
  - Absence of atypia, necrosis, infiltrative borders, and brisk mitoses
  - Negative Alcian blue stain at pH 2.5
- Apoplectic leiomyoma
  - History of exogenous progestin use or recent pregnancy
  - Classic areas of leiomyoma
  - Multiple stellate zones of hemorrhage surrounded by a hypercellular rim
  - Myxoid material often in areas of "drop-out"
- Myxoid leiomyoma
  - Exceedingly rare entity
  - Well-circumscribed nodule without infiltrative borders
  - Lacks tumor cell necrosis
  - At most mild atypia or ≤ 1 mitosis/2.4 mm^2
  - Diagnosis should be rendered with caution and only after extensive sampling
- Low-grade endometrial stromal sarcoma, myxoid/fibromyxoid variant
  - Classic low-grade component present
  - CD10+, ER+, PR+
  - No *BCOR/BCORL1* alterations or *ALK* fusions
- Other myxoid soft tissue neoplasms
  - Exceedingly rare
  - Should harbor molecular alterations classic to the entity
    - Myxoid liposarcoma–*FUS/DDIT3*
    - Myxoid-rich solitary fibrous tumor–*NAB2-STAT6*
    - Epithelioid sarcoma–*INI* loss
    - Extraskeletal myxoid chondrosarcoma–*NR4A3* rearrangement
  - No *BCOR/BCORL1* alterations or *ALK* fusions

Fig. 10. Myxoid leiomyosarcoma. Infiltrative growth (*A*). Fascicles of spindle cells percolating through a myxoid matrix (*B*). Moderate cytologic atypia and rare mitoses (*C, encircled*).

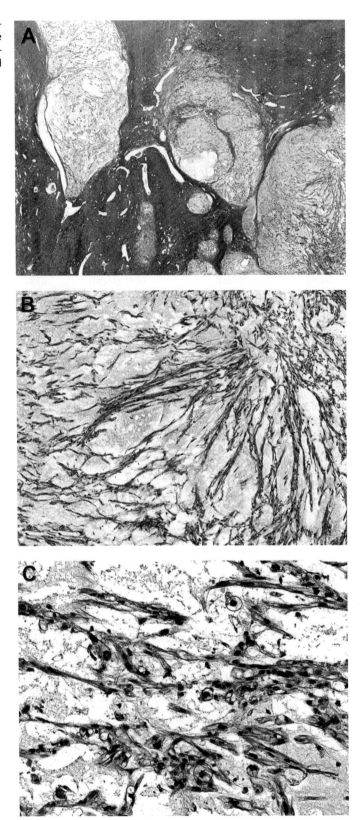

Table 3
Key morphologic, immunohistochemical, and molecular findings of myxoid mesenchymal neoplasms

	ZC3H7B-BCOR High-Grade Endometrial Stromal Sarcoma	*BCOR* ITD High-Grade Endometrial Stromal Sarcoma	Inflammatory Myofibroblastic Tumor	Myxoid Leiomyosarcoma
Age, range (median)	23–79 (54) y	14–62 (44) y	6–78 (38) y	33–77 (52) y
Morphology	• Haphazard fascicles • Myxoid background • Uniformly atypical spindle cells	• High-grade round cells • High-grade spindle cells • Low-grade spindle cells	• Myxoid, compact/ fascicular, hyalinized patterns • Spindle cells • Inflammatory cells (often lymphoplasmacytic)	• Paucicellular • Nodular or diffuse growth • Spindle cells in a myxoid background
Desmin	5% (focal)	60% (focal)	67%–91%	84%–100%
SMA	30% (focal)	0%	67%–89%	100%
Caldesmon	6% (focal)	0%	42%–67%	40%–89%
CD10	100%	83%	74%–100%	67%–75%
ER	22%	50%	60%–83%	29%–75%
PR	27%	25%	75%–83%	NT
Cyclin D1 (diffuse staining)	85%	100%	NT	NT
BCOR (diffuse staining)	50%	100%	0%	0%
ALK	0%	N/A	95%	0%
Molecular	• *ZC3H7B-BCOR* fusion • Activation of cyclin D1-CDK4 kinase (65%) • *MDM2* amplification (45%–100%)	• *BCOR* internal tandem duplication of exon 15 • *CDKN2A/2B* homozygous deletions (20%)	• *ALK* fusions (*TIMP3* and *THBS1* most common partners in pregnancy) • *ROS1*, *RET*, *NTRK* fusions rare	• Subset with *PLAG1* fusions • *TP53* and *CDKN2A* alterations appear infrequent

Abbreviation: NT, not tested.

ACKNOWLEDGMENTS

The authors would like to thank the following pathologists for sharing digital whole slide images for the article: Drs. David Kolin, Brigham and Womens' Hospital (see **Figs.** 3D, E, **4C, 7C**), Brooke Howitt, Stanford University (see **Fig.** 3F), Esther Oliva, Massachusetts General Hospital (see **Fig.** 6D), and Andre Pinto, University of Miami (see **Figs.** 7A, B, **9C, D**).

DISCLOSURE

The authors have nothing to disclose.

REFERENCES

1. Yamamoto E, Ino K, Sakurai M, et al. Fertility-sparing operation for recurrence of uterine cervical perivascular epithelioid cell tumor. Rare Tumors 2010;2(2):e26.
2. Bradshaw MJ, Folpe AL, Croghan GA. Perivascular epithelioid cell neoplasm of the uterine cervix: an unusual tumor in an unusual location. Rare Tumors 2010;2(4):e56.
3. Zhang C, Pan F, Qiao J, et al. Perivascular epithelioid cell tumor of the cervix with malignant potential. Int J Gynaecol Obstet 2013;123(1):72–3.
4. Kovac O, Babal P, Kajo K, et al. Perivascular epithelioid cell tumor (PEComa) of the uterine

cervix: a case report of a 43-Yr-Old woman with abnormal uterine bleeding treated with hysterectomy. Int J Gynecol Pathol 2018;37(5):492–6.

5. Schoolmeester JK, Howitt BE, Hirsch MS, et al. Perivascular epithelioid cell neoplasm (PEComa) of the gynecologic tract: clinicopathologic and immunohistochemical characterization of 16 cases. Am J Surg Pathol 2014;38(2):176–88.

6. Folpe AL, Mentzel T, Lehr HA, et al. Perivascular epithelioid cell neoplasms of soft tissue and gynecologic origin: a clinicopathologic study of 26 cases and review of the literature. Am J Surg Pathol 2005;29(12):1558–75.

7. Cho HJ, Lee MK, Kang BM, et al. A 6-year-old girl with vaginal spotting who was diagnosed with perivascular epithelioid cell neoplasm after vaginoscopic resection. Obstet Gynecol Sci 2014;57(5):409–11.

8. Fink D, Marsden DE, Edwards L, et al. Malignant perivascular epithelioid cell tumor (PEComa) arising in the broad ligament. Int J Gynecol Cancer 2004;14(5):1036–9.

9. Kim WK, Alvarez X, Fisher J, et al. CD163 identifies perivascular macrophages in normal and viral encephalitic brains and potential precursors to perivascular macrophages in blood. Am J Pathol 2006;168(3):822–34.

10. Rys J, Karolewski K, Pudelek J, et al. Perivascular epithelioid tumor (PEComa) of the falciform/broad ligament. Pol J Pathol 2008;59(4):211–5.

11. Lee SE, Choi YL, Cho J, et al. Ovarian perivascular epithelioid cell tumor not otherwise specified with transcription factor E3 gene rearrangement: a case report and review of the literature. Hum Pathol 2012;43(7):1126–30.

12. LeGallo RD, Stelow EB, Sukov WR, et al. Melanotic xp11.2 neoplasm of the ovary: report of a unique case. Am J Surg Pathol 2012;36(9):1410–4.

13. Westaby JD, Magdy N, Fisher C, et al. Primary ovarian malignant PEComa: a case report. Int J Gynecol Pathol 2017;36(4):400–4.

14. Tazelaar HD, Batts KP, Srigley JR. Primary extrapulmonary sugar tumor (PEST): a report of four cases. Mod Pathol 2001;14(6):615–22.

15. Tasaka R, Hashiguchi Y, Kasai M, et al. Perivascular epithelioid cell tumor of vulva: a rare case. Eur J Gynaecol Oncol 2019;40(1):148–50.

16. Bennett JA, Braga AC, Pinto A, et al. Uterine PEComas: a morphologic, Immunohistochemical, and molecular analysis of 32 tumors. Am J Surg Pathol 2018;42(10):1370–83.

17. Greene LA, Mount SL, Schned AR, et al. Recurrent perivascular epithelioid cell tumor of the uterus (PEComa): an immunohistochemical study and review of the literature. Gynecol Oncol 2003;90(3):677–81.

18. Lim GS, Oliva E. The morphologic spectrum of uterine PEC-cell associated tumors in a patient with tuberous sclerosis. Int J Gynecol Pathol 2011;30(2):121–8.

19. Froio E, Piana S, Cavazza A, et al. Multifocal PEComa (PEComatosis) of the female genital tract associated with endometriosis, diffuse adenomyosis, and endometrial atypical hyperplasia. Int J Surg Pathol 2008;16(4):443–6.

20. Liang SX, Pearl M, Liu J, et al. Malignant" uterine perivascular epithelioid cell tumor, pelvic lymph node lymphangioleiomyomatosis, and gynecological pecomatosis in a patient with tuberous sclerosis: a case report and review of the literature. Int J Gynecol Pathol 2008;27(1):86–90.

21. Agaram NP, Sung YS, Zhang L, et al. Dichotomy of genetic abnormalities in PEComas with therapeutic implications. Am J Surg Pathol 2015;39(6):813–25.

22. Vang R, Kempson RL. Perivascular epithelioid cell tumor ('PEComa') of the uterus: a subset of HMB-45-positive epithelioid mesenchymal neoplasms with an uncertain relationship to pure smooth muscle tumors. Am J Surg Pathol 2002;26(1):1–13.

23. Hornick JL, Fletcher CD. Sclerosing PEComa: clinicopathologic analysis of a distinctive variant with a predilection for the retroperitoneum. Am J Surg Pathol 2008;32(4):493–501.

24. Schoolmeester JK, Dao LN, Sukov WR, et al. TFE3 translocation-associated perivascular epithelioid cell neoplasm (PEComa) of the gynecologic tract: morphology, immunophenotype, differential diagnosis. Am J Surg Pathol 2015;39(3):394–404.

25. Longacre TA, Hendrickson MR, Kapp DS, et al. Lymphangioleiomyomatosis of the uterus simulating high-stage endometrial stromal sarcoma. Gynecol Oncol 1996;63(3):404–10.

26. Valencia-Guerrero A, Pinto A, Anderson WJ, et al. PNL2: A Useful Adjunct Biomarker to HMB45 in the Diagnosis of Uterine Perivascular Epithelioid Cell Tumor (PEComa). Int J Gynecol Pathol 2020;39(6):529–36.

27. Bennett JA, Ordulu Z, Pinto A, et al. Uterine PEComas: correlation between melanocytic marker expression and TSC alterations/TFE3 fusions. Mod Pathol 2021.

28. Gulavita P, Fletcher CDM, Hirsch MS. PNL2: an adjunctive biomarker for renal angiomyolipomas and perivascular epithelioid cell tumours. Histopathology 2018;72(3):441–8.

29. Chang KL, Folpe AL. Diagnostic utility of microphthalmia transcription factor in malignant melanoma and other tumors. Adv Anat Pathol 2001;8(5):273–5.

30. Valencia-Guerrero A, Pinto A, Anderson WJ, et al. PNL2: a useful adjunct biomarker to HMB45 in the diagnosis of uterine perivascular epithelioid

cell tumor (PEComa). Int J Gynecol Pathol 2020;
39(6):529–36.

31. Argani P, Aulmann S, Illei PB, et al. A distinctive subset of PEComas harbors TFE3 gene fusions. Am J Surg Pathol 2010;34(10):1395–406.

32. Pan CC, Chung MY, Ng KF, et al. Constant allelic alteration on chromosome 16p (TSC2 gene) in perivascular epithelioid cell tumour (PEComa): genetic evidence for the relationship of PEComa with angiomyolipoma. J Pathol 2008;214(3):387–93.

33. Crino PB, Nathanson KL, Henske EP. The tuberous sclerosis complex. N Engl J Med 2006;355(13):1345–56.

34. Goncharova EA, Goncharov DA, Eszterhas A, et al. Tuberin regulates p70 S6 kinase activation and ribosomal protein S6 phosphorylation. A role for the TSC2 tumor suppressor gene in pulmonary lymphangioleiomyomatosis (LAM). J Biol Chem 2002;277(34):30958–67.

35. Wagner AJ, Malinowska-Kolodziej I, Morgan JA, et al. Clinical activity of mTOR inhibition with sirolimus in malignant perivascular epithelioid cell tumors: targeting the pathogenic activation of mTORC1 in tumors. J Clin Oncol 2010;28(5):835–40.

36. Dickson MA, Schwartz GK, Antonescu CR, et al. Extrarenal perivascular epithelioid cell tumors (PEComas) respond to mTOR inhibition: clinical and molecular correlates. Int J Cancer 2013;132(7):1711–7.

37. Sanfilippo R, Jones RL, Blay JY, et al. Role of chemotherapy, VEGFR inhibitors, and mTOR inhibitors in advanced perivascular epithelioid cell tumors (PEComas). Clin Cancer Res 2019;25(17):5295–300.

38. Wagner AJ, Ravi V, Ganjoo KN, et al. ABI-009 (nab-sirolimus) in advanced malignant perivascular epithelioid cell tumors (PEComa): Preliminary efficacy, safety, and mutational status from AMPECT, an open label phase II registration trial. J Clin Oncol 2019;37(15s):11005.

39. Wagner AJ, Ravi V, Riedel RF, et al. Long-term follow-up for duration of response (DoR) after weekly nab-sirolimus in patients with advanced malignant perivascular epithelioid cell tumors (PEComa): results from a registrational open-label phase II trial, AMPECT. J Clin Oncol 2020;38(15s):11516.

40. Selenica P, Conlon N, Gonzalez C, et al. Genomic profiling aids classification of diagnostically challenging uterine mesenchymal tumors with myomelanocytic differentiation. Am J Surg Pathol 2021;45(1):77–92.

41. Doyle LA, Nowak JA, Nathenson MJ, et al. Characteristics of mismatch repair deficiency in sarcomas. Mod Pathol 2019;32(7):977–87.

42. Perera RM, Di Malta C, Ballabio A. MiT/TFE family of transcription factors, lysosomes, and cancer. Annu Rev Cancer Biol 2019;3:203–22.

43. Bennett JA, Oliva E. Perivascular epithelioid cell tumors (PEComa) of the gynecologic tract. Genes Chromosomes Cancer 2021;60(3):168–79.

44. Selenica P, Conlon N, Gonzalez C, et al. Genomic profiling aids classification of diagnostically challenging uterine mesenchymal tumors with myomelanocytic differentiation. Am J Surg Pathol 2021;45(1):77–92.

45. Malinowska I, Kwiatkowski DJ, Weiss S, et al. Perivascular epithelioid cell tumors (PEComas) harboring TFE3 gene rearrangements lack the TSC2 alterations characteristic of conventional PEComas: further evidence for a biological distinction. Am J Surg Pathol 2012;36(5):783–4.

46. Stacchiotti S, Marrari A, Dei Tos AP, et al. Targeted therapies in rare sarcomas: IMT, ASPS, SFT, PEComa, and CCS. Hematol Oncol Clin North Am 2013;27(5):1049–61.

47. Schoffski P, Wozniak A, Kasper B, et al. Activity and safety of crizotinib in patients with alveolar soft part sarcoma with rearrangement of TFE3: European Organization for Research and Treatment of Cancer (EORTC) phase II trial 90101 'CREATE. Ann Oncol 2018;29(3):758–65.

48. WHO classification of tumours female genital organs. Lyon: World Health Organization; 2020.

49. Clement PB, Scully RE. Uterine tumors resembling ovarian sex-cord tumors. A clinicopathologic analysis of fourteen cases. Am J Clin Pathol 1976;66(3):512–25.

50. Irving JA, Carinelli S, Prat J. Uterine tumors resembling ovarian sex cord tumors are polyphenotypic neoplasms with true sex cord differentiation. Mod Pathol 2006;19(1):17–24.

51. de Leval L, Lim GS, Waltregny D, et al. Diverse phenotypic profile of uterine tumors resembling ovarian sex cord tumors: an immunohistochemical study of 12 cases. Am J Surg Pathol 2010;34(12):1749–61.

52. Lee CH, Kao YC, Lee WR, et al. Clinicopathologic characterization of GREB1-rearranged uterine sarcomas with variable sex-cord differentiation. Am J Surg Pathol 2019;43(7):928–42.

53. Segala D, Gobbo S, Pesci A, et al. Tamoxifen related uterine tumor resembling ovarian sex cord tumor (UTROSCT): a case report and literature review of this possible association. Pathol Res Pract 2019;215(5):1089–92.

54. Moore M, McCluggage WG. Uterine tumour resembling ovarian sex cord tumour: first report of a large series with follow-up. Histopathology 2017;71(5):751–9.

55. Goebel EA, Hernandez Bonilla S, Dong F, et al. Uterine tumor resembling ovarian sex cord tumor (UTROSCT): a morphologic and molecular study of 26 cases confirms recurrent NCOA1-3 rearrangement. Am J Surg Pathol 2020;44(1):30–42.

56. Brunetti M, Panagopoulos I, Gorunova L, et al. RNA-sequencing identifies novel GREB1-NCOA2 fusion gene in a uterine sarcoma with the chromosomal translocation t(2;8)(p25;q13). Genes Chromosomes Cancer 2018;57(4):176–81.

57. Croce S, Lesluyes T, Delespaul L, et al. GREB1-CTNNB1 fusion transcript detected by RNA-sequencing in a uterine tumor resembling ovarian sex cord tumor (UTROSCT): A novel CTNNB1 rearrangement. Genes Chromosomes Cancer 2019; 58(3):155–63.

58. Staats PN, Garcia JJ, Dias-Santagata DC, et al. Uterine tumors resembling ovarian sex cord tumors (UTROSCT) lack the JAZF1-JJAZ1 translocation frequently seen in endometrial stromal tumors. Am J Surg Pathol 2009;33(8):1206–12.

59. Chiang S, Staats PN, Senz J, et al. FOXL2 mutation is absent in uterine tumors resembling ovarian sex cord tumors. Am J Surg Pathol 2015;39(5):618–23.

60. Kabbani W, Deavers MT, Malpica A, et al. Uterine tumor resembling ovarian sex-cord tumor: report of a case mimicking cervical adenocarcinoma. Int J Gynecol Pathol 2003;22(3):297–302.

61. Nogales FF, Stolnicu S, Harilal KR, et al. Retiform uterine tumours resembling ovarian sex cord tumours. A comparative immunohistochemical study with retiform structures of the female genital tract. Histopathology 2009;54(4):471–7.

62. Hurrell DP, McCluggage WG. Uterine tumour resembling ovarian sex cord tumour is an immunohistochemically polyphenotypic neoplasm which exhibits coexpression of epithelial, myoid and sex cord markers. J Clin Pathol 2007; 60(10):1148–54.

63. Bennett JA, Lastra RR, Barroeta JE, et al. Uterine tumor resembling ovarian sex cord stromal tumor (UTROSCT): a series of 3 cases with extensive rhabdoid differentiation, malignant behavior, and ESR1-NCOA2 fusions. Am J Surg Pathol 2020; 44(11):1563–72.

64. Dickson BC, Childs TJ, Colgan TJ, et al. Uterine tumor resembling ovarian sex cord tumor: a distinct entity characterized by recurrent NCOA2/3 gene fusions. Am J Surg Pathol 2019;43(2):178–86.

65. Grither WR, Dickson BC, Fuh KC, et al. Detection of a somatic GREB1-NCOA1 gene fusion in a uterine tumor resembling ovarian sex cord tumor (UTROSCT). Gynecol Oncol Rep 2020;34:100636.

66. Croce S, de Kock L, Boshari T, et al. Uterine tumor resembling ovarian sex cord tumor (UTROSCT) commonly exhibits positivity with sex cord markers FOXL2 and SF-1 but lacks FOXL2 and DICER1 mutations. Int J Gynecol Pathol 2016;35(4):301–8.

67. Nucci MR, Schoolmeester JK, Sukov WR, et al. Uterine tumors resembling ovarian sex cord tumor (UTROSCT) lack rearrangment of PHF1 by FISH. Mod Pathol 2014;27:298A.

68. Devereaux KA, Kertowidjojo E, Natale K, et al. GTF2A1-NCOA2-Associated uterine tumor resembling ovarian sex cord tumor (UTROSCT) shows focal rhabdoid morphology and aggressive behavior. Am J Surg Pathol 2021;45(12):1725–8.

69. Ye S, Wu J, Yao L, et al. Clinicopathological characteristics and genetic variations of uterine tumours resembling ovarian sex cord tumours. J Clin Pathol 2021.

70. Kommoss FKF, Stichel D, Schrimpf D, et al. DNA methylation-based profiling of uterine neoplasms: a novel tool to improve gynecologic cancer diagnostics. J Cancer Res Clin Oncol 2020;146(1):97–104.

71. Chen Z, Lan J, Chen Q, et al. A novel case of uterine tumor resembling ovarian sex-cord tumor (UTROSCT) recurrent with GREB1-NCOA2 fusion. Int J Gynaecol Obstet 2021;152(2):266–8.

72. Chang B, Bai Q, Liang L, et al. Recurrent uterine tumors resembling ovarian sex-cord tumors with the growth regulation by estrogen in breast cancer 1-nuclear receptor coactivator 2 fusion gene: a case report and literature review. Diagn Pathol 2020;15(1):110.

73. Chapel DB, Nucci MR, Quade BJ, et al. Epithelioid leiomyosarcoma of the uterus: modern outcome-based appraisal of diagnostic criteria in a large institutional series. Am J Surg Pathol 2022;46(4):464–75.

74. Kurman RJ, Norris HJ. Mesenchymal tumors of the uterus. VI. Epithelioid smooth muscle tumors including leiomyoblastoma and clear-cell leiomyoma: a clinical and pathologic analysis of 26 cases. Cancer 1976;37(4):1853–65.

75. Prayson RA, Goldblum JR, Hart WR. Epithelioid smooth-muscle tumors of the uterus: a clinicopathologic study of 18 patients. Am J Surg Pathol 1997; 21(4):383–91.

76. Chiang S, Samore W, Zhang L, et al. PGR gene fusions identify a molecular subset of uterine epithelioid leiomyosarcoma with rhabdoid features. Am J Surg Pathol 2019;43(6):810–8.

77. Chiang S, Lee CH, Stewart CJR, et al. BCOR is a robust diagnostic immunohistochemical marker of genetically diverse high-grade endometrial stromal sarcoma, including tumors exhibiting variant morphology. Mod Pathol 2017;30(9):1251–61.

78. Marino-Enriquez A, Lauria A, Przybyl J, et al. BCOR internal tandem duplication in high-grade uterine sarcomas. Am J Surg Pathol 2018;42(3):335–41.

79. Cotzia P, Benayed R, Mullaney K, et al. Undifferentiated uterine sarcomas represent under-recognized high-grade endometrial stromal sarcomas. Am J Surg Pathol 2019;43(5):662–9.

80. Juckett LT, Lin DI, Madison R, et al. A pan-cancer landscape analysis reveals a subset of endometrial stromal and pediatric tumors defined by internal tandem duplications of BCOR. Oncology 2019; 96(2):101–9.

81. Lin DI, Hemmerich A, Edgerly C, et al. Genomic profiling of BCOR-rearranged uterine sarcomas reveals novel gene fusion partners, frequent CDK4 amplification and CDKN2A loss. Gynecol Oncol 2020;157(2):357–66.

82. Brahmi M, Franceschi T, Treilleux I, et al. Molecular classification of endometrial stromal sarcomas using RNA sequencing defines nosological and prognostic subgroups with different natural history. Cancers (Basel) 2020;12(9):2604.

83. Lewis N, Soslow RA, Delair DF, et al. ZC3H7B-BCOR high-grade endometrial stromal sarcomas: a report of 17 cases of a newly defined entity. Mod Pathol 2018;31(4):674–84.

84. Hoang LN, Aneja A, Conlon N, et al. Novel high-grade endometrial stromal sarcoma: a morphologic mimicker of myxoid leiomyosarcoma. Am J Surg Pathol 2017;41(1):12–24.

85. Lu B, Chen J, Shao Y, et al. Two cases of ZC3H7B-BCOR high grade endometrial stromal sarcoma with an extension on its morphological features. Pathology 2020;52(6):708–12.

86. Dickson BC, Lum A, Swanson D, et al. Novel EPC1 gene fusions in endometrial stromal sarcoma. Genes Chromosomes Cancer 2018;57(11):598–603.

87. Ondic O, Bednarova B, Ptakova N, et al. ZC3H7B-BCOR high-grade endometrial stromal sarcoma may present as myoma nascens with cytoplasmic signet ring cell change. Virchows Arch 2020; 476(4):615–9.

88. Kommoss FK, Chang KT, Stichel D, et al. Endometrial stromal sarcomas with BCOR-rearrangement harbor MDM2 amplifications. J Pathol Clin Res 2020;6(3):178–84.

89. Nagaputra JC, Gooh RCH, Kuick CH, et al. ZC3H7B-BCOR high-grade endometrial stromal sarcoma with osseous metaplasia: Unique feature in a recently defined entity. Hum Pathol Case Rep 2019;15:54–8.

90. Lee CH, Marino-Enriquez A, Ou W, et al. The clinicopathologic features of YWHAE-FAM22 endometrial stromal sarcomas: a histologically high-grade and clinically aggressive tumor. Am J Surg Pathol 2012;36(5):641–53.

91. Mansor S, Kuick CH, Lim SL, et al. ZC3H7B-BCOR-rearranged endometrial stromal sarcomas: a distinct subset merits its own classification? Int J Gynecol Pathol 2019;38(5):420–5.

92. Momeni-Boroujeni A, Mohammad N, Wolber R, et al. Targeted RNA expression profiling identifies high-grade endometrial stromal sarcoma as a clinically relevant molecular subtype of uterine sarcoma. Mod Pathol 2021;34(5):1008–16.

93. Mohammad N, Stewart CJR, Chiang S, et al. p53 immunohistochemical analysis of fusion-positive uterine sarcomas. Histopathology 2021;78(6):805–13.

94. Huynh KD, Fischle W, Verdin E, et al. BCoR, a novel corepressor involved in BCL-6 repression. Genes Dev 2000;14(14):1810–23.

95. Astolfi A, Fiore M, Melchionda F, et al. BCOR involvement in cancer. Epigenomics 2019;11(7):835–55.

96. Panagopoulos I, Thorsen J, Gorunova L, et al. Fusion of the ZC3H7B and BCOR genes in endometrial stromal sarcomas carrying an X;22-translocation. Genes Chromosomes Cancer 2013;52(7):610–8.

97. Micci F, Gorunova L, Agostini A, et al. Cytogenetic and molecular profile of endometrial stromal sarcoma. Genes Chromosomes Cancer 2016;55(11):834–46.

98. Micci F, Heim S, Panagopoulos I. Molecular pathogenesis and prognostication of "low-grade" and "high-grade" endometrial stromal sarcoma. Genes Chromosomes Cancer 2021;60(3):160–7.

99. Lin DI, Huang RSP, Mata DA, et al. Clinicopathological and genomic characterization of BCORL1-driven high-grade endometrial stromal sarcomas. Mod Pathol 2021;34(12):2200–10.

100. Bennett JA, Nardi V, Rouzbahman M, et al. Inflammatory myofibroblastic tumor of the uterus: a clinicopathological, immunohistochemical, and molecular analysis of 13 cases highlighting their broad morphologic spectrum. Mod Pathol 2017; 30(10):1489–503.

101. Parra-Herran C, Quick CM, Howitt BE, et al. Inflammatory myofibroblastic tumor of the uterus: clinical and pathologic review of 10 cases including a subset with aggressive clinical course. Am J Surg Pathol 2015;39(2):157–68.

102. Banet N, Ning Y, Montgomery EA. Inflammatory myofibroblastic tumor of the placenta: a report of a novel lesion in 2 patients. Int J Gynecol Pathol 2015;34(5):419–23.

103. Schoolmeester JK, Sukov WR. ALK-rearranged inflammatory myofibroblastic tumor of the placenta, with observations on site of origin. Int J Gynecol Pathol 2017;36(3):228–9.

104. Ladwig NR, Schoolmeester JK, Weil L, et al. Inflammatory myofibroblastic tumor associated with the placenta: short tandem repeat genotyping confirms uterine site of origin. Am J Surg Pathol 2018;42(6):807–12.

105. Cheek EH, Fadra N, Jackson RA, et al. Uterine inflammatory myofibroblastic tumors in pregnant women with and without involvement of the placenta: a study of 6 cases with identification of a novel TIMP3-RET fusion. Hum Pathol 2020;97:29–39.

106. Devereaux KA, Fitzpatrick MB, Hartinger S, et al. Pregnancy-associated Inflammatory myofibroblastic tumors of the uterus are clinically distinct and

highly enriched for TIMP3-ALK and THBS1-ALK fusions. Am J Surg Pathol 2020;44(7):970–81.

107. Makhdoum S, Nardi V, Devereaux KA, et al. Inflammatory myofibroblastic tumors associated with the placenta: a series of 9 cases. Hum Pathol 2020; 106:62–73.

108. Schoolmeester JK, Minn K, Sukov WR, et al. Uterine inflammatory myofibroblastic tumor involving the decidua of the extraplacental membranes: report of a case with a TIMP3-ROS1 gene fusion. Hum Pathol 2020;100:45–6.

109. Haimes JD, Stewart CJR, Kudlow BA, et al. Uterine inflammatory myofibroblastic tumors frequently harbor ALK fusions with IGFBP5 and THBS1. Am J Surg Pathol 2017;41(6):773–80.

110. Bennett JA, Croce S, Pesci A, et al. Inflammatory myofibroblastic tumor of the uterus: an immunohistochemical study of 23 cases. Am J Surg Pathol 2020;44(11):1441–9.

111. Collins K, Ramalingam P, Euscher ED, et al. Uterine inflammatory myofibroblastic neoplasms with aggressive behavior, including an epithelioid inflammatory myofibroblastic sarcoma: a clinicopathologic study of 9 cases. Am J Surg Pathol 2022; 46(1):105–17.

112. Rabban JT, Zaloudek CJ, Shekitka KM, et al. Inflammatory myofibroblastic tumor of the uterus: a clinicopathologic study of 6 cases emphasizing distinction from aggressive mesenchymal tumors. Am J Surg Pathol 2005;29(10):1348–55.

113. Marino-Enriquez A, Wang WL, Roy A, et al. Epithelioid inflammatory myofibroblastic sarcoma: an aggressive intra-abdominal variant of inflammatory myofibroblastic tumor with nuclear membrane or perinuclear ALK. Am J Surg Pathol 2011;35(1): 135–44.

114. Lee JC, Li CF, Huang HY, et al. ALK oncoproteins in atypical inflammatory myofibroblastic tumours: novel RRBP1-ALK fusions in epithelioid inflammatory myofibroblastic sarcoma. J Pathol 2017; 241(3):316–23.

115. Fang H, Langstraat CL, Visscher DW, et al. Epithelioid inflammatory myofibroblastic sarcoma of the ovary with RANB2-ALK fusion: report of a case. Int J Gynecol Pathol 2018;37(5):468–72.

116. Mohammad N, Haimes JD, Mishkin S, et al. ALK is a specific diagnostic marker for inflammatory myofibroblastic tumor of the uterus. Am J Surg Pathol 2018;42(10):1353–9.

117. Pickett JL, Chou A, Andrici JA, et al. Inflammatory myofibroblastic tumors of the female genital tract are under-recognized: a low threshold for ALK immunohistochemistry is required. Am J Surg Pathol 2017;41(10):1433–42.

118. Taheri D, Zahavi DJ, Del Carmen Rodriguez M, et al. For staining of ALK protein, the novel D5F3 antibody demonstrates superior overall performance in terms of intensity and extent of staining in comparison to the currently used ALK1 antibody. Virchows Arch 2016;469(3):345–50.

119. Parra-Herran C. ALK Immunohistochemistry and Molecular Analysis in Uterine Inflammatory Myofibroblastic Tumor: Proceedings of the ISGyP Companion Society Session at the 2020 USCAP Annual Meeting. Int J Gynecol Pathol 2021;40(1):28–31.

120. Schaefer IM, Hornick JL, Sholl LM, et al. Abnormal p53 and p16 staining patterns distinguish uterine leiomyosarcoma from inflammatory myofibroblastic tumour. Histopathology 2017; 70(7):1138–46.

121. Devereaux KA, Kunder CA, Longacre TA. ALK-rearranged tumors are highly enriched in the STUMP subcategory of uterine tumors. Am J Surg Pathol 2019;43(1):64–74.

122. Zarei S, Abdul-Karim FW, Chase DM, et al. Uterine inflammatory myofibroblastic tumor showing an atypical ALK signal pattern by FISH and DES-ALK fusion by RNA sequencing: a case report. Int J Gynecol Pathol 2020;39(2):152–6.

123. Fuehrer NE, Keeney GL, Ketterling RP, et al. ALK-1 protein expression and ALK gene rearrangements aid in the diagnosis of inflammatory myofibroblastic tumors of the female genital tract. Arch Pathol Lab Med 2012;136(6):623–6.

124. Takahashi A, Kurosawa M, Uemura M, et al. Anaplastic lymphoma kinase-negative uterine inflammatory myofibroblastic tumor containing the ETV6-NTRK3 fusion gene: a case report. J Int Med Res 2018;46(8):3498–503.

125. Bennett JA, Wang P, Wanjari P, et al. Uterine inflammatory myofibroblastic tumor: first report of a ROS1 fusion. Genes Chromosomes Cancer 2021;46(1):105–17.

126. Kwak EL, Bang YJ, Camidge DR, et al. Anaplastic lymphoma kinase inhibition in non-small-cell lung cancer. N Engl J Med 2010;363(18):1693–703.

127. Butrynski JE, D'Adamo DR, Hornick JL, et al. Crizotinib in ALK-rearranged inflammatory myofibroblastic tumor. N Engl J Med 2010;363(18):1727–33.

128. Mosse YP, Voss SD, Lim MS, et al. Targeting ALK With crizotinib in pediatric anaplastic large cell lymphoma and inflammatory myofibroblastic tumor: a children's oncology group study. J Clin Oncol 2017;35(28):3215–21.

129. Alan O, Kuzhan O, Koca S, et al. How long should we continue crizotinib in ALK translocation-positive inflammatory myofibroblastic tumors? Long-term complete response with crizotinib and review of the literature. J Oncol Pharm Pract 2020;26(4):1011–8.

130. Kyi C, Friedman CF, Mueller JJ, et al. Uterine mesenchymal tumors harboring ALK fusions and response to ALK-targeted therapy. Gynecol Oncol Rep 2021;37:100852.

131. Busca A, Parra-Herran C. Myxoid mesenchymal tumors of the uterus: an update on classification,

definitions, and differential diagnosis. Adv Anat Pathol 2017;24(6):354–61.

132. Wang WL, Soslow R, Hensley M, et al. Histopathologic prognostic factors in stage I leiomyosarcoma of the uterus: a detailed analysis of 27 cases. Am J Surg Pathol 2011;35(4):522–9.

133. Abeler VM, Royne O, Thoresen S, et al. Uterine sarcomas in Norway. A histopathological and prognostic survey of a total population from 1970 to 2000 including 419 patients. Histopathology 2009;54(3): 355–64.

134. Parra-Herran C, Schoolmeester JK, Yuan L, et al. Myxoid leiomyosarcoma of the uterus: A clinicopathologic analysis of 30 cases and review of the literature with reappraisal of its distinction from other uterine myxoid mesenchymal neoplasms. Am J Surg Pathol 2016;40(3):285–301.

135. Yoon JY, Marino-Enriquez A, Stickle N, et al. Myxoid smooth muscle neoplasia of the uterus: comprehensive analysis by next-generation sequencing and nucleic acid hybridization. Mod Pathol 2019;32(11):1688–97.

136. Arias-Stella JA 3rd, Benayed R, Oliva E, et al. Novel PLAG1 gene rearrangement distinguishes a subset of uterine myxoid leiomyosarcoma from other uterine myxoid mesenchymal tumors. Am J Surg Pathol 2019;43(3):382–8.

137. Thiryayi SA, Turashvili G, Latta EK, et al. PLAG1-rearrangment in a uterine leiomyosarcoma with myxoid stroma and heterologous differentiation. Genes Chromosomes Cancer 2021;60(10):713–7.

138. Van Dyck F, Declercq J, Braem CV, et al. PLAG1, the prototype of the PLAG gene family: versatility in tumour development (review). Int J Oncol 2007; 30(4):765–74.

139. Zheng Y, Xu L, Hassan M, et al. Bayesian modeling identifies PLAG1 as a key regulator of proliferation and survival in rhabdomyosarcoma cells. Mol Cancer Res 2020;18(3):364–74.

140. Hensen K, Van Valckenborgh IC, Kas K, et al. The tumorigenic diversity of the three PLAG family members is associated with different DNA binding capacities. Cancer Res 2002;62(5): 1510–7.

141. Kas K, Voz ML, Roijer E, et al. Promoter swapping between the genes for a novel zinc finger protein and beta-catenin in pleomorphic adenomas with t(3;8)(p21;q12) translocations. Nat Genet 1997; 15(2):170–4.

142. Voz ML, Astrom AK, Kas K, et al. The recurrent translocation t(5;8)(p13;q12) in pleomorphic adenomas results in upregulation of PLAG1 gene expression under control of the LIFR promoter. Oncogene 1998;16(11):1409–16.

Update on Mesenchymal Lesions of the Lower Female Genital Tract

Sabrina Croce, MD, PhD[a,b,*], Raul Perret, MD[a,b],
François Le Loarer, MD, PhD[a,b,c]

KEYWORDS

- Sarcoma • Mesenchymal lesions • Cervix • Vulva • Vagina • NTRK
- Lipoblastoma-like tumor of the vulva • SMARCA4 • SMARCB1

Key points: SMARCB1-deficient vulvar sarcomas

- These tumors overlap with epithelioid sarcomas, myoepithelial carcinomas, and, to a lesser extent, malignant rhabdoid tumors

- SMARCB1 loss is mostly secondary to genomic deletions

- Epithelioid sarcomas diffusely express cytokeratins; CD34 is positive in half of the cases

- Myoepithelial carcinomas with SMARCB1 loss display a neural and epithelial phenotype along with an abundant myxoid matrix.

- Malignant rhabdoid tumors occur mostly in infancy

- The so-called primary yolk sac tumor of the vulva are also associated with *SMARCB1* loss

- These tumors are aggressive and have a propensity to invade lymph nodes

---

ABSTRACT

This article provides an update of the recent developments in mesenchymal tumors of lower genital tract. We focus on the characterization of recurrent molecular events in certain genital stromal tumors, for instance angiomyofibroblastomas and superficial myofibroblastomas. Moreover, fusions involving Tyrosine-kinases receptors (*NTRK, FRFR1, RET, COL1A1-PDGFB*) have been demonstrated in an emerging group of mesenchymal tumors characterized by a fibrosarcoma-like morphology and a predilection for uterine cervix of premenopausal women. We also cover the topic of smooth muscle tumors of the lower genital tract, which can be now classified using the same diagnostic criteria than their uterine counterpart..

OVERVIEW

This article provides an update of the recent developments in mesenchymal tumors of lower genital tract. We focus on the characterization of recurrent molecular events in certain genital stromal tumors, for instance angiomyofibroblastomas and superficial myofibroblastomas. Moreover, fusions involving Tyrosine-kinases receptors (*NTRK, FRFR1, RET, COL1A1-PDGFB*) have been demonstrated in an emerging group of mesenchymal tumors characterized by a fibrosarcoma-like morphology and a predilection for uterine cervix

---

[a] Biopathology Department, Anticancer Center, Institut Bergonié, Bordeaux, France; [b] INSERM U 1218, Action Unit, Bordeaux, France; [c] University of Bordeaux, Talence, France
* Corresponding author. Biopathology Department, Comprehensive cancer center, Institut Bergonié, Bordeaux, France.
E-mail address: s.croce@bordeaux.unicancer.fr

Surgical Pathology 15 (2022) 341–367
https://doi.org/10.1016/j.path.2022.02.009

Box 1
Lower genital (uterine cervix, vagina, and vulva) mesenchymal tumors

Site specific:

- Deep angiomyxoma

- Superficial angiomyxoma

- Angiomyofibroblastoma

- Cellular angiofibroma

- Superficial myofibroblastoma

- Myofibroblastoma

- Lipoblastomalike tumor of the vulva

Non-site specific:

- Smooth muscle tumors

- Rhabdomyosarcoma (embryonal and other subtypes)

- Fibroblastic tumors
  - Solitary fibrous tumor
- Tumors of uncertain origin or differentiation
  - *NTRK* fusion sarcomas
  - *COL1A1-PDFGFB* fusion sarcoma
  - *FGFR1* fusion sarcoma
  - *RET* fusion sarcomas
  - *MEIS1-NCOA* fusion sarcoma
  - SMARC-deficient sarcomas

---

of premenopausal women. We also cover the topic of smooth muscle tumors of the lower genital tract, which can be now classified using the same diagnostic criteria than their uterine counterpart. (**Box 1**).

SITE-SPECIFIC GENITAL MESENCHYMAL TUMORS

Originating from the subepithelial stromal cells of the mesenchyme, genital stromal tumors are located in the lower gynecologic tract (from the uterine cervix to the vulva). Because these tumors share some morphologic and immunohistochemical features, the diagnosis relies on clinical-morphologic and radiologic correlations rather than on immunohistochemistry alone. The most important diagnostic findings are (1) location (superficial vs deep), (2) size (often >10 cm for deep angiomyxoma [DA] and ≤10 cm for all other benign entities), and (3) presence of infiltration of adjacent structures (present in DA, absent in others). Although all these site-specific entities are indolent, it is important to recognize DA because of its tendency for local recurrence and

infiltration, sometimes requiring debilitating pelvic-peritoneal surgery[1] (**Table 1**).

DEEP (AGGRESSIVE) ANGIOMYXOMA

Deep (aggressive) angiomyxoma is a locally aggressive genital stromal tumor located in the deep soft tissues of the genital-pelvic-perineal region. DA occurs in a large spectrum of ages but most frequently in the fourth decade.[1–3] Although not associated with distant spread, this tumor has a high rate of local recurrence (close to 40%)[2,4–6] and shows infiltrating borders with frequent invasion of adjacent soft tissues (**Fig. 1**A, B).

Histologically, this tumor is uniformly paucicellular composed of delicate ovoid, spindle cells with unipolar or bipolar cytoplasmic processes embedded in a copious myxoid stroma with loose fibrillary collagen. An evenly distributed vascular component encompassing thin to large and thick-walled vessels is present, often associated with a cuffing of smooth muscle fibers and perivascular collagen condensation.[2,6] Atypia and brisk mitotic counts are absent. The tumor infiltrates adjacent anatomic structures, often in a deceptive

Table 1
Clinicopathological and molecular features of genital stromal tumors

Lesion	Location	Age	Macroscopy/Size	Microscopy	IHC	Molecular Events	Prognosis
Deep angiomyxoma	Deep • Vulva • Vagina • Pelvic and perineal regions	Reproductive age Fourth decade	• Gelatinous • Ill-defined • Infiltrative borders • Large • >10 cm	• Uniformly paucicellular • Infiltration of adjacent structures • Ovoid, spindle cells with cytoplasmic processes • Myxoid stroma • Prominent vasculature • Perivascular cuffing of smooth muscle cells	• ER/PR positive • Desmin and CD34 variably positive • HMGA2 positive (68%–90%) • RB1 retained	• HMGA2 rearrangement (~30%) • *HMGA2-YAP1* fusion	• Benign • Recurrence up to 30%–40%
Superficial angiomyxoma	Superficial subcutis • Vulva, groin	Reproductive age	• Polypoid exophytic • Gelatinous • Well limited	• Poorly delineated but noninfiltrating myxoid lobules • Spindle ovoid nuclei • Curvilinear thin vessels • Polymorpho-nucleated infiltrate • Overline skin or adnexa	• ER/RP positive • HMGA2 positive • Desmin negative • CD34 frequently positive • RB1 retained		• Benign • Recurrence up to 30%–40%

(continued on next page)

Table 1
(continued)

Lesion	Location	Age	Macroscopy/Size	Microscopy	IHC	Molecular Events	Prognosis
Angiomyofibroblastoma	Vulvovaginal region	Reproductive age (fourth–fifth decade)	• Pink-tan brown • Size<5 cm	• Well circumscribed • Hypocellular and hypercellular areas • Spindle and epithelioid stromal cells • Edematous/collagenous matrix	• ER and PR positive • Desmin positive • Actin negative • CD34 variable positive • RB1 retained • CYP2E1 positivity	*MTG1-CYP2E1* fusion	• Benign • No recurrence
Cellular angiofibroma	Vulvovaginal region	Reproductive age (fourth–fifth decade)	• Well limited • Mean size 2.8 cm	• Uniform spindle or ovoid cells • Scant cytoplasm • abundant vasculature of all size vessels from small to medium to thick	• ER and PR positive • CD34 variable positive • Desmin rarely positive (20%) • RB1 loss of expression	RB1 deletions	• Benign • Low risk of recurrence
Superficial myofibroblastoma	Cervicovaginal	Reproductive age (5th decade)	• Polyps • Nodule • Size <5 cm	• Superficial • Well limited • Grenz zone • Uniform spindle, ovoid or stellate cells • Collagenous stroma • Sieve, reticular, or patternless architecture	• ER and PR positive • CD34 and desmin positive • RB1 loss of expression	RB1 deletions	• Benign • No recurrence

	Location	Age	Macroscopy	Microscopy	IHC	Molecular	Behavior
Mammary-type genital myofibroblastoma	Vulva, vagina perineum	Wide range (fifth–sixth decade)	• Well limited • Median size 6.6 cm	• Well limited • Hypo/hypercellular • Spindle cells • Short fascicles band of collagen hyalinized	• ER and PR positive • CD34 and desmin positive • RB1 loss of expression	RB1 deletions	• Benign • Low risk of recurrence
Lipoblastoma-like tumor of the vulva	Vulva-surrounding tissues	Reproductive age (peak third decade)	• Well circumscribed • Gelatinous cut surface • Variable size (2–15 cm)	• Multilobular • Mature adipocytes, lipoblasts, and bland spindle cells • Myxoid stroma-rich ramified capillaries • Uniform distribution of the cellular density	• Variable CD34 and S100 expression • RB1 loss or mosaic expression • PLAG1, HMGA2, and MDM2 negative	• Simple genomic profiles • Lacks DDIT3 and PLAG1 rearrangements	• Benign • Low risk of local recurrence

Abbreviation: IHC, immunohistochemistry.

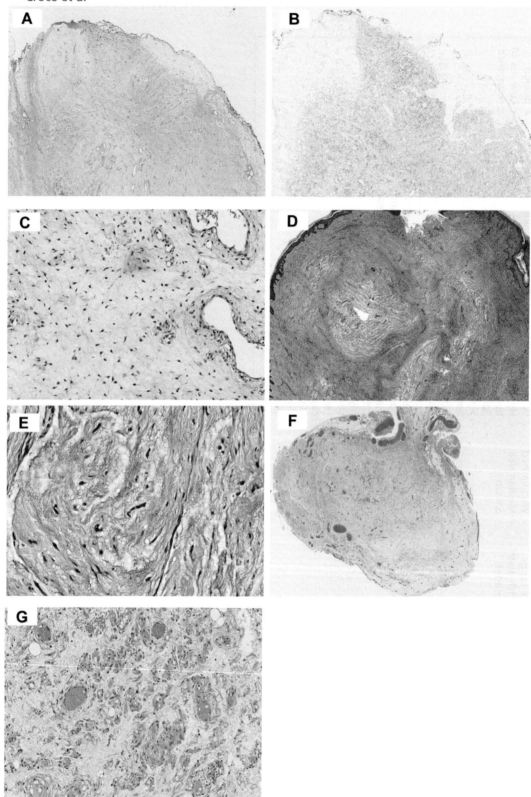

Fig. 1. Deep angiomyxoma showing infiltrative borders (*A*). The tumor strongly expresses HMGA2 nuclear staining (*B*). Edematous and myxoid stroma with uniform ovoid or spindle cells with unipolar or bipolar cytoplasmic processes with mild atypia (*C*). Superficial angiomyxoma. Multiple subcutaneous myxoid and hypocellular nodules (*D*) made of spindle or ovoid bland nuclei (*E*). Angiomyofibroblastoma alternates hypocellular with hypercellular areas (*F*). Spindle and plumped cells with plasmacytoid appearance, without atypia, arranged around thin-walled vessels (*G*). (*Courtesy of* Dr Carlos Parra-Herran.)

fashion given the paucicellular nature of the neoplasm (**Fig.** 1A, B, C).

Recently, rare morphologic features have been described in a subset of DA: neurofibroma-like appearance, hypercellular areas, microcystic and reticular stromal changes, nodular leiomyomatosis-like differentiation, and extensive collagenous/fibrosclerotic stroma.[7] These features can be diffuse in the tumor, but a classic morphology of DA, at least focal, was present and it was essential for the diagnosis.[2]

DA expresses Estrogen receptors (ER) and Progesterone receptors (PR), with variable CD34 and desmin positivity. Nuclear RB1 staining is retained. HMGA2 is expressed in 68% to 90% of cases[8,9]; unfortunately, this marker lacks specificity because it may also be positive in other mesenchymal tumors (44% of smooth muscle tumors, 19% of fibroepithelial polyps).[8] Despite this limitation, HMGA2 immunostaining can be useful to assess the tumor extent and the status of the margins (see **Fig.** 1B). HMGA2 expression is related in some cases to HMGA2 rearrangements (reported in one-third of DAs)[10–12] or by deregulated expression with an intact gene. Recently a new HMGA2-YAP1 fusion has been reported in a DA.[13] The chimeric gene is the result of the fusion between the first 3 exons of HMGA2 juxtaposed to exon 2 of whole YAP1 gene. The oncogenic mechanism of HMGA2-YAP1 fusion seems to be related to the immunohistochemical expression of HMGA2.[14] In the reported case, the immunohistochemical expression of HMGA2 or YAP1 was not described.[13]

SUPERFICIAL ANGIOMYXOMA

First described by Allen and colleagues[15] in 1988 in the cutaneous and subcutaneous tissues of the head and neck, superficial angiomyxoma has also been described in the dermis and subcutis of the vulva and groin. This benign tumor mostly occurs during reproductive age, especially in the fourth decade.

Grossly, superficial angiomyxoma frequently shows polypoid exophytic growth. Histologically, it is made of multiple non-infiltrative myxoid and hypocellular nodules containing spindle cells with ovoid bland nuclei and a delicate vasculature made of curvilinear vessels[16] (**Fig.** 1D, E). In case of absence of overlying skin in the sample, the presence of adnexal structures engulfed by the tumor guides the diagnosis. An inflammatory infiltrate rich in neutrophils is frequently associated to the tumor. Immunohistochemically HMGA2, ER, PR, and desmin are negative, CD34 is frequently positive.[16] Recently a loss of expression of PRKAR1A protein (1-alpha

regulatory subunit of protein kinase A) has been observed in 80% (12 of 15) of superficial angiomyxomas.[17]

Superficial angiomyxoma can recur but not in a destructive manner.[16] Multifocality should raise suspicion for an underlying Carney complex.[18]

ANGIOMYOFIBROBLASTOMA

First described by Fletcher and colleagues[19] in 1992, angiomyofibroblastoma is a well-delimited myofibroblastic tumor, usually smaller than 5 cm, arising especially in the vulva and less frequently in the vagina in reproductive age women (fourth to fifth decade).[20–22] The tumor is well circumscribed and shows alternating hypocellular with hypercellular areas of bland spindle and plumped cells with plasmacytoid appearance arranged around thin-walled vessels and capillaries; the matrix is edematous and collagenous, typically more prominent in hypocellular areas (**Fig.** 1F,G). A lipomatous pattern, with variable amount of mature adipocytes, has been reported.[23] The immunohistochemical profile is nonspecific with heterogeneous expression of desmin, ER, and PR, and inconstant CD34 positivity. RB1 expression is intact.

CELLULAR ANGIOFIBROMA

First described by Nucci and colleagues[24] in 1997, cellular angiofibroma is a benign well-circumscribed tumor located in the vulvovaginal region and more rarely in the peritoneum, occurring at reproductive age, especially in the fourth decade.[25,26] The tumor is variably but evenly cellular. The tumor is composed of uniform spindle to ovoid cells with inconspicuous nucleoli and scant cytoplasm embedded in a myxoid or hyalinized stroma. The vasculature is abundant and made of a mixture of variably sized vessels. A variable fatty component can be present, and the stroma can be hyalinized or show abundant wispy collagenous fibers[25–27] (**Fig.** 2A–C). Immunohistochemically, the tumor shows variable expression of CD34 (30%–60%) and desmin (20%) with frequent expression of ER and PR. Notably, RB1 staining is lost,[28,29] a finding related to 13q14 deletion.[29] An atypical "pseudosarcomatous" variant with aberrant expression of p53 has been described especially in the vulva without recurrence or metastasis.[25,30,31]

SUPERFICIAL MYOFIBROBLASTOMA

This entity, first described by Laskin and colleagues[32] in 2001, presents as a well-circumscribed tumor in the cervicovaginal area, separated of the overlying epithelium by a Grenz zone. The tumor occurs in a large age range but

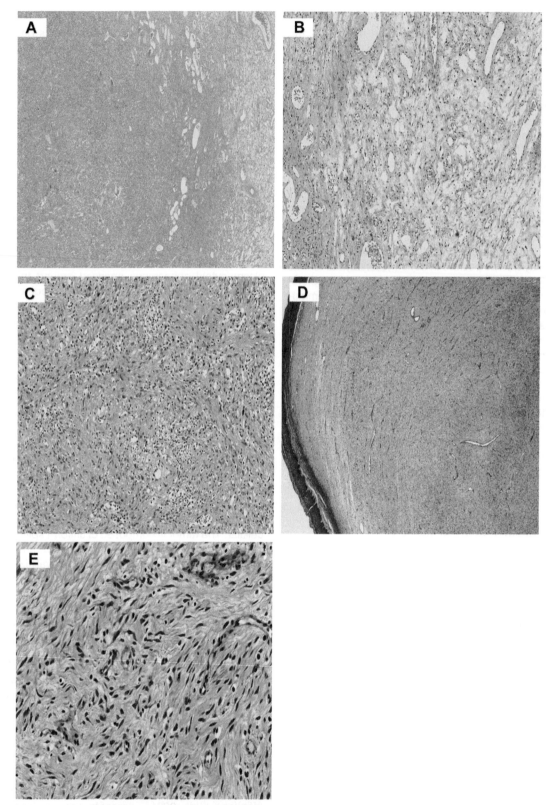

Fig. 2. Cellular angiofibroma. Cellular proliferation of spindle cells in hyalinized stroma with abundant vasculature (*A*) alternating with edematous stroma (*B*) rich in inflammatory infiltrate (*C*). Mammary-type genital myofibroblastoma. Dense subcutaneous lesion with delicate vasculature and variable cellularity (*D*) made of spindle myofibroblastic cells without atypia separated by collagen bands (*E*). (*Courtesy of* Dr Carlos Parra-Herran.)

especially in the fifth decade.[33] The tumor is made of uniform spindle, ovoid, or stellate cells embedded in a collagenous stroma. The cells may be arranged in sieve, reticular, or haphazard growth patterns.[32,34] On immunohistochemistry, the tumor cells express ER, PR, CD34, and desmin. RB1 staining has not been thoroughly studied. Superficial myofibroblastoma has significant morphologic and immunophenotype with myofibroblastoma (see later discussion). It is conceivable that both entities represent the same lesion; however, there are certain differences. Unlike myofibroblastoma, superficial myofibroblastoma shows a Grenz zone and a more frequent sievelike or lacelike arrangement of the cells; it also lacks an adipocytic component, which is often seen in myofibroblastoma. The investigators favoring the existence of superficial myofibroblastoma as a distinct entity also highlight its occurrence in a young age group and suggest a link with tamoxifen therapy.[33]

Recently, a MTG1-CYP2E1 fusion was present in 5 tested cases of angiomyofibroblastoma and in 60% (3 of 5) of superficial myofibroblastomas. The fusion was absent in potential mimickers such as DA, cellular angiofibroma, and fibroepithelial stromal polyp.[35] This fusion involves a 125-kb-long microdeletion in 10q26.3 which is not detectable by fluorescence in situ hybridization (FISH). The gene fusion derives from the assembling of the first 9 exons of the MTG1 gene juxtaposed to the 5' regulatory region of CYP2E1 gene followed by the entire sequence of the CYP2E1 gene.[35] The result is that CYP2E1, which is normally expressed only in the liver, is under the promoter of MTG1, which is ubiquitous. The MTG1-CYP2E1 fusion then leads to CYP2E1 overexpression, which can be highlighted by immunohistochemistry. Strong granular cytoplasmic staining is highly specific for the presence of the fusion. Conversely, MTG1 staining seems less specific because it was detected also in tumors lacking the MTG1-CYP2E1 fusion.[35]

MYOFIBROBLASTOMA (SO-CALLED MAMMARY TYPE)

Similar to myofibroblastoma of the breast, genital myofibroblastoma is a benign well-circumscribed tumor made of spindle myofibroblastic cells arranged in short fascicles separated by a band of ropy hyalinized collagen (especially in old lesions). The tumor is variably cellular with abundant collagen bands (Fig. 2D, E). Atypia and mitoses are absent. A fatty component is often seen, although in variable proportions, and can be scant.[36–38] Immunohistochemically, most of the myofibroblastomas express desmin and CD34.[37] Nearly 90% of the tumors lose the RB1 nuclear expression.[28,37]

Loss of heterozygosity of the region 13q14 including RB1 and FOXO1 genes is a recurrent event in cellular angiofibroma (up to 91% of reported cases)[25,28,29,39–43] and mammary-type myofibroblastoma (from 60% to 100%)[34] as well as spindle cell lipoma of soft tissue[28] suggesting that these entities are neoplastic variations of a single cytogenetic aberration.

LIPOBLASTOMA-LIKE TUMOR OF THE VULVA

Lipoblastoma-like tumor of the vulva (LLTV) is a benign mesenchymal tumor initially described in 2003 by Lae and colleagues.[44] This rare neoplasm typically presents as a variably sized mass in the genital region of young females (median age 29 years, range 13–56 years). Most cases follow a benign clinical course with rare local recurrences after complete surgical excision.[44–46] Notably, rare examples arising in the male population have also been reported.[47] Macroscopically, these lesions are generally well circumscribed and have a gelatinous cut surface. Histologically, they are composed of multiple lobules associated with a variable proportion of mature adipocytes, univacuolated or multivacuolated lipoblasts, and spindle cells (Fig. 3A–C). Importantly, the cells are uniformly distributed within the lobules and surrounded by an abundant myxoid matrix rich in ramified capillaries. Tumor cell nuclei are typically uniform, round to ovoid, and with fine chromatin. Mitotic activity is very low, and necrosis is absent. LLTV shows a nonspecific immunophenotype with variable CD34 and S100 expression (Fig. 3D, E). HMGA2, MDM2, and PLAG1 are negative in the vast majority of cases. RB1 may show a complete loss or a mosaic pattern of expression. Genetically, LLTV lacks PLAG1 and DDIT3 gene rearrangements and shows a "silent" genomic profile without significant variation in gene copy number (Fig. 3F).

Tumors in the differential diagnosis of LLTV include myxoid liposarcoma, spindle cell lipoma, atypical spindle cell lipomatous tumor, and lipoblastoma. Although histologically similar to LLTV, myxoid liposarcoma rarely arises in the genital region and often shows stromal mucin pools and increased cellularity at the periphery of the lobules. In challenging cases, the detection of DDIT3 rearrangements by molecular analysis can be used to confirm the diagnosis of myxoid liposarcoma. Similar to LLTV, spindle cell lipoma comprises a variable proportion of spindle cells, myxoid

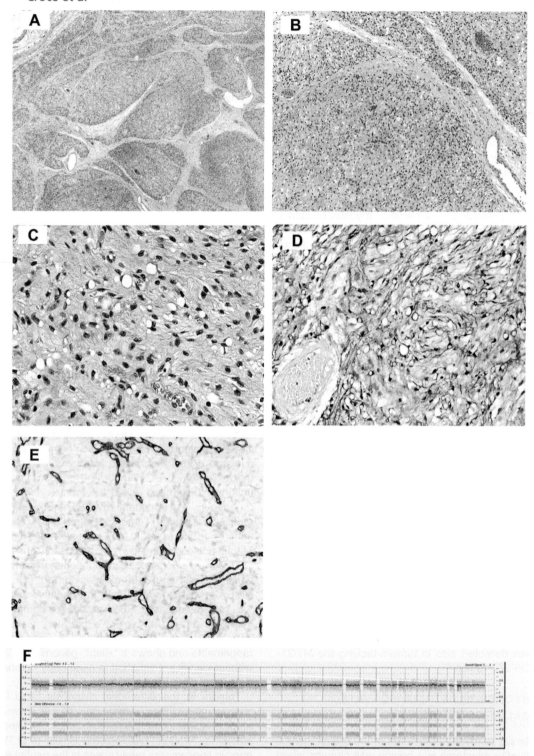

Fig. 3. Lipoblastoma-like tumor of the vulva. Typical low-power histology showing multiple tumor lobules separated by fibrous septa of variable thickness (*A*). The lobules show a homogeneous distribution of the cellularity. (*B*) High-power histology showing a mixture of univacuolated lipoblasts and spindle cells without nuclear atypia. The spindle cells have inconspicuous cytoplasm and uniform round to ovoid nuclei with fine chromatin. The stroma is myxoid and rich in ramified capillaries (*C*). S100 and CD34 expression are variable in LLTV. This case is diffusely and strongly positive with S100 (*D*) and negative with CD34 (*E*). Genomic copy number analysis of a case of lipoblastoma-like tumor of the vulva showing a normal diploid profile without genomic gains and losses. Chromosomes 1 to X/Y are plotted on the x-axis, whereas copy number alterations (*upper panel*) and B allele frequency (*lower panel*) are plotted on the y-axis (*F*).

stroma, and fat cells. Moreover, both lesions can show loss of RB1 staining. However, spindle cell lipoma predominantly arises in the back and shoulder of adult males and lacks the multilobular architecture and the arborizing capillary vasculature seen in LLTV. Atypical spindle cell lipomatous tumor is a recently described lesion composed of a variable proportion of atypical spindle cells, mature adipocytes, and lipoblasts embedded in a fibrous to myxoid stroma.[48] Atypical spindle cell lipomatous tumor can be distinguished from LLTV by the presence of atypical hyperchromatic spindle cells. Finally, lipoblastoma can closely mimic LLTV on histology, but it predominantly affects infants (<10 years) and rarely occurs in the genitals.[49,50] Moreover, most lipoblastomas harbor rearrangements of *PLAG1*, resulting in protein overexpression, which can be demonstrated with immunohistochemistry.

Key Points
SITE-SPECIFIC GENITAL MESENCHYMAL TUMORS

- Wide spectrum of indolent tumors with overlapping morphologic and immunohistochemical features.
- It is important to diagnose DA because of risk of local recurrence (up to 40%)
- *Deep angiomyxoma*
  ○ Located deep in genito-pelvi-perineal tissues
  ○ Infiltrative borders
  ○ Paucicellular myxoid tumor without atypia and low mitotic activity
  ○ Immunohistochemistry: expression of HMGA2 (68%–90%)
- *Superficial angiomyxoma*
  ○ Located in dermis or hypodermis of vulva and vagina
  ○ Noninfiltrative myxoid and hypocellular nodules
  ○ Loss of expression of PRKAR1A protein (in sporadic tumors as well as in Carney complex)
- *Angiomyofibroblastoma*
  ○ Located in vulva and vagina
  ○ Hypocellular and hypercellular foci of spindle and plumped cells disposed around vessels
  ○ *MTG1-CYP2E1* fusion (seen in 100% angiomyofibroblastomas and 60% of superficial myofibroblastomas)

  ○ CYP2E1 cytoplasmic immunostaining in the presence of the fusion
- *Lipoblastomalike tumor of the vulva*
  ○ Young females
  ○ Benign tumor with rare recurrences
  ○ Well-circumscribed gelatinous nodules
  ○ Mature adipocytes, lipoblasts, and spindle cells
  ○ Immunohistochemistry: nonspecific (variable CD34 and S100 expression)

NON-SITE-SPECIFIC MESENCHYMAL LESIONS

SMOOTH MUSCLE TUMORS

Among the lesions that are not site specific, smooth muscle tumors are the most frequent in the vulvovaginal region. Cervical uterine smooth muscle lesions are diagnosed according to uterine diagnostic criteria.[51,52] Until now, 2 classification systems coexisted, one for vulvar smooth muscle tumors[53,54] and one for the vagina.[55] According to the Tavassoli and Norris[55] classification systems published in 1979, a smooth muscle tumor of the vagina was classified as a leiomyosarcoma in the presence of either infiltrative margins or both of the following: (1) moderate to severe cytologic atypia and (2) greater than or equal to 5 mitoses/10 high-power field (HPF). According to the 1996 revised criteria, a vulvar leiomyosarcoma was diagnosed with 3 of 4 diagnostic features: (1) size greater than or equal to 5 cm, (2) moderate to severe cytologic atypia, (3) greater than or equal to 5 mitoses/10HPF, and (4) infiltrative margins.[54]

Recently the diagnostic criteria of uterine smooth muscle tumors have been applied to the lower genital tract and compared with the other classification systems in a large series of 71 smooth muscle tumors (53 vaginal and 18 vulvar).[56] The uterine smooth muscle tumor criteria were equally sensitive and more specific than site-specific criteria.[56] The uterine smooth muscle tumors criteria have the advantage of a pure morphologic classification, which allows to be free from macroscopic and clinical data, which are often difficult to assess (eg, margins status in conservative surgeries). Furthermore, the uterine criteria are based on histomorphology alone without taking into account the tumor size, which is practical because vulvovaginal leiomyosarcomas are often resected only partially or can be received fragmented.[57]

Using uterine criteria, 2 or 3 morphologic features warrant the diagnosis of a vulvar or a vaginal spindle cell leiomyosarcoma: diffuse moderate to severe atypia, greater than or equal to 4 mitoses/mm^2 (10 mitoses/10 HPF) or tumor cell necrosis (**Box 2**). Interestingly, this classification also demonstrated its diagnostic value when applied to leiomyoma variants and smooth muscle tumors of uncertain malignant potential.[57] While using uterine smooth muscle criteria, lesions with only 1 worrisome feature should be treated with caution, especially if the tumor size and border status are unknown or known to be worrisome (size $\geq$ 5 cm, infiltrative margins). In these situations, a diagnosis of leiomyoma can be favored, but ensuring completeness of excision and continuing monitoring can also be recommended. As myxoid and epithelioid variants of smooth muscle tumors are rare, the scheme needs to be further validated on larger series in this setting.

SOLITARY FIBROUS TUMOR

Solitary fibrous tumor (SFT) is known to occur in soft tissues, pleura, pelviperitoneum, and abdominal wall.[58–60] In the gynecologic tract, vulva is the most frequent site followed by vagina and uterine cervix.[61] In the lower genital tract, SFT tends to affect younger patients than in the upper genital tract (mean 48 vs 61) and the mean size in the lower genital tract is variable (5–6 cm).[61,62]

SFT is defined as a fibroblastic tumor with prominent thin-walled staghorn vasculature and *NAB2-STAT6* gene rearrangement.[63] In general, SFT shows well-circumscribed borders and is associated with patternless, trabecular, fascicular, or nested architectures. The cells are spindle to ovoid in shape, embedded in a collagenous stroma containing an abundant staghorn, hemangiopericytomalike vasculature[61] (**Fig. 4A, B**).

In published series, SFT of the female genital tract expresses CD34 (90%–95%).[61] ER and PR show a variable positivity (43% and 33%, respectively). STAT6 antibody (**Fig. 4C**) shows a high sensitivity varying from 90% to 100% in SFT of the gynecologic tract as in other sites.[61] It should be emphasized that STAT6 staining may be rarely seen in other soft tissue tumors, including 12% of dedifferentiated liposarcomas, 12% of unclassified sarcomas, and 8% of desmoid tumors,[64] as well as a subset of sex cord and stromal ovarian tumors (5% of ovarian fibromas and 33% of ovarian sclerosing stromal tumors)[61] and 33% of gynecologic inflammatory myofibroblastic tumors.

The Demicco multivariate risk stratification system helps in predicting the risk of adverse clinical outcome (in particular risk of metastasis). The system takes into account 4 features (1) patient age (<55 or $\geq$55 years), (2) tumor size (<5 cm, 5–10 cm, 10<15 cm, or >15 cm), (3) mitotic rate (0, 1–3, or $\geq$4 per 10 HPFs), and (4) presence or absence of necrosis.[59] This novel system has been shown to be superior in predicting the risk of metastasis compared with a univariate model assessing only the number of mitoses[62] (**Table 2**).

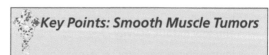

Key Points: Smooth Muscle Tumors

- Uterine morphologic diagnostic criteria are validated for lower genital tract smooth muscle tumors.

Any 2 of 3 of these criteria warrant the diagnosis of conventional (spindle cell) leiomyosarcoma.
- Moderate to severe cytologic atypia

- Greater than or equal to 4 mitoses/mm^2/$\geq$10 mitoses/10HPF

- Tumor cell necrosis

LOWER GENITAL TRACT SARCOMAS WITH KINASE-RELATED FUSIONS

Rare and until recently poorly understood, the repertoire of genetic alterations of fibrosarcoma-

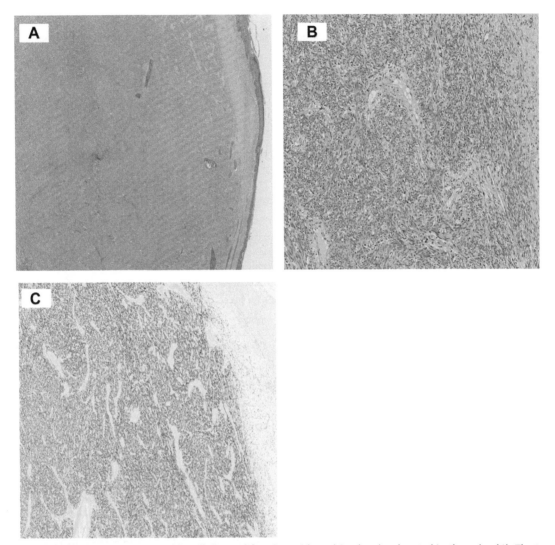

Fig. 4. Solitary fibrous tumor. Highly cellular proliferation with pushing borders located in the vulva (*A*). The tumor is highly cellular with staghorn vessels and ovoid to spindle-shaped cells arranged in a patternless architecture (*B*). STAT6 nuclear staining (*C*).

like tumors of the female genital tract has widened considerably due to the accessibility of RNA/DNA sequencing techniques applied to uterine (cervical) sarcomas. Furthermore, the involvement of tyrosine kinases in the fusions has sparked excitement because they may represent targetable alterations.[65–74] Fibrosarcoma-like tumors tend to present in the cervix of premenopausal or young women and are associated with variable morphologies and immunohistochemical profiles. Common characteristics include moderate cellularity, a spindle cell appearance (fibrosarcoma-like), frequent stromal and perivascular hyalinization, as well as a lymphoplasmacytoid infiltrate.

The emerging entities can be grouped as spindle cell tumors with *NTRK* fusions, *FGFR1*-

TACC1 fusion, *RET-SPECCIL* fusion, and *COL1A1-PDGFB* fusion. Tumors associated with *ALK* fusions (involved in inflammatory myofibroblastic tumors) can also occur in the cervix (see the article "Update on Uterine Mesenchymal Neoplasms" in this issue). This list is not exhaustive because new driver gene fusions are being continuously discovered.

NTRK-Fused Sarcomas/Spindle Cell Tumors with NTRK Fusion

The definition of these tumors is still an open debate: in gynecologic pathology they are reported as *NTRK* fusion-positive uterine sarcomas,[65,66,71,72,75] whereas in the soft tissue

Table 2
Modified four-variable risk stratification model for development of metastasis in solitary fibrous tumors

Risk Factor	Score
Age (y)	
<55	0
≥55	1
Tumor size (cm)	
<5	0
5 to <10	1
10 to <15	2
≥15	3
Mitotic count (/10 high-power fields)	
0	0
1–3	1
≥4	2
Tumor necrosis	
<10%	0
≥10%	1
Risk class	Total score
Low	0–3
Intermediate	4–5
High	6–7

Data from Demicco EG, Wagner MJ, Maki RG, et al. Risk assessment in solitary fibrous tumors: validation and refinement of a risk stratification model. *Mod Pathol*. 2017;30(10):1433-1442.[59]

the provisional terminology is spindle cell tumors with *NTRK* fusion.[70] The nomenclature will probably evolve in the future.

This tumor was first described by Mills and colleagues,[76] who in 2011 reported 3 spindle cell neoplasms of the uterine cervix arranged in a fascicular and herringbone pattern with CD34 and S100 expression. Subsequently, Chiang and colleagues[65] first reported their association with underlying *NTRK* fusions. In all reported *NTRK* rearrangements the oncogenic mechanism is similar: the 3′ *NTRK* region, which contains the kinase domain, is juxtaposed to the 5′ genomic region of the partner gene, which may be located in the same or a different chromosome than the *NTRK* genes (**Fig. 5E**). The chimeric protein results in ligand-independent constitutive activation of the kinase activity resulting in the promotion of cell proliferation, differentiation, and survival.[77]

NTRK-rearranged uterine sarcomas occur in young women (mean age 35 years, range 23–60 years) with a recent case occurring in a 13-year-old teenager.[78] These sarcomas are preferentially located in the cervix and are limited to the uterus at the moment of the diagnosis (stage I).[71] Microscopically, they tend to have a "fibrosarcoma-like" morphology with spindle cells arranged in fascicles or with a herringbone or patternless architecture. The vasculature is quite variable with thick hyalinized or thin vessels, sometimes showing a hemangiopericytoma-like pattern. An inflammatory lymphocytic infiltrate is seen in 70% of cases. The proliferation can entrap the endocervical glands mimicking an adenosarcoma. The cells are spindle shaped and uniform with scant cytoplasm, clumped chromatin, and mild-to-moderate nuclear atypia (**Fig. 5A, B**). The mitotic activity is highly variable (from 0 to 50 mitoses).

On immunohistochemistry these tumors are negative for smooth muscle markers (desmin and h-caldesmon) and for hormonal receptors. CD34 staining is variable (positive in 61% of the cases reported in the literature) and S100 protein is often positive (either diffuse or focal); however, experience is still limited owing to the low number of cases (**Fig. 5C, D**). Pan-TRK antibodies are strongly and diffusely expressed, showing a cytoplasmic, a nuclear or a cytoplasmic and perinuclear pattern of staining, depending on the partner gene. Pan-Trk staining is useful to differentiate *NTRK*-fused sarcoma from adenosarcomas.[75] Nonetheless, some caveats have been recently highlighted about

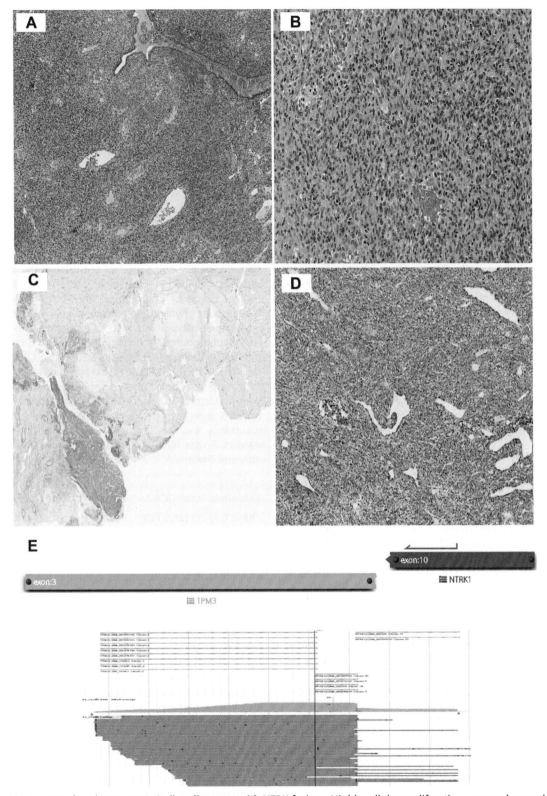

Fig. 5. NTRK-fused sarcomas/spindle cell tumors with NTRK fusions. Highly cellular proliferation arranged around cervical normal crypts mimicking an adenosarcoma (*A*). Uniform monotonous spindle cell tumor with brisk mitotic activity (*B*). CD34 staining can be heterogeneous and focal (*C*). panTrk shows strong and diffuse cytoplasmic staining (*D*). Fusion transcript between the exon 3 of *TMP3* and exon 10 of *NTRK1* by targeted RNA sequencing (*E*). Image E courtesy of Dr I Hostein.

pan-Trk specificity[65,79,80] because this marker may stain up to 91% of high-grade endometrial stromal sarcomas, with a sensitivity and a specificity of pan-Trk immunostaining of 80% and 74%, respectively.[79] For this reason, pan-Trk positivity by immunohistochemistry needs to be confirmed by the detection of the NTRK fusion by molecular techniques as RNA sequencing.

Because these tumors can recur, and 1 patient died of disease, they should be regarded as potentially malignant.[71] In pediatric and soft tissue NTRK-fused sarcomas, the mitotic count, the presence of marked atypia, and the involvement of NTRK3 correlate with unfavorable clinical course.[70] No prognostic factor has been identified in cervical NTRK fusion sarcomas due to the limited amount of available evidence. Because NTRK-fused sarcomas belong to the family of sarcomas with "simple genomic profile,"[66] it is possible that increased genomic complexity may be acquired or present in aggressive cases as recently suggested by Vargas and colleagues on a series of 6 NTRK fusion sarcomas (5 fibrosarcomalike tumors located in soft tissue, lung, thyroid, and liver and 1 in uterine cervix).[81] Further studies are required to confirm this hypothesis.

SARCOMAS WITH *FGFR1-TACC1* FUSION

A cervical sarcoma with FGFR1-TACC1 fusion has been recently reported in a single case report of cervical "fibrosarcoma-like" sarcoma.[72] The tumor occurred in a 48-year-old patient presenting with a 5.3-cm large cervical mass.[72] The tumor showed moderate cellularity and was composed of spindle cell appearance with moderate atypia and associated with an inflammatory infiltrate. On immunohistochemistry the tumor expressed diffusely CD34 and S100 protein and showed patchy positivity for CD10 and panTrk despite the absence of an NTRK fusion. The patient developed pelvic and lung metastases 15 months later.[72]

The fusion between FGFR1 (fibroblast growth factor receptor 1), which is a tyrosine kinase receptor, and TACC1 (transforming acidic coiled-coil1) has also been described in glioblastomas and GIST where this fusion is responsible for alteration of chromosome segregation during the mitosis contributing to the acquisition of aneuploidy.[82,83] This fusion is of great interest because it may be targeted with FGRF inhibitors, even if currently the efficacy of FGFR inhibitors seems to be low.[84]

Sarcomas with *RET-SPECC1L* Fusion

The recently reported RET-SPECC1L fusion enriches and expands the genomic spectrum of fibrosarcoma-like tumors of the cervix. In analogy to pediatric spindle cell tumors of the soft tissue, RET fusion seems to represent an alternative to NTRK gene fusion.[85] The oncogenic mechanism lies in the fusion between the exon 12 of RET (rearranged during transfection), which conserves the tyrosine kinase activity, and the exon 9 of SPECC1L (sperm antigen with calponin homology and coiled-coil domains), which preserves the dimerization coiled-coil motifs.[85] This fusion results in the constitutive activation of RET, which belongs to the superfamily of tyrosine kinase receptors, and the subsequent activation of downstream signaling pathway.[86–88]

The lesion occurred in a 20-year-old woman presenting with a 3.4-cm large cervical mass microscopically composed of monotonous spindle cells arranged in a fascicular pattern with infiltrative borders. The tumor showed marked perivascular hyalinization and a herringbone vasculature. Atypia was mild to moderate with a low mitotic count (4 mitoses/10 HPF). The tumor diffusely expressed CD34 and S100 but SOX10, desmin, RE, PR, and BCOR, were negative. Pan-TRK was not contributory. Total hysterectomy was performed following a prior conization with positive margins. The patient did not develop recurrence and was alive without evidence of disease at 2-year follow-up without complementary adjuvant therapy.[74]

Sarcomas with *COL1A1-PDGFB* Fusion

These tumors have been recently described in the uterine corpus and in the cervix.[66,89] These tumors share the same cytogenetic alteration with dermatofibrosarcoma protuberans (including vulvar dermatofibrosarcoma) as well as pediatric giant cell fibroblastoma.[90–95] The oncogenic mechanism consists in the activation of PDGFB (platelet-derived growth factor B), which belongs to the tyrosine kinase family, via fusion that places PDGFB under the control of the COL1A1 (collagen type 1 alpha 1 chain) promoter.[91] COL1A1-PDGFB sarcomas are rare and may be localized both in the cervix and in the uterine corpus. Affected patients are older than patients with NTRK-fused sarcomas (mean age 58 years).[66,71,89] Among the 5 patients reported in the literature, 1 died of disease (after 60 months), 1 was alive with disease at 2 months, 1 was alive without disease at 10 months, 1 was a recent case, and 1 was alive with lung metastases, which responded to imatinib therapy.[66,72,89]

Microscopically the tumors appear "blue," arranged in a storiform or herringbone pattern of growth with infiltrative borders (**Fig. 6**A). The cells are uniformly spindle or ovoid with scant

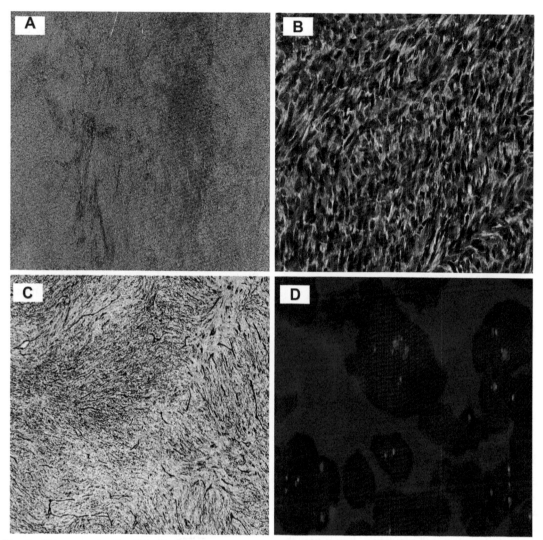

Fig. 6. *COL1A1-PDGFB* fused sarcoma. Highly cellular "blue" tumor showing a storiform and solid pattern of growth (*A*). Uniform ovoid cells with scant cytoplasm (*B*). Positive CD34 staining (*C*). FISH dual fusion highlighting the orange/green fusion signal between *COL1A1* and *PDGFB* genes (*D*).

cytoplasm (**Fig.** 6B). At the immunohistochemical level, the cells are positive for CD34, which could be lost in the setting of fibrosarcoma transformation.[66] On the contrary, S100, ER, PR, and smooth muscle markers are negative (**Fig.** 6C). There are contradictory data about panTrk staining across 2 distinct studies because this antibody was negative in the first 4 cases reported in the literature[66] and patchy positive in another study,[72] using 2 different antibodies. The *COL1A1-PDGFB* fusion was detected by dual fusion FISH (**Fig.** 6D) and/ or RNA sequencing.

Interestingly, *COL1A1-PDGFB* fusion sarcoma may be targeted, although indirectly, with imatinib. In fact, a complete clinical response was reported in a stage IV *COL1A1-PDGFB* sarcoma of the cervix.[89]

Key Points
SARCOMAS WITH KINASE-RELATED FUSIONS (*NTRK, RET, FGFR1, COL1A1-PDGB*)

○ Rare tumors

○ Young women (older for *COL1A1-PDGFB*-associated sarcomas)

○ More often cervical (less frequently uterine corpus, especially for NTRK-associated sarcomas)

○ Morphology: fibrosarcoma-like appearance, monotonous spindle cells with variable atypia and mitotic count; fascicular, herringbone, or patternless architecture

- ○ Immunohistochemistry
  - ■ *NTRK*: panTrk cytoplasmic staining
    - • ER, PR, and smooth muscle markers negative
    - • CD34 variable expression (61% positive)
    - • S100 positive (can be focal)
  - ■ *FGRF1*
    - • ER, PR, and smooth muscle markers negative
    - • CD34 and S100 positive
    - • Pan-Trk can be weak and patchy
  - ■ *RET*
    - • ER, PR, and smooth muscle markers negative
    - • CD34 and S100 positive
  - ■ *COL1A1-PDGFB*
    - • CD34 positive (could be lost in the setting of fibrosarcoma transformation)
    - • S100 negative
    - • Pan-Trk discordant results (negative in one series,[66] weakly positive in another[72])
  - ○ RNA sequencing essential to detect the fusions

SARCOMAS WITH *MEIS1-NCOA1-2* Fusion

Recently, a series of spindle cell sarcomas arising in the genitourinary tract harboring *MEIS1-NCOA1/2* gene fusions has been reported.[96,97] *MEIS1* (myeloid ecotropic viral integration site) is implicated in stem cell regulation, tumor growth, and myocardial regeneration.[98] *NCOA* (nuclear receptor coactivator) genes encode nuclear hormone receptor transcriptional coactivators, which facilitate chromatin remodeling and transcription.[99] The gene fusions occur between the exons 6 or 7 of *MEIS1* gene and the exons 12 or 13 of *NCOA1/2*[96,97]; the oncogenic mechanisms of the fusion remain unknown.

Reported tumors were located in the kidney, scrotum, pararectal tissues, vagina, and uterine corpus. We have also encountered this lesion in the vulva (unpublished case). Interestingly, *MEIS* seems to share similar anatomic predilection with *BCOR* and *YWHAE*-fused sarcomas.

Microscopically, the lesions shared a common morphology: tumor cells displayed monomorphic nuclei and were spindle or ovoid in shape arranged in short fascicles with alternating hypercellular and hypocellular areas in the presence of a myxoid to hyalinized stroma.[96] The immunohistochemical profile is nonspecific, with CD10 expression, cyclin D1 focal positivity, and BCOR negativity. ER is negative or weakly positive. Two tumors were described in the uterine corpus mimicking an undifferentiated uterine sarcoma uniform type, one showing aggregates of primitive cells and the second showing sheets of benign adipocytes.[96,97] The first tumor had been initially classified as a low-grade endometrial stromal sarcoma.

Because local recurrences were seen in this series, *MEIS1-NCOA1/2* fusion sarcomas should be considered at least as having a low malignant potential. More detailed clinicopathological and genetic data are needed.

RHABDOMYOSARCOMAS OF THE LOWER GENITAL TRACT

Rhabdomyosarcomas are malignant mesenchymal tumors that, by definition, display striated muscle differentiation. These tumors are highly heterogeneous at the microscopic and genetic levels and cannot be extensively covered in this review (for a recent review, refer to Leiner and colleagues[100]). Nonetheless, a specific subtype of rhabdomyosarcomas with a predilection for the lower female genital tract is discussed: rhabdomyosarcomas with *DICER1* mutations (DICER1-RMS).[101,102]

At the morphologic level, DICER1-RMS are undistinguishable from other embryonal rhabdomyosarcomas (eRMS). DICER1-RMS share a similar predilection for the perineal region; therefore, a DICER1-RMS should be systematically suspected before rendering a diagnosis of eRMS in the genitourinary tract. Moreover, near 100% of eRMS of the cervix harbor *DICER1* mutations, whereas eRMS of the vagina are all *DICER1* wild-type, as well as most cervical adenosarcomas that enter in the differential diagnosis.[103,104] Cervical müllerian adenosarcoma is the main differential diagnosis because it may contain a heterologous component of rhabdomyosarcoma. The distinction between an adenosarcoma with a heterologous eRMS component and a pure eRMS may be extremely arduous to make and has potentially tremendous clinical consequences. Practically, in the absence of a *DICER1* mutation, a diagnosis of cervical adenosarcoma should be favored over the diagnosis of an eRMS.[103,104] Clinically, patient's age varies widely with a reported median age of 36 years.[105] On microscopy, the presence of cartilaginous foci (**Fig. 7**A) or more rarely of ossification hints toward a DICER1-RMS. Apart from this, they display the classical features of eRMS, composed of thin spindle cells with variable rhabdomyoblastic differentiation (**Fig. 7**B–E). These tumors are heterogeneous,

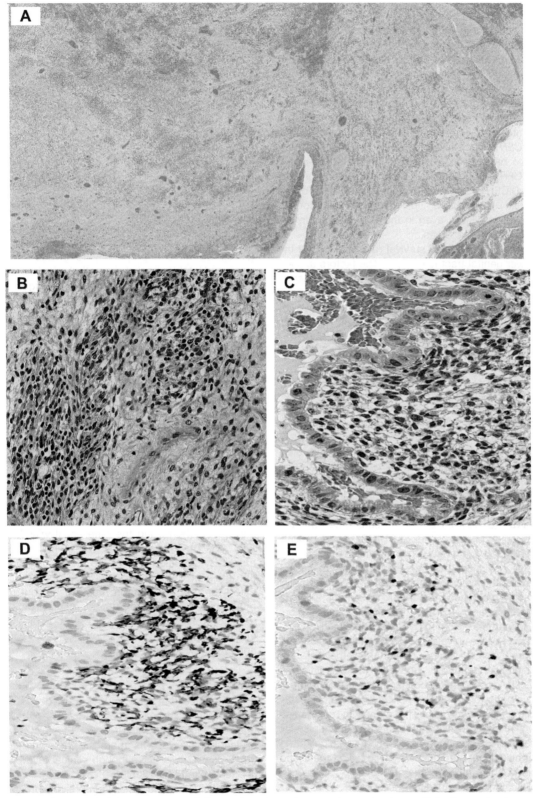

Fig. 7. Embryonal rhabdomyosarcoma of the cervix. Polypoid tumor alternating hypocellular hemorrhagic areas with hypercellular foci of spindle or ovoid immature cells (*A, B*). The neoplastic cells condense underneath the epithelium forming a cambium layer (*C*). Tumor cells show strong and diffuse expression of desmin (*D*) but focal expression of myogenin (*E*).

showing variation of cellularity, especially in cases abutting the mucosa, in which a distinct rim of hypercellular tumor cells is seen immediately underneath the epithelium, a phenomenon referred to as the "cambium layer" (see **Fig. 7**C).

At the molecular level, these tumors show inactivating mutations of *DICER1,* which encodes a protein involved in the biogenesis of micro-RNAs. *DICER1* mutations are mostly somatic but can also be germline in the setting of the so-called DICER1 syndrome.[106,107] The methylation profiles of DICER1-RMS seem to differ from those of the other subfamilies of rhabdomyosarcomas, including eRMS, even in those developed in the same anatomic areas.[105]

The 5-year overall survival rate of eRMS of the lower genital tract is 68%.[108] The factors associated with a better survival are young age, absence of distant metastasis, negative lymph node, complete surgery,[109] and *DICER1* mutation.[105]

SARCOMAS WITH DEFICIENCY OF BAF COMPLEXES

BAF (BRG1-associated factors, also known as SWI/SNF) complexes are multiprotein complexes involved in the regulation of gene transcription. *SMARCB1* and *SMARCA4* subunits are the most frequently mutated subunits of these complexes, yielding to aggressive tumors that develop preferentially in the ovary and uterus (*SMARCA4*-deficient uterine sarcomas[108] and small cell carcinomas of the ovary, hypercalcemic type, which are not discussed in this review) and in the vulva (*SMARCB1*-deficient sarcomas of the vulva[110]). In soft tissue, *SMARCB1* loss is mainly seen in 3 tumor subtypes: epithelioid sarcomas (ES), malignant rhabdoid tumors, and malignant myoepithelioma (also referred to as myoepithelial carcinoma). These tumors are ubiquitous and can therefore also occur in the vulvoperineal region. The features harbored by *SMARCB1*-deficient sarcomas of the vulva are somewhat intermediate between these tumor types. Nonetheless, the differential diagnosis between these entities is mostly gnoseological because all share an aggressive behavior. Altogether, *SMARCB1*-deficient sarcomas of the vulva seem to comply in most cases with the diagnostic criteria of ES or myoepithelial carcinomas. The morphologic nuances highlighted in this subset of tumors may only reflect the tissue context in which the tumors develop rather than clinically meaningful differences.

Malignant Rhabdoid Tumors

These tumors were the first human malignancies linked to *SMARCB1* inactivation[111] and mostly seen in the pediatric population. These tumors may harbor varied cytomorphology ranging from rounded to epithelioid or rhabdoid appearances. On immunohistochemistry, tumor cells express focally cytokeratins and/or EMA; nuclear SMARCB1 expression is lost (absent). These tumors display flat diploid genetic profiles that are distinct from those of ES.[112,113]

Epithelioid Sarcomas

ES affects primarily young adults and has been described in varied anatomic locations except the central nervous system. ES are malignant tumors associated with a protracted course with high rates of recurrence (70%) and metastasis (50%). ES have a propensity to invade lymph nodes. Notably, a clinicopathological series focused on vulvar counterparts of ES suggests a similarly aggressive clinical behavior.[110]

At the morphologic level, ES have 2 main presentations. First, they have a heterogeneous hybrid appearance with admixed epithelioid and spindle cell components, embedded in a fibrous stroma that often contains an abundant inflammatory infiltrate. This morphologic presentation has been referred to as the classical type of ES. ES may also present as solid deep tumor masses that harbor striking epithelioid and rhabdoid cytomorphology (**Fig. 8**A, B). ES cells typically harbor large ovoid vesicular nuclei, with limited, if any, anisokaryosis. All ES strongly express cytokeratins and/or EMA (**Fig. 8**D) but not squamous cell markers (p63 and p40). In rare cases, the expression of keratins or EMA can be patchy raising the differential with MRT (Fig. 8C, D).CD34 is expressed in half of the cases. By definition, SMARCB1 is lost in virtually all cases of ES (**Fig. 8**E). *SMARCB1* is inactivated through deletions in most cases, but not mutations.[113,114] These tumors display diploid genetic profiles with few recurrent copy number alterations apart from deletions of *SMARCB1* and *CDKN2A* locus.[113]

SMARCB1-Deficient Myoepithelial Carcinomas

It is estimated that 10% to 20% of myoepithelial carcinomas, also called malignant myoepitheliomas, are associated with SMARCB1 loss.[115] Their clinical behavior seems aggressive, keeping with outcomes seen in ES, although clinical follow-up is often limited in available series.

By definition, myoepithelial tumors coexpress at least one epithelial marker among AE1/E3, EMA, p63, and one neural marker (among SOX10, S100, or GFAP). These tumors display heterogeneous intratumor and intertumor morphologies;

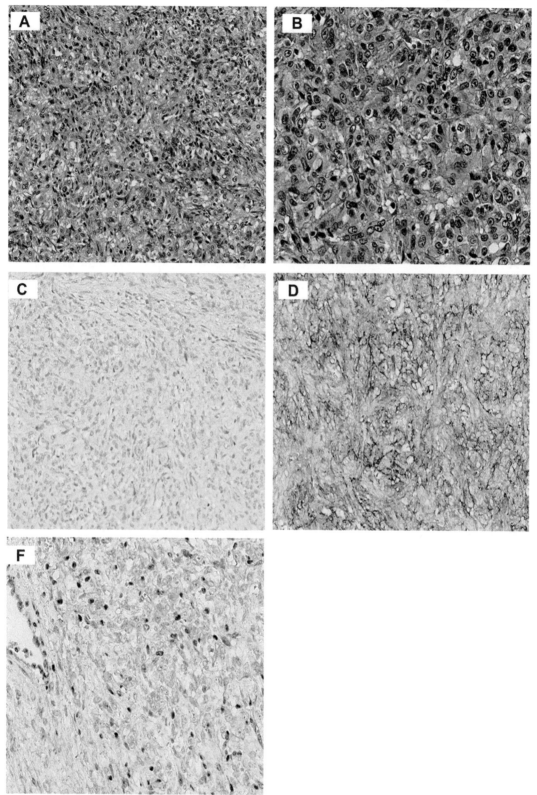

Fig. 8. SMARCB1-deficient vulvar sarcoma/epithelioid sarcoma. This SMARCB1-deficient vulvar sarcoma developed in the vulvoperineal area of a 52-year female. The tumor has a solid architecture composed of sheets of epithelioid cells with scant accompanying stroma (*A*). At high-power magnification (X40), tumor cells display large vesicular nuclei devoid of pleomorphism along with a large eosinophilic cytoplasm (*B*). Tumor cells are negative for pan-cytokeratins (*C*) but express diffusely EMA (*D*) and have loss of SMARCB1 nuclear expression, whereas normal cells retain its signal (*E*).

they display an abundant stroma that may be hyaline or myxoid, in which the tumor cells arrange in trabeculae, nests, or cords. In this subtype of tumors, the nuclei are large and atypical with large nucleoli; there is brisk mitotic activity and tumor necrosis. On immunohistochemistry, tumor cells commonly express smooth muscle actin. Loss of SMARCB1 expression is seen in 10% of myoepithelial tumors, with strong predilection for myoepithelial carcinoma.[115] This loss seems mostly related to genomic deletions as in ES.[113]

SMARCB1-Deficient Sarcomas of the Vulva

This descriptive term has been proposed to account for SMARCB1-deficient tumors that do not harbor the typical features of ES or myoepithelial carcinomas.[110] Nonetheless, only 3 of 14 SMARCB1-deficient tumors of the vulva did fall into this category after a comprehensive review.[110] The tumors falling into this "wastebasket" category had a hybrid appearance, admixing spindled, epithelioid, and rhabdoid components (**Fig. 9**). On immunohistochemistry, tumor cells expressed focally cytokeratins, EMA, and CD34.

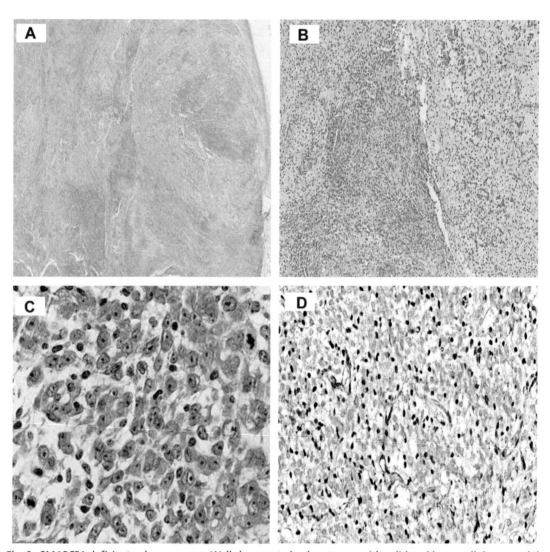

Fig. 9. *SMARCB1*-deficient vulvar sarcoma. Well-demarcated vulvar tumor with solid and loose cellular areas (*A*). Solid areas are made of sheets of epithelioid cells contrasting with areas rich in myxoid stroma. In these areas the tumor cells are spindle to epithelioid (*B, C*). There is diffuse loss of SMARCB1 (INI1, BAF47) (*D*). Tumor cells do not express neural markers; cytokeratins and EMA were focally positive (not shown). The absence of the typical phenotype seen in epithelioid sarcomas and myoepithelioid carcinoma yielded to the diagnosis of SMARCB1-deficient vulvar sarcoma.

Recent evidence suggests that the so-called primary yolk sac tumors of the vulva (PYSTV) may represent a morphologic variant of SMARCB1-deficient sarcomas of the vulva.[116] Historically it is known that PYSTV is associated with elevated levels of alfa fetoprotein (AFP). Moreover, they largely resemble their ovarian counterpart because they have the typical architecture of microcysts, papillae, glands, and/or cords, sometimes with distinct "Shiller-Duval bodies." PYSTV have an immunoprofile otherwise typical of yolk sac tumors, which includes diffuse expression of SALL4, glypican 3, and cytokeratins. PYSTV have recently been shown to be associated with recurrent SMARCB1 loss, thus suggesting that they are not bona fide yolk sac tumors and represent instead SMARCB1-deficient vulvar sarcomas. These preliminary findings need to be further confirmed with larger series.

In SMARCB1-deficient vulvar sarcomas, SMARCB1 is inactivated through genomic deletions.[110] Vulvar "Yolk sac-like" tumors are also associated with SMARCB1 deletions, whereas the common genetic alterations of germ cell tumors are not present.[116]

Myoepithelioma-like Tumors of the Vulva

These tumors are extremely rare with only one small clinicopathological series available describing these tumors,[117] mostly in Asian populations.[118,119] These tumors seem to represent a benign counterpart of SMARCB1-deficient neoplasms of the vulva because only local recurrence has been reported in these tumors[117]; they are superficial, located in the subcutis, presenting with a multinodular pattern.[117] These tumors are well delineated with pushing borders, distinct from the infiltrative pattern seen in ES and myoepithelial carcinomas. At first glance, the tumor has a worrisome epithelioid to rhabdoid cytomorphology. However, careful examination confirms the absence of mitotic activity and tumor necrosis. The tumors contain a variable amount of myxoid stroma, in which the cells may have reticular or trabecular arrangements. The nuclei are rather monotonous without overt pleomorphism; their morphology is especially reminiscent of myoepitheliomas, but the tumor cells do not express neural markers such as S100 protein and GFAP. CD34 is also negative. Cytokeratins are positive in only a subset of cases, whereas SMARCB1 is always lost. These tumors express consistently estrogen and progesterone receptors, which is rarely seen in ES and myoepitheliomas.[117] The molecular mechanism underlying SMARCB1 inactivation has not been studied yet, although it is known

that these tumors lack EWSR1 and NR4A3 rearrangements.[117]

DISCLOSURE

The authors declare no conflict of interest.

REFERENCES

1. Schoolmeester JK, Fritchie KJ. Genital soft tissue tumors. J Cutan Pathol 2015;42(7):441–51.
2. Fetsch JF, Laskin WB, Lefkowitz M, et al. Aggressive angiomyxoma: a clinicopathologic study of 29 female patients. Cancer 1996;78(1):79–90.
3. Chapel DB, Cipriani NA, Bennett JA. Mesenchymal lesions of the vulva. Semin Diagn Pathol 2021; 38(1):85–98.
4. Steeper TA, Rosai J. Aggressive angiomyxoma of the female pelvis and perineum. Report of nine cases of a distinctive type of gynecologic soft-tissue neoplasm. Am J Surg Pathol 1983;7(5): 463–75.
5. Begin LR, Clement PB, Kirk ME, et al. Aggressive angiomyxoma of pelvic soft parts: a clinicopathologic study of nine cases. Hum Pathol 1985;16(6): 621–8.
6. Granter SR, Nucci MR, Fletcher CD. Aggressive angiomyxoma: reappraisal of its relationship to angiomyofibroblastoma in a series of 16 cases. Histopathology 1997;30(1):3–10.
7. Magro G, Angelico G, Michal M, et al. The Wide Morphological Spectrum of Deep (Aggressive) Angiomyxoma of the Vulvo-Vaginal Region: A Clinicopathologic Study of 36 Cases, including Recurrent Tumors. Diagnostics (Basel) 2021;11(8).
8. Harkness R, McCluggage WG. HMGA2 Is a Useful Marker of Vulvovaginal Aggressive Angiomyxoma But May Be Positive in Other Mesenchymal Lesions at This Site. Int J Gynecol Pathol 2021;40(2):185–9.
9. Dreux N, Marty M, Chibon F, et al. Value and limitation of immunohistochemical expression of HMGA2 in mesenchymal tumors: about a series of 1052 cases. Mod Pathol 2010;23(12):1657–66.
10. Nucci MR, Weremowicz S, Neskey DM, et al. Chromosomal translocation t(8;12) induces aberrant HMGIC expression in aggressive angiomyxoma of the vulva. Genes Chromosomes Cancer 2001; 32(2):172–6.
11. Medeiros F, Erickson-Johnson MR, Keeney GL, et al. Frequency and characterization of HMGA2 and HMGA1 rearrangements in mesenchymal tumors of the lower genital tract. Genes Chromosomes Cancer 2007;46(11):981–90.
12. Micci F, Panagopoulos I, Bjerkehagen B, et al. Deregulation of HMGA2 in an aggressive angiomyxoma with t(11;12)(q23;q15). Virchows Arch 2006;448(6):838–42.

13. Lee MY, da Silva B, Ramirez DC, et al. Novel HMGA2-YAP1 fusion gene in aggressive angiomyxoma. BMJ Case Rep 2019;12(5).

14. Mansoori B, Mohammadi A, Ditzel HJ, et al. HMGA2 as a Critical Regulator in Cancer Development. Genes (Basel) 2021;12(2).

15. Allen PW, Dymock RB, MacCormac LB. Superficial angiomyxomas with and without epithelial components. Report of 30 tumors in 28 patients. Am J Surg Pathol 1988;12(7):519–30.

16. Fetsch JF, Laskin WB, Tavassoli FA. Superficial angiomyxoma (cutaneous myxoma): a clinicopathologic study of 17 cases arising in the genital region. Int J Gynecol Pathol 1997;16(4):325–34.

17. Hafeez F, Krakowski AC, Lian CG, et al. Sporadic superficial angiomyxomas demonstrate loss of PRKAR1A expression. Histopathology 2021;80(6):1001–3.

18. Kirschner LS, Carney JA, Pack SD, et al. Mutations of the gene encoding the protein kinase A type I-alpha regulatory subunit in patients with the Carney complex. Nat Genet 2000;26(1):89–92.

19. Fletcher CD, Tsang WY, Fisher C, et al. Angiomyofibroblastoma of the vulva. A benign neoplasm distinct from aggressive angiomyxoma. Am J Surg Pathol 1992;16(4):373–82.

20. Nielsen GP, Rosenberg AE, Young RH, et al. Angiomyofibroblastoma of the vulva and vagina. Mod Pathol 1996;9(3):284–91.

21. Hisaoka M, Kouho H, Aoki T, et al. Angiomyofibroblastoma of the vulva: a clinicopathologic study of seven cases. Pathol Int 1995;45(7):487–92.

22. Laskin WB, Fetsch JF, Tavassoli FA. Angiomyofibroblastoma of the female genital tract: analysis of 17 cases including a lipomatous variant. Hum Pathol 1997;28(9):1046–55.

23. Cao D, Srodon M, Montgomery EA, et al. Lipomatous variant of angiomyofibroblastoma: report of two cases and review of the literature. Int J Gynecol Pathol 2005;24(2):196–200.

24. Nucci MR, Granter SR, Fletcher CD. Cellular angiofibroma: a benign neoplasm distinct from angiomyofibroblastoma and spindle cell lipoma. Am J Surg Pathol 1997;21(6):636–44.

25. Flucke U, van Krieken JH, Mentzel T. Cellular angiofibroma: analysis of 25 cases emphasizing its relationship to spindle cell lipoma and mammary-type myofibroblastoma. Mod Pathol 2011;24(1):82–9.

26. Iwasa Y, Fletcher CD. Cellular angiofibroma: clinicopathologic and immunohistochemical analysis of 51 cases. Am J Surg Pathol 2004;28(11):1426–35.

27. McCluggage WG, Ganesan R, Hirschowitz L, et al. Cellular angiofibroma and related fibromatous lesions of the vulva: report of a series of cases with a morphological spectrum wider than previously described. Histopathology 2004;45(4):360–8.

28. Chen BJ, Marino-Enriquez A, Fletcher CD, et al. Loss of retinoblastoma protein expression in spindle cell/pleomorphic lipomas and cytogenetically related tumors: an immunohistochemical study with diagnostic implications. Am J Surg Pathol 2012;36(8):1119–28.

29. Maggiani F, Debiec-Rychter M, Vanbockrijck M, et al. Cellular angiofibroma: another mesenchymal tumour with 13q14 involvement, suggesting a link with spindle cell lipoma and (extra)-mammary myofibroblastoma. Histopathology 2007;51(3):410–2.

30. Chen E, Fletcher CD. Cellular angiofibroma with atypia or sarcomatous transformation: clinicopathologic analysis of 13 cases. Am J Surg Pathol 2010;34(5):707–14.

31. Kandil DH, Kida M, Laub DR, et al. Sarcomatous transformation in a cellular angiofibroma: a case report. J Clin Pathol 2009;62(10):945–7.

32. Laskin WB, Fetsch JF, Tavassoli FA. Superficial cervicovaginal myofibroblastoma: fourteen cases of a distinctive mesenchymal tumor arising from the specialized subepithelial stroma of the lower female genital tract. Hum Pathol 2001;32(7):715–25.

33. Ganesan R, McCluggage WG, Hirschowitz L, et al. Superficial myofibroblastoma of the lower female genital tract: report of a series including tumours with a vulval location. Histopathology 2005;46(2):137–43.

34. Magro G, Caltabiano R, Kacerovska D, et al. Vulvovaginal myofibroblastoma: expanding the morphological and immunohistochemical spectrum. A clinicopathologic study of 10 cases. Hum Pathol 2012;43(2):243–53.

35. Maggiani F, Debiec-Rychter M, Verbeeck G, et al. Extramammary myofibroblastoma is genetically related to spindle cell lipoma. Virchows Arch 2006;449(2):244–7.

36. Howitt BE, Fletcher CD. Mammary-type Myofibroblastoma: Clinicopathologic Characterization in a Series of 143 Cases. Am J Surg Pathol 2016;40(3):361–7.

37. McMenamin ME, Fletcher CD. Mammary-type myofibroblastoma of soft tissue: a tumor closely related to spindle cell lipoma. Am J Surg Pathol 2001;25(8):1022–9.

38. Panagopoulos I, Gorunova L, Bjerkehagen B, et al. Loss of chromosome 13 material in cellular angiofibromas indicates pathogenetic similarity with spindle cell lipomas. Diagn Pathol 2017;12(1):17.

39. Uehara K, Ikehara F, Shibuya R, et al. Molecular Signature of Tumors with Monoallelic 13q14 Deletion: a Case Series of Spindle Cell Lipoma and Genetically-Related Tumors Demonstrating a Link Between FOXO1 Status and p38 MAPK Pathway. Pathol Oncol Res 2018;24(4):861–9.

40. Chien YC, Mokanszki A, Huang HY, et al. First Glance of Molecular Profile of Atypical Cellular Angiofibroma/Cellular Angiofibroma with Sarcomatous Transformation by Next Generation Sequencing. Diagnostics (Basel) 2020;10(1).

41. Fritchie KJ, Carver P, Sun Y, et al. Solitary fibrous tumor: is there a molecular relationship with cellular angiofibroma, spindle cell lipoma, and mammary-type myofibroblastoma? Am J Clin Pathol 2012;137(6):963–70.

42. Cordaro A, Haynes HR, Murigu T, et al. A report of a patient presenting with three metachronous 13q14LOH mesenchymal tumours: spindle cell lipoma, cellular angiofibroma and mammary myofibroblastoma. Virchows Arch 2021;479(3):631–5.

43. Tajiri R, Shiba E, Iwamura R, et al. Potential pathogenetic link between angiomyofibroblastoma and superficial myofibroblastoma in the female lower genital tract based on a novel MTG1-CYP2E1 fusion. Mod Pathol 2021;34(12):2222–8.

44. Lae ME, Pereira PF, Keeney GL, et al. Lipoblastoma-like tumour of the vulva: report of three cases of a distinctive mesenchymal neoplasm of adipocytic differentiation. Histopathology 2002;40(6):505–9.

45. Schoolmeester JK, Michal M, Steiner P, et al. Lipoblastoma-like tumor of the vulva: a clinicopathologic, immunohistochemical, fluorescence in situ hybridization and genomic copy number profiling study of seven cases. Mod Pathol 2018;31(12):1862–8.

46. Mirkovic J, Fletcher CD. Lipoblastoma-like tumor of the vulva: further characterization in 8 new cases. Am J Surg Pathol 2015;39(9):1290–5.

47. Droop E, Orosz Z, Michal M, et al. A lipoblastoma-like tumour of the paratesticular region - male counterpart of lipoblastoma-like tumour of the vulva. Histopathology 2020;76(4):628–30.

48. Marino-Enriquez A, Nascimento AF, Ligon AH, et al. Atypical Spindle Cell Lipomatous Tumor: Clinicopathologic Characterization of 232 Cases Demonstrating a Morphologic Spectrum. Am J Surg Pathol 2017;41(2):234–44.

49. Coffin CM, Lowichik A, Putnam A. Lipoblastoma (LPB): a clinicopathologic and immunohistochemical analysis of 59 cases. Am J Surg Pathol 2009;33(11):1705–12.

50. Collins MH, Chatten J. Lipoblastoma/lipoblastomatosis: a clinicopathologic study of 25 tumors. Am J Surg Pathol 1997;21(10):1131–7.

51. Bell SW, Kempson RL, Hendrickson MR. Problematic uterine smooth muscle neoplasms. A clinicopathologic study of 213 cases. Am J Surg Pathol 1994;18(6):535–58.

52. PC I. Uterine leiomyoma and leiomyomatosis. IARC Lyon; 2020.

53. Tavassoli FA, Norris HJ. Smooth muscle tumors of the vulva. Obstet Gynecol 1979;53(2):213–7.

54. Nielsen GP, Rosenberg AE, Koerner FC, et al. Smooth-muscle tumors of the vulva. A clinicopathological study of 25 cases and review of the literature. Am J Surg Pathol 1996;20(7):779–93.

55. Tavassoli FA, Norris HJ. Smooth muscle tumors of the vagina. Obstet Gynecol 1979;53(6):689–93.

56. Sayeed S, Xing D, Jenkins SM, et al. Criteria for Risk Stratification of Vulvar and Vaginal Smooth Muscle Tumors: An Evaluation of 71 Cases Comparing Proposed Classification Systems. Am J Surg Pathol 2018;42(1):84–94.

57. Swanson AA, Howitt BE, Schoolmeester JK. Criteria for risk stratification of vulvar and vaginal smooth muscle tumors: a follow-up study with application to leiomyoma variants, smooth muscle tumors of uncertain malignant potential, and leiomyosarcomas. Hum Pathol 2020;103:83–94.

58. Demicco EG, Park MS, Araujo DM, et al. Solitary fibrous tumor: a clinicopathological study of 110 cases and proposed risk assessment model. Mod Pathol 2012;25(9):1298–306.

59. Demicco EG, Wagner MJ, Maki RG, et al. Risk assessment in solitary fibrous tumors: validation and refinement of a risk stratification model. Mod Pathol 2017;30(10):1433–42.

60. Salas S, Resseguier N, Blay JY, et al. Prediction of local and metastatic recurrence in solitary fibrous tumor: construction of a risk calculator in a multicenter cohort from the French Sarcoma Group (FSG) database. Ann Oncol 2017;28(8):1979–87.

61. Yang EJ, Howitt BE, Fletcher CDM, et al. Solitary fibrous tumour of the female genital tract: a clinicopathological analysis of 25 cases. Histopathology 2018;72(5):749–59.

62. Devins KM, Young RH, Croce S, et al. Solitary Fibrous Tumors of the Female Genital Tract: A Study of 27 Cases Emphasizing Nonvulvar Locations, Variant Histology, and Prognostic Factors. Am J Surg Pathol 2022;1(46):363–75.

63. Howitt BEaDEG. Solitary fibrous Tumour of the lower genital tract. 2020;WHO Classifications of Female genital tumours.

64. Demicco EG, Harms PW, Patel RM, et al. Extensive survey of STAT6 expression in a large series of mesenchymal tumors. Am J Clin Pathol 2015;143(5):672–82.

65. Chiang S, Cotzia P, Hyman DM, et al. NTRK Fusions Define a Novel Uterine Sarcoma Subtype With Features of Fibrosarcoma. Am J Surg Pathol 2018;42(6):791–8.

66. Croce S, Hostein I, Longacre TA, et al. Uterine and vaginal sarcomas resembling fibrosarcoma: a clinicopathological and molecular analysis of 13 cases showing common NTRK-rearrangements and the description of a COL1A1-PDGFB fusion novel to

uterine neoplasms. Mod Pathol 2019;32(7): 1008–22.

67. Cheek EH, Fadra N, Jackson RA, et al. Uterine inflammatory myofibroblastic tumors in pregnant women with and without involvement of the placenta: a study of 6 cases with identification of a novel TIMP3-RET fusion. Hum Pathol 2020;97: 29–39.

68. Cocco E, Scaltriti M, Drilon A. NTRK fusion-positive cancers and TRK inhibitor therapy. Nat Rev Clin Oncol 2018;15(12):731–47.

69. Knezevich SR, McFadden DE, Tao W, et al. A novel ETV6-NTRK3 gene fusion in congenital fibrosarcoma. Nat Genet 1998;18(2):184–7.

70. Antonescu CR. Emerging soft tissue tumors with kinase fusions: An overview of the recent literature with an emphasis on diagnostic criteria. Genes Chromosomes Cancer 2020;59(8):437–44.

71. Croce S, Hostein I, McCluggage WG. NTRK and other recently described kinase fusion positive uterine sarcomas: A review of a group of rare neoplasms. Genes Chromosomes Cancer 2021;60(3): 147–59.

72. Devereaux KA, Weiel JJ, Mills AM, et al. Neurofibrosarcoma Revisited: An Institutional Case Series of Uterine Sarcomas Harboring Kinase-related Fusions With Report of a Novel FGFR1-TACC1 Fusion. Am J Surg Pathol 2021;45(5):638–52.

73. Haimes JD, Stewart CJR, Kudlow BA, et al. Uterine Inflammatory Myofibroblastic Tumors Frequently Harbor ALK Fusions With IGFBP5 and THBS1. Am J Surg Pathol 2017;41(6):773–80.

74. Weisman PS, Altinok M, Carballo EV, et al. Uterine Cervical Sarcoma With a Novel RET-SPECC1L Fusion in an Adult: A Case Which Expands the Homology Between RET-rearranged and NTRK-rearranged Tumors. Am J Surg Pathol 2020;44(4): 567–70.

75. Rabban JT, Devine WP, Sangoi AR, et al. NTRK fusion cervical sarcoma: a report of three cases, emphasising morphological and immunohistochemical distinction from other uterine sarcomas, including adenosarcoma. Histopathology 2020; 77(1):100–11.

76. Mills AM, Karamchandani JR, Vogel H, et al. Endocervical fibroblastic malignant peripheral nerve sheath tumor (neurofibrosarcoma): report of a novel entity possibly related to endocervical CD34 fibrocytes. Am J Surg Pathol 2011;35(3): 404–12.

77. Amatu A, Sartore-Bianchi A, Bencardino K, et al. Tropomyosin receptor kinase (TRK) biology and the role of NTRK gene fusions in cancer. Ann Oncol 2019;30(Suppl_8), viii5-viii15.

78. Goulding EA, Morreau P, De Silva M, et al. Case report: NTRK1-rearranged cervical sarcoma with fibrosarcoma like morphology presenting in a 13-year-old managed with a neo-adjuvant TRK-inhibitor and surgical excision. Gynecol Oncol Rep 2021;37:100845.

79. Chiang S. S100 and Pan-Trk Staining to Report NTRK Fusion-Positive Uterine Sarcoma: Proceedings of the ISGyP Companion Society Session at the 2020 USCAP Annual Meeting. Int J Gynecol Pathol 2021;40(1):24–7.

80. Momeni-Boroujeni A, Mohammad N, Wolber R, et al. Targeted RNA expression profiling identifies high-grade endometrial stromal sarcoma as a clinically relevant molecular subtype of uterine sarcoma. Mod Pathol 2021;34(5):1008–16.

81. Vargas AC, Ardakani NM, Wong DD, et al. Chromosomal imbalances detected in NTRK-rearranged sarcomas by the use of comparative genomic hybridisation. Histopathology 2021;78(7):932–42.

82. Singh D, Chan JM, Zoppoli P, et al. Transforming fusions of FGFR and TACC genes in human glioblastoma. Science 2012;337(6099):1231–5.

83. Shi E, Chmielecki J, Tang CM, et al. FGFR1 and NTRK3 actionable alterations in "Wild-Type" gastrointestinal stromal tumors. J Transl Med 2016;14(1): 339.

84. Napolitano A, Ostler AE, Jones RL, et al. Fibroblast Growth Factor Receptor (FGFR) Signaling in GIST and Soft Tissue Sarcomas. Cells 2021;10(6).

85. Antonescu CR, Dickson BC, Swanson D, et al. Spindle Cell Tumors With RET Gene Fusions Exhibit a Morphologic Spectrum Akin to Tumors With NTRK Gene Fusions. Am J Surg Pathol 2019;43(10): 1384–91.

86. Takahashi M, Ritz J, Cooper GM. Activation of a novel human transforming gene, ret, by DNA rearrangement. Cell 1985;42(2):581–8.

87. Wang X. Structural studies of GDNF family ligands with their receptors-Insights into ligand recognition and activation of receptor tyrosine kinase RET. Biochim Biophys Acta 2013;1834(10):2205–12.

88. Li AY, McCusker MG, Russo A, et al. RET fusions in solid tumors. Cancer Treat Rev 2019;81:101911.

89. Grindstaff SL, DiSilvestro P, Quddus MR. COL1A1-PDGFB fusion uterine sarcoma and its response to Imatinib therapy. Gynecol Oncol Rep 2020;34: 100653.

90. Pedeutour F, Simon MP, Minoletti F, et al. Translocation, t(17;22)(q22;q13), in dermatofibrosarcoma protuberans: a new tumor-associated chromosome rearrangement. Cytogenet Cell Genet 1996; 72(2–3):171–4.

91. Simon MP, Pedeutour F, Sirvent N, et al. Deregulation of the platelet-derived growth factor B-chain gene via fusion with collagen gene COL1A1 in dermatofibrosarcoma protuberans and giant-cell fibroblastoma. Nat Genet 1997;15(1):95–8.

92. Karanian M, Perot G, Coindre JM, et al. Fluorescence in situ hybridization analysis is a helpful

test for the diagnosis of dermatofibrosarcoma protuberans. Mod Pathol 2015;28(2):230–7.

93. Maire G, Martin L, Michalak-Provost S, et al. Fusion of COL1A1 exon 29 with PDGFB exon 2 in a der(22) t(17;22) in a pediatric giant cell fibroblastoma with a pigmented Bednar tumor component. Evidence for age-related chromosomal pattern in dermatofibrosarcoma protuberans and related tumors. Cancer Genet Cytogenet 2002;134(2):156–61.

94. Jahanseir K, Xing D, Greipp PT, et al. PDGFB Rearrangements in Dermatofibrosarcoma Protuberans of the Vulva: A Study of 11 Cases Including Myxoid and Fibrosarcomatous Variants. Int J Gynecol Pathol 2018;37(6):537–46.

95. Edelweiss M, Malpica A. Dermatofibrosarcoma protuberans of the vulva: a clinicopathologic and immunohistochemical study of 13 cases. Am J Surg Pathol 2010;34(3):393–400.

96. Kao YC, Bennett JA, Suurmeijer AJH, et al. Recurrent MEIS1-NCOA2/1 fusions in a subset of low-grade spindle cell sarcomas frequently involving the genitourinary and gynecologic tracts. Mod Pathol 2021;34(6):1203–12.

97. Kommoss FKF, Kolsche C, Mentzel T, et al. Spindle Cell Sarcoma of the Uterine Corpus With Adipose Metaplasia: Expanding the Morphologic Spectrum of Neoplasms With MEIS1-NCOA2 Gene Fusion. Int J Gynecol Pathol 2021;23. https://doi.org/10.1097/PGP.0000000000000803.

98. Jiang M, Xu S, Bai M, et al. The emerging role of MEIS1 in cell proliferation and differentiation. Am J Physiol Cell Physiol 2021;320(3):C264–9.

99. Szwarc MM, Lydon JP, O'Malley BW. Reprint of "Steroid receptor coactivators as therapeutic targets in the female reproductive system. J Steroid Biochem Mol Biol 2015;153:144–50.

100. Leiner J, Le Loarer F. The current landscape of rhabdomyosarcomas: an update. Virchows Arch 2020;476(1):97–108.

101. McCluggage WG, Foulkes WD. DICER1-associated sarcomas at different sites exhibit morphological overlap arguing for a unified nomenclature. Virchows Arch 2021;479(2):431–3.

102. McCluggage WG, Foulkes WD. DICER1-sarcoma: an emerging entity. Mod Pathol 2021;34(12):2096–7.

103. de Kock L, Yoon JY, Apellaniz-Ruiz M, et al. Significantly greater prevalence of DICER1 alterations in uterine embryonal rhabdomyosarcoma compared to adenosarcoma. Mod Pathol 2020;33(6):1207–19.

104. Apellaniz-Ruiz M, McCluggage WG, Foulkes WD. DICER1-associated embryonal rhabdomyosarcoma and adenosarcoma of the gynecologic tract: Pathology, molecular genetics, and indications for molecular testing. Genes Chromosomes Cancer 2021;60(3):217–33.

105. Kommoss FKF, Stichel D, Mora J, et al. Clinicopathologic and molecular analysis of embryonal rhabdomyosarcoma of the genitourinary tract: evidence for a distinct DICER1-associated subgroup. Mod Pathol 2021;34(8):1558–69.

106. Nasioudis D, Alevizakos M, Chapman-Davis E, et al. Rhabdomyosarcoma of the lower female genital tract: an analysis of 144 cases. Arch Gynecol Obstet 2017;296(2):327–34.

107. Bauer AJ, Stewart DR, Kamihara J, et al. DICER1 and Associated Conditions: Identification of At-risk Individuals and Recommended Surveillance Strategies-Response. Clin Cancer Res 2019;25(5):1689–90.

108. Schultz KAP, Williams GM, Kamihara J, et al. DICER1 and Associated Conditions: Identification of At-risk Individuals and Recommended Surveillance Strategies. Clin Cancer Res 2018;24(10):2251–61.

109. Kolin DL, Quick CM, Dong F, et al. SMARCA4-deficient Uterine Sarcoma and Undifferentiated Endometrial Carcinoma Are Distinct Clinicopathologic Entities. Am J Surg Pathol 2020;44(2):263–70.

110. Folpe AL, Schoolmeester JK, McCluggage WG, et al. SMARCB1-deficient Vulvar Neoplasms: A Clinicopathologic, Immunohistochemical, and Molecular Genetic Study of 14 Cases. Am J Surg Pathol 2015;39(6):836–49.

111. Versteege I, Sevenet N, Lange J, et al. Truncating mutations of hSNF5/INI1 in aggressive paediatric cancer. Nature 1998;394(6689):203–6.

112. Lee RS, Stewart C, Carter SL, et al. A remarkably simple genome underlies highly malignant pediatric rhabdoid cancers. J Clin Invest 2012;122(8):2983–8.

113. Le Loarer F, Zhang L, Fletcher CD, et al. Consistent SMARCB1 homozygous deletions in epithelioid sarcoma and in a subset of myoepithelial carcinomas can be reliably detected by FISH in archival material. Genes Chromosomes Cancer 2014;53(6):475–86.

114. Sullivan LM, Folpe AL, Pawel BR, et al. Epithelioid sarcoma is associated with a high percentage of SMARCB1 deletions. Mod Pathol 2013;26(3):385–92.

115. Hollmann TJ, Hornick JL. INI1-deficient tumors: diagnostic features and molecular genetics. Am J Surg Pathol 2011;35(10):e47–63.

116. Kolin DL, Konstantinopoulos PA, Campos SM, et al. Vulvar Yolk Sac Tumors Are Somatically Derived SMARCB1 (INI-1)-Deficient Neoplasms. Am J Surg Pathol 2022;46(2):169–78.

117. Yoshida A, Yoshida H, Yoshida M, et al. Myoepithelioma-like Tumors of the Vulvar Region: A Distinctive Group of SMARCB1-deficient Neoplasms. Am J Surg Pathol 2015;39(8):1102–13.

118. Xu Y, Gao H, Gao JL. Myoepithelioma-like tumor of the vulvar region: a case report in China and review of the literature. Diagn Pathol 2020;15(1):3.

119. Zhang HZ, Wang SY. Myoepithelioma-like tumour of the vulvar region. Pathology 2019;51(6):665–8.

Squamous and Glandular Epithelial Tumors of the Cervix

A Pragmatical Review Emphasizing Emerging Issues in Classification, Diagnosis, and Staging

Simona Stolnicu, MD, PhD[a],*, Robert A. Soslow, MD[b]

KEYWORDS

• Human papillomavirus • Classification • Pattern of invasion • Stage • Prognosis

---

Key points

• Both invasive endocercvical adenocarcinoma and squamous cell carcinoma and their precursors are currently classified based on HPV-status, with prognostic and predictive value

• Immunohistochemistry and HPV testing should be used only in difficult cases for invasive adenocarcinomas while for squamous cell carcinomas, these tests are mandatory when evaluating HPV-status as no morphologic criteria can reliably differentiate between HPVAs and HPVIs SCCs.

• Various issues related to FIGO staging and prognostic parameters will be elucidated by ongoing studies

---

ABSTRACT

Squamous cell carcinoma is the most frequent epithelial malignant tumor of the cervix and among the most frequent neoplasm in women worldwide. Endocervical adenocarcinoma is the second most common malignancy. Both tumors and their precursors are currently classified based on human papillomavirus status, with prognostic and predictive value. Various prognostic biomarkers and alternative morphologic parameters have been recently described and could be used in the management of these patients. This pragmatical review highlights recent developments, emerging issues as well as controversial areas regarding the cause-based classification, diagnosis, staging, and prognostic parameters of epithelial malignant tumors of the cervix.

OVERVIEW

Cervical cancer is the fourth most common malignancy to affect women worldwide, and although national screening programs as well as vaccination programs are running effectively in high-income countries, the incidence and the associated mortality are still increasing in middle- and low-income countries, with highest incidence and mortalities found in sub-Saharan Africa, followed by southeastern Asia and South America.[1,2] In Europe, Romania has the highest incidence and mortality owing to cervical cancer.[1]

Conflicts of interest: The authors have no conflicts of interest to disclose.

Funding: No funding

[a] Department of Pathology, University of Medicine, Pharmacy, Sciences and Technology of Targu Mures, 38 Gheorghe Marinescu Street, Targu Mures 540139, Romania; [b] Department of Pathology, Memorial Sloan Kettering Cancer Center, 1275 York Ave, New York, NY 10065, USA

* Corresponding author.

E-mail address: stolnicu@gmx.net

surgpath.theclinics.com

Most cervical cancers are of epithelial origin and represented by human papillomavirus-associated (HPVA) squamous cell carcinoma (SCC) (75%–80%), endocervical adenocarcinoma (ECA) (25%), and rarely by other epithelial malignant tumors. Historically, HPV infection has been considered necessary for the development of all cervical cancers. However, it has become recently recognized that a significant proportion of cervical adenocarcinomas is not associated with persistent high-risk human papillomavirus infection. Most of the recent studies focused on ECAs report that approximately 85% of ECAs are HPVA, whereas 10% to 15% are human papillomavirus-independent (HPVI).[3] In contrast to many recent advances in ECAs, less information on SCCs has been published, with a few studies and case reports indicating that HPVI SCCs very rarely occur.[4] In both tumor types, HPV status is a prognostic and predictive factor. HPVA tumors have a better prognosis and a better response to treatment compared with HPVI tumors.[3,5,6] For this reason and to harmonize the classification of all lower genital tract tumors, both SCCs and ECAs and their precursors are currently classified by the latest World Health Organization (WHO) 2020 classification into HPVA and HPVI.[7]

The purpose of the present review is to highlight emerging issues regarding the cause-based classification, diagnosis, staging, and prognostic parameters in SCC and ECAs.

EVOLUTION IN CLASSIFICATION OF CERVICAL EPITHELIAL NEOPLASIA

SCC was defined by WHO 2014 classification as invasive epithelial neoplasia composed of squamous cells of varying degrees of differentiation.[8] The precursor lesion proposed by 2014 WHO in virtually all cases of SCC was high grade squamous intraepithelial lesion (HSIL), driven by high-risk HPV infection.[8] Cytoarchitectural features and the extent of squamous keratinization were taken into account when grading these tumors, but the prognostic and predictive relevance remains controversial.

Histologic types of SCC, all thought to be HPV-driven (such as basaloid, verrucous, warty, papillary, squamotransitional, and lymphoepithelioma-like carcinoma), were described by 2014 WHO, which speculated that the histologic variation in the appearance may be related to the location of HSIL in the cervix, variation of HSIL histology, and patterns of genes activated in the progression of the disease from precursor to invasive rather than the cause.[8] In retrospect, it appears that

subtyping these carcinomas based on basaloid features and keratinization was meaningless; indeed, National Comprehensive Cancer Network 2019 suggests a universal approach to cervical cancer treatment.[9]

In a similar fashion, ECAs were previously classified by vague and descriptive morphologic features (eg, mucinous, endometrioid, villoglandular), largely lacking specific quantitative criteria.[8] The lack of correlation between morphologic subtypes and clinical behavior encountered in squamous carcinoma also plagued the classification of ECAs.

The 2020 WHO Classification shifts the basis of the categorization of SCC and ECA from morphology to HPV status, most importantly because the HPVA and HPVI pathways are both biologically different and clinically relevant in cervical cancer (**Table 1**).[7] In addition, the definitions of certain subtypes of endometrioid and serous carcinomas were significantly changed to provide clarity, either quantitation of morphologic features required for diagnosis (eg, usual, mucinous ECA) or the entire redefinition of the concept mostly based on HPV status (eg, endometrioid, serous ECA). This is in line with recent classification for vulvar tumors or other organs such as oropharynx, all based on cause.[7]

INVASIVE SQUAMOUS CELL CARCINOMA

HUMAN PAPILLOMAVIRUS-ASSOCIATED SQUAMOUS CELL CARCINOMA OF THE CERVIX

This tumor is related to high-risk HPV subtypes, most commonly of 16 and 18 subtypes, underlying 70% of all HPVA SCCs, but also 31, 33, 35, 39, 45, 51, 52, 56, 58 and 59.[10] Possible oncogenic subtypes as well as low-risk HPV subtypes (6 and 11) have been also identified.[11,12] HSIL is the first manifestation of the disease and represents a non-obligate precursor to SCC. HPVA SCC develops from HSIL as a consequence of additional genetic alterations and associated factors (such as immune microenvironment), a process that takes usually more than 10 years. More recently, genomic alterations of PI3K/MAPK and TGF-β signaling pathways as well as *ERBB3* (HER3), *CASP8*, *HLA-A*, *SHKBP1*, and *TGFBR2* mutated genes have been reported.[13,14] Epstein-Barr virus is no longer thought to be involved in the pathogenesis of cervical lymphoepithelioma-like carcinomas, as evidence has shown that these tumors are also HPV-driven.[15,16]

Median age for HPVA SCC at diagnosis is 51 years old, but note that 30% of tumors develop under the age of 35. Cervical cytology screening

Table 1
Comparison of 2014 and 2020 World Health Organization classification of epithelial malignant tumors of the cervix

2014 WHO Classification	2020 WHO Classification
SCC usual type	SCC, HPVA
Keratinizing	SCC, HPVI
Nonkeratinizing	SCC, NOS
Papillary	HPVA ECA
Basaloid	Usual adenocarcinoma
Warty	Mucinous adenocarcinoma (NOS, intestinal, signet-ring cell,
Verrucous	ISMC)
Squamotransitional	Adenocarcinoma NOS
Lymphoepithelioma-like	HPVI ECA
ECA, usual type	Gastric adenocarcinoma
Mucinous carcinoma NOS	Clear cell adenocarcinoma
Mucinous carcinoma, gastric	Mesonephric adenocarcinoma
Mucinous carcinoma, intestinal	Endometrioid adenocarcinoma
Mucinous carcinoma, signet ring cell	Adenocarcinoma NOS
Villoglandular carcinoma	Other epithelial tumors
Mesonephric carcinoma	Carcinosarcoma
Serous carcinoma	Adenosquamous carcinoma and mucoepidermoid
Clear cell carcinoma	carcinomas
Endometrioid carcinoma	Adenoid basal carcinoma
Adenocarcinoma NOS	Carcinoma of the uterine cervix, unclassifiable
Other epithelial tumors	
Adenosquamous carcinoma	
Adenoid basal carcinoma	
Adenoid cystic carcinoma	
Undifferentiated carcinoma	

plays an important part in recognizing precursor and invasive lesions, which is especially useful when the lesion is microscopic. Clinically visible tumors are associated with vaginal and postcoital bleeding, discharge, and pelvic pain. Patients with advanced staged tumors may also present with urinary symptoms, pelvic pain, or rectovaginal or vesicovaginal fistulas. The tumor usually develops at the transformation zone. Small tumors may occur as a red and erosive area, whereas large tumors can be either exophytic (polypoid or papillary), or endophytic, in which case the tumor enlarges the cervix often in the absence of a visible lesion. The endophytic pattern of growth is infiltrative into the cervical wall, sometimes resulting in a barrel-shaped cervix if the tumor involves most of the cervical wall circumference (**Fig. 1**). On the cut surface, the tumor has a white-gray color, hard consistency, and necrosis, and in advanced cases, when examining the hysterectomy specimens, the tumor infiltrates beyond the cervix into parametrium, vagina, or corpus.

The morphologic spectrum of invasive SCC is shown in **Fig. 2**. The most common morphology is represented by irregularly shaped and sized nests, cords, or sheets of tumor cells infiltrating

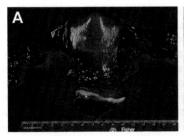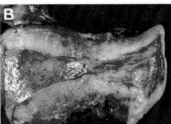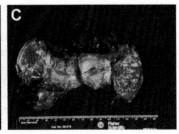

Fig. 1. SCC: at gross examination, tumors with a large diameter can be either exophytic (*A*) or endophytic, enlarging the cervix in the absence of a visible lesion (*B*), sometimes resulting in a barrel-shaped cervix (*C*). (*Courtesy* of Dr Kay Park, MD, New York, NY).

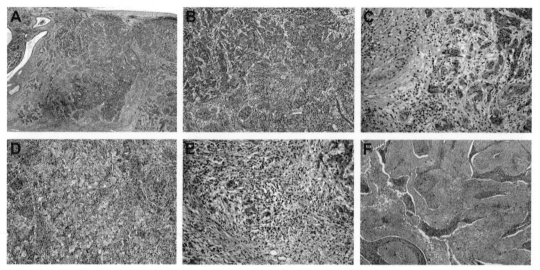

Fig. 2. Spectrum of stromal invasion in SCC: irregular shaped and sized nests infiltrating the stroma (*A*), composed of tumor cells with squamous differentiation at higher power magnification (*B*); cords of tumor cells infiltrating the cervical stroma (*C*); solid sheets of tumor cells (*D*); single tumor cells can be found, usually as a minor component (*E*); stromal invasion with a papillary architecture (*F*).

the cervical stroma. Single-tumor cells can also be found, usually as a minor component. The tumor cells are large, polygonal, with atypical nuclei and variable number of mitotic figures. Paradoxic maturation of epithelial cells, loss of polarity, and basal palisading are features associated with stromal invasion. Occasionally, the tumor cells have marked clearing of the cytoplasm, owing to the presence of abundant glycogen. Focal intracytoplasmic mucin can be encountered (positive for Mucicarmin, Alcian blue, or PAS-D); the authors accept this finding in a primarily SCC if it is focal and most of the tumor shows definitive squamous differentiation with keratin pearls and/or intercellular bridges. The presence of focal cytoplasmic mucin in SCC should not be interpreted as adenosquamous carcinoma (in which one should see 2 different infiltrative malignant components, one with malignant squamous and one with malignant glandular morphology on hematoxylin-eosin [H&E] -stained slides) or invasive stratified mucin-producing carcinoma (ISMC; in which definitive squamous differentiation is absent and the glandular differentiation can be shown using immunohistochemistry; see later discussion). The stroma surrounding the tumor cells is desmoplastic and may present inflammatory infiltrates and fibromyxoid changes. Necrosis is also frequently found in the center of tumor nests, whereas a foreign body giant cell reaction may be present in association with extracellular keratin. When encountered, giant cell reaction also evokes the possibility of previous biopsy or excision site, and it is important to consider the possibility that

epithelial elements in this site may represent displacement owing to the procedure rather than true invasion. The morphology of the epithelium, especially the presence of invasive features (paradoxic maturation, desmoplasia), is important in this distinction. Lymphovascular invasion (LVI) is most often detected at the periphery of the tumor.

At present, distinguishing between different histologic growth patterns and the presence of keratinization is no longer the basis for subclassification. More studies are needed to understand the interplay between HPV infection, degree of keratinization, basaloid features, and invasion patterns on one hand and clinical outcomes on the other hand. Until such evidence emerges, including these morphologic variations in the report, it may still be prudent as a way to gather evidence and because the morphology may be instrumental in the workup of subsequent tumor recurrences or metastasis in the same patient. In the following paragraphs, the authors present a discussion of the morphologic patterns of SCC, so the pathologist is able to make an accurate diagnosis and evoke an appropriate differential.

The *keratinizing pattern* features keratin pearls, rounded nests of squamous cells arranged in concentric circles surrounding a central focus of acellular keratin. The tumor cells are usually large, polygonal, with intercellular bridges with ample dense and eosinophilic cytoplasm, keratohyaline granules, and cytoplasmic keratinization, whereas the nuclei show variable pleomorphism and coarse, clumped chromatin (**Fig. 3**). This pattern

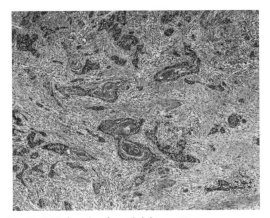

Fig. 3. SCC showing keratinizing pattern.

usually has a well-differentiated and mature morphologic appearance.

The *nonkeratinizing pattern* is represented by neoplastic squamous cells growing in nests or sheets but with an absence of keratin pearls and keratohyalin granules. Features of squamous differentiation persist with individual cell keratinization and intercellular bridges (**Fig. 4**). This pattern is usually moderately to poorly differentiated, and nuclear pleomorphism is often marked. Occasionally, the tumor cells can be markedly pleomorphic or acquire spindle morphology, sometimes in association with osteoclast-like multinucleated cells that merge with areas of more classic SCC morphology. Immunohistochemically, the atypical spindle cells can express vimentin and actin (which is a pitfall, as these stains are not specific), but fortunately are also positive for keratin and Epithelial membrane antigen (EMA) and overexpress p16, which are helpful in excluding a true mesenchymal lesion (eg, leiomyosarcoma). The terms "sarcomatoid" or "pseudosarcomatous" should be avoided to minimize confusion with sarcoma or carcinosarcoma. When present, however,

spindled patterns should be described in the report.

In the *basaloid pattern*, rounded nests of smaller, immature, and basal-type squamous atypical cells, similar to basaloid HSIL, invade the stroma. There is a high nuclear:cytoplasmic ratio (**Fig. 5**). Areas of comedo-like necrosis may be present. The tumor can mimic an HSIL or a minimally invasive carcinoma in biopsy material or when superficial. Attention to the architecture is important: markedly irregular, confluent, and/or infiltrative nests should be suspected to be invasive; stromal desmoplasia is often helpful in confirming invasion.

The *warty pattern* (also called condylomatous) is characterized by the presence of tumor cells with koilocytic features involving the deep infiltrative component as well as the superficial component, which is frequently exophytic. The superficial component is represented by papillary structures with fibrovascular cores, lined by koilocytes (**Fig. 6**). The infiltrative part is of typically invasive SCC morphology.

Similarly, *papillary SCC* has exophytic architecture with or without endophytic destructive stromal invasion. Such tumors, even when lacking destructive stromal invasion, can be diagnosed as "carcinoma" (without stromal invasion) because of the abnormal exophytic architecture, often correlating with the presence of a visible mass on clinical examination (**Fig. 7**). Of note, the extent and size of the complicated papillary architecture required for a diagnosis of "papillary SCC" (vs HSIL with papillary growth) are not included in the WHO 2020 classification, so it is left to the judgment of the pathologist. In the authors' opinion, a diagnosis of papillary SCC is warranted when the lesion is large enough to be seen clinically or macroscopically (for example, the clinical diagnosis is "cervical mass" or "cervical lesion").

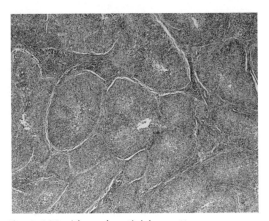

Fig. 4. SCC with nonkeratinizing pattern.

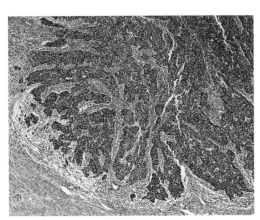

Fig. 5. Basaloid pattern in SCC.

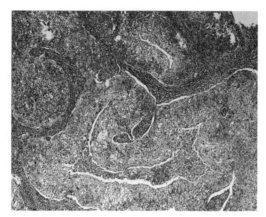

Fig. 6. Warty pattern in SCC.

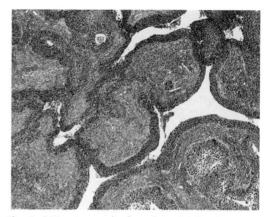

Fig. 8. SCC composed of nonkeratinizing immature squamous epithelium resembling urothelial mucosa (previously diagnosed as squamotransitional carcinoma).

On a biopsy, papillary SCC may be seen as only surface exophytic growth without stromal invasion; in this setting, the authors use the diagnosis "papillary SCC" followed by a comment informing the treating clinicians that the lesion is entirely exophytic and that stromal invasion may or may not be found on excision.

A related term found in the literature, "squamotransitional carcinoma," is no longer recommended by 2020 WHO. The term has been used to describe papillary SCC composed of nonkeratinizing immature squamous epithelium resembling urothelial mucosa (**Fig. 8**). Immunohistochemically, lesions with squamotransitional morphology are cytokeratin 7-positive and cytokeratin 20-negative, this profile being more characteristic of cervical SCC rather than a transitional (urothelial) carcinoma. More recent literature has demonstrated that "squamotransitional features" are usually associated with low-risk HPV subtypes, such as 6 and 11[12]; therefore, they can be negative for p16 overexpression by immunohistochemistry.

Tumors diagnosed by 2014 WHO classification as *verrucous carcinoma* are very rarely encountered in the cervix (they are more common, and better characterized, in the vulva). Studies have shown that verrucous carcinoma lacks lymph node metastases (LNM) and may recur in up to 50% of cases.[17,18] WHO 2020 classification no longer includes the verrucous growth pattern in the morphology of cervical SCC.[7]

The *lymphoepithelioma-like pattern* is represented by tumor cells forming invasive nests associated with a massive inflammatory infiltrate, composed of lymphocytes, plasma cells, and eosinophils and occasionally with formation of lymphoid follicles without germinal centers. The cells are undifferentiated, nonkeratinized, with a moderate amount of eosinophilic cytoplasm and large vesicular nuclei, with prominent nucleoli. The tumor borders are typically indistinct, and the tumor nests look syncytial (**Fig. 9**).

SCC is not a difficult diagnosis for a surgical pathologist, in general. However, difficult situations may occur in the following circumstances:

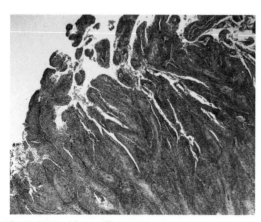

Fig. 7. SCC with papillary pattern.

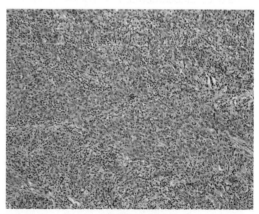

Fig. 9. SCC with lymphoepithelioma-like growth pattern.

- Distinguishing between in situ and invasive carcinomas. Note that occasional invasive carcinomas have a deceptively benign pattern of invasion with very well-circumscribed nests and no stromal desmoplasia. Invasion can be suggested or diagnosed when appreciating that the normal architecture is lost and no residual benign endocervical cells are admixed. Even if focal, invasive nests showing paradoxic maturation and associated desmoplastic, inflamed stroma are sufficient to diagnose an invasive carcinoma in this context. SCC can also have an HSIL-like morphology; invasive carcinoma can be recognized when HSIL-like trabeculae are arranged back to back in association with loss of polarity of basal epithelial cells. Such foci are seen deeper and out of the plane of usual endocervical crypts. These cases are particularly difficult to differentiate from true HSIL involving endocervical crypts and difficult to interpret on biopsy material.
- Differentiating between a benign or reactive lesion (such as stromal decidual changes, placental site nodule, reactive atypia, postirradiation changes, and SCC): in this scenario, p16 and Ki67 are very helpful, with p16 blocklike positivity and high Ki67 index favoring SCC. Keratin expression can also help excluding ectopic decidua.
- Exophytic benign (ie, condyloma acuminatum or papilloma) versus malignant tumor (ie, warty or papillary SCC); evaluation of the tumor interface with the surrounding stroma is critical, as exophytic malignant tumors will more often be accompanied by an invasive component. In addition, significant full-thickness atypia and loss of maturation are expected in malignant tumors and not in condyloma or papilloma, which should have retained maturation and a bland basal cell layer. p16 and HPV testing are of great help.

P16, as a surrogate marker for the presence of high-risk HPV infection, shows diffuse blocklike positivity (every single tumor cell) in HPVA SCCs. Note that p16 overexpression can be found in other tumor types of female genital tract carcinomas, particularly serous carcinomas, unrelated to HPV infection. Exceptionally, p16 can be negative in HPVA tumors, owing to various technical issues, antigen preservation in old blocks, and p16 silencing. High-risk HPV (HR-HPV) messenger RNA (mRNA) in situ hybridization has better sensitivity and specificity for HR-HPV infection compared with polymerase chain reaction method and superior sensitivity, specificity, and positive

and negative predictive values compared with p16 HPVA.[3] Importantly, negative p16 and HR-HPV detection studies can be due to infection by a low-risk HPV. This instance is exceedingly rare, again associated with papillary/squamotransitional lesions.

P63 and p40 are diffusely nuclear positive and may help in differential diagnosis with endometrioid carcinoma with extensive squamous differentiation. Cytokeratin 7 and EMA are positive in all cases. Anti-PD-1 checkpoint inhibitor pembrolizumab has been approved for treatment of recurrent and advanced cervical SCC resistant to other therapy. Patient candidacy for this drug is based on the predictive PD-L1 biomarker positivity, performed by immunohistochemistry.[19] Interpretation of this marker rests on a combined positive score (of 1 or more), based on the total number of PD-L1–positive tumor cells, macrophages, and lymphocytes, divided by the total number of tumor cells present, multiplied by 100. Using this score, most tumors would qualify for the treatment. Checkpoint inhibitor-based immunotherapy has recently demonstrated some promising results in patients with SCCs.[19–21]

HPVA tumors have a better prognosis than HPVI tumors.[5] In a multivariate analysis, HPVI status and International Federation of Gynecology and Obstetrics (FIGO) stage were the only predictors of increased risk of progression and mortality,[5,6] but it should be noted that only very few HPV-negative carcinomas were SCCs. Stage not only represents the most important prognostic indicator for cervical SCC but also an important tool for establishing the management. LNM together with stage were the most important prognostic parameters in determining patient outcome in 1 study.[22] Size, depth of invasion (DOI), LVI, and direct infiltration into parametrium are all adverse prognostic factors. Tumor grade is included in pathologic reports for both SCC and ECAs, but its clinical value is uncertain, and no particular grading system has achieved universal acceptance.[23] Indeed, the International Collaboration on Cancer Reporting (ICCR) does not recommend grading SCCs.[24] Patterns of stromal invasion may hold more importance. Jesinghaus and colleagues[25] investigated a novel 3-tiered histopathological grading system, based on "tumor budding and cell nest size" (TBNS) (Table 2). The following patterns have been identified: buds and tonguelike invasion (irregular protrusions of paradoxically mature cells), confluent (rounded nests associated with pushing border), or papillary. An independent validation study showed an association between the 3-tiered TBNS system, and overall, disease-specific and disease-free survival, independent

Table 2
Tumor budding and nest size grading system for cervical squamous cell carcinoma

Parameter		Score	Description
Tumor Budding Activity/ 10 HPF[a]	No Budding	1	No Budding
	<15 budding foci	2	Low budding activity
	≥15 budding foci	3	High budding activity
Smallest cell nest size within the tumor[b]	>15 cells	1	Large
	5–15 cells	2	Intermediate
	2–4 cells	3	Small
	Single-cell invasion	4	Single-cell invasion
TBNS grade	G1	2 or 3	Well differentiated
Total score (sum of [a] and [b] scores)	G2	4 or 5	Moderately differentiated
	G3	6 or 7	Poorly differentiated

[a] Tumor Budding Activity/10 HPF
[b] Smallest cell nest size within the tumor
From Jesinghaus M, Strehl J, Boxberg M, et al. Introducing a novel highly prognostic grading scgeme based on tumor budding and cell nest size for SCC of the utetine cervix. J Pathol Clin Res 2018; 4(2): 93 to 102.

of patient age, pathologic stage, and regional lymph node status.[26] Several studies reported that tumors with confluent or papillary type of invasion had a better prognosis than tumors with tumor buds and/or "spraylike" invasion.[22,25–27] Further studies are needed to better define the importance of invasion patterns on clinical outcomes.

HUMAN PAPILLOMAVIRUS-INDEPENDENT SQUAMOUS CELL CARCINOMA OF THE CERVIX

This is a recently described entity, and its incidence is generally unknown. Negative high-risk HPV results were previously interpreted as largely attributable to technical artifacts or to cases positive for low-risk HPV subtypes.[28] Recent studies with more sensitive techniques for high-risk HPV detection showed, however, that about 5% to 7% of cervical SCCs are HPV-negative.[5,6] The cause is unknown, but there are reports that these tumors show a high frequency of abnormal p53 immunostaining, suggestive of mutation.[6] Also, mutations in genes, such as *KRAS*, *ARID1A*, and *PTEN*, have been described in association with squamous carcinoma.[14] Patients with HPVI tumors are older that those with HPVA tumors and, similar to ECAs, the mean age at presentation is 60 years old. Clinical symptoms and macroscopic appearance are similar to the ones found in HPVA tumors.

HPVI tumors have been described to be keratinizing and well differentiated with numerous keratin pearls.[29] Verrucous carcinoma has been described, but most of them as case reports.[6] WHO 2020 mentions that any histologic growth pattern can be seen in the HPVI category, as no morphologic criteria can reliably differentiate HPVA from HPVI SCCs, and that ancillary testing is required to make this diagnostic distinction.[7] P16 and p53 immunohistochemistry, as well as HR-HPV mRNA in situ hybridization (ISH), may become important diagnostic adjuncts if clinical management becomes reliant upon HPV status.

Molecular testing for HPV is negative in all HPVI SCCs; p16 can show focal and patchy staining, but not diffuse staining. P63, p40, and cytokeratin 7 are positive in virtually all cases. So far, no predictive biomarkers have been demonstrated for HPVI SCCs. Differential diagnosis is similar to HPVA tumors.

It has been suggested that HPVI SCC have a worse prognosis than that of HPVA tumors: recent series have shown that HPVI cervical carcinomas have a higher rate of LNM, and disease-free survival and overall survival are worse that in HPVA tumors.[5,6,30] However, outcome analysis in these studies was not restricted to HPVI SCCs and also included HPVI ECAs, which have been analyzed separately in multiple studies and are known to have worse behavior (see next section). Thus, it remains to be determined whether HPVI SCC of the cervix is, by itself, a more aggressive neoplasm compared with HPVA squamous counterparts.

HUMAN PAPILLOMAVIRUS-NOT OTHERWISE SPECIFIED SQUAMOUS CELL CARCINOMA OF THE CERVIX

This is an SCC for which HPV status cannot be assessed in the absence of p16 and/or molecular HPV testing. Routinely performing these ancillary techniques on all cervical carcinomas is expensive or not feasible in many pathology laboratories. Thus, a diagnosis of SCC not otherwise specified (NOS) is an acceptable alternative.

INVASIVE ENDOCERVICAL ADENOCARCINOMA

The absolute and relative incidence of invasive ECAs has increased in the last decades, now representing about 25% of all cervical cancers. ECAs represent a heterogeneous spectrum of tumors with respect to cause (about 15% of them are HPVI), morphology, and prognosis.

Having reviewed more than 500 cases of ECAs, the authors have observed that HPVA ECAs consistently display easily recognizable apical mitotic figures and basal apoptosis. Conversely, absent or limited apical mitotic activity was equated with an HPVI ECA.[3] These principles formed the basis for the International ECA Criteria and Classification (IECC), which were adopted by new classification of ECAs in 2020 WHO.[3,7] The excellent predictive value of this morphologic approach for positive HPV status was validated using HR-HPV mRNA ISH in the authors' initial study[3] and subsequently in an external cohort.[31]

WHO 2020 has also mandated dichotomized classification (HPVA or HPVI) for ECA precursor lesions. Endocervical in situ adenocarcinoma and stratified mucin-producing intraepithelial lesions are glandular precursors of HPVA ECAs, whereas in situ gastric-type adenocarcinoma and atypical lobular endocervical glandular hyperplasia (LEGH) are precursors of invasive HPVI gastric-type adenocarcinoma.[7] At present, very little is known about precursors of other HPVI ECAs.[32]

HUMAN PAPILLOMAVIRUS-ASSOCIATED ENDOCERVICAL ADENOCARCINOMA

All HPVA ECAs are high-risk HPV related, with HPV 18, 16, and 45 subtypes being the most prevalent.[1,7] Risk factors are similar to those of cervical SCC. Mean age at presentation is 50 years, similar to the one for SCC, and it has been demonstrated that HPVA ECAs occur in younger patients than HPVI ones.[3] The cellular origin of ECA is hypothesized to be a population of pluripotent subcolumnar reserve cells in the squamocolumnar junction. Most ECAs develop within the transformation zone with a minority of cases located within the endocervical canal, adjacent to the lower uterine segment. In most cases, the symptoms are vaginal bleeding and/or discharge. The tumor can be visible on clinical examination (exophytic,

ulcerated mass, or, less frequently, thickening of the cervical wall with a barrel shape), but in settings with robust cervical cancer screening, most cervical cancers are small and microscopic. HPVA ECA is further subdivided in several categories. Many existed before IECC and 2020 WHO, but now count with refined criteria, as follows.

USUAL TYPE

The vast majority (80%) of HPVA ECAs are "usual type" (endocervical type) and architecturally represented by glands of various sizes and shapes lined by columnar epithelium with intracytoplasmic variable mucin depletion (**Fig. 10**). This mucin-depleted population represents most of the tumor, but up to 50% of tumor cells may contain intracytoplasmic mucin.[3] The nuclei are elongated and hyperchromatic. Morphologic variations, such as microglandular, macrocystic, and papillary, may be encountered. Villoglandular and the more recently described micropapillary growth patterns are currently considered variants of usual-type ECA. The *villoglandular* variant is considered a relatively indolent form by virtue of its predominant exophytic growth often with no or only minimal stromal invasion. Conversely, the *micropapillary* variant appears to be aggressive, as emerging evidence has shown that any amount of micropapillary pattern is associated with LNM and worse behavior[33,34]; thus, a comment regarding its presence should be included in the final pathology report. Micropapillary growth can also be present in HPVIs.[33]

With only occasional exceptions, all HPVAs, including the most common "usual type," stain similarly: "block" positivity for p16 (defined as strong, nuclear, and cytoplasmic staining within the lesional epithelium) and positive nuclear and/or cytoplasmic signals for HR-HPV mRNA ISH.[3] Of note, both HPV in situ hybridization and p16

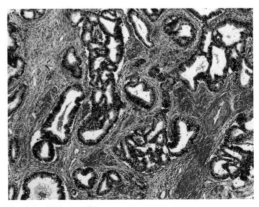

Fig. 10. ECA usual type.

can be negative (defined as completely p16 negative or patchy non–block-type immunoreactivity) in poorly fixed tissues and older paraffin blocks.[3] Usual-type ECAs may contain variable amounts of benign squamous metaplasia, which should be differentiated from adenosquamous carcinoma in which both glandular and squamous components are malignant. Of interest, this situation is rarely encountered, and when present, the squamous metaplasia is located at the superficial part of the tumor, not intermixed with glandular malignant component. Usual-type ECA with mucin depletion should be distinguished from endometrioid adenocarcinoma (p16, ER, and PR can assist). Usual-type ECA with a papillary or micropapillary architecture and highly atypical nuclei should not be diagnosed as primary cervical serous carcinoma, which is exceedingly rare and arguably not existent because drop metastases from the endometrium or upper genital tract are more likely and should be excluded first (which may require deferral to hysterectomy and salpingo-oophorectomy evaluation). p53 and HPV testing should provide the correct diagnosis, whereas p16 should be avoided for this differential diagnosis (both will show overexpression).

MUCINOUS TYPE

This group includes the patterns formerly known as mucinous NOS (**Fig. 11**), intestinal (**Fig. 12**), and signet-ring ECA (**Fig. 13**); definitions require more than 50% of tumor cells with intracytoplasmatic mucin, goblet cell, or signet-ring morphology, respectively, whereas generally retaining the apical mitotic activity and apoptosis seen in usual-type ECA. ISMC, a new entity within this group of mucinous HPVA ECA,[35] contains nests of columnar cells with a variable amount of intracytoplasmic mucin and peripheral nuclear palisading (**Fig. 14**).[3,35] In any percentage, ISMC

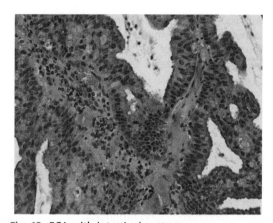

Fig. 12. ECA with intestinal pattern.

is associated with a worse prognosis, early recurrent disease, and a substantial risk of distant metastatic disease, especially to the lungs.[36] Mucinous-type HPVA should be differentiated from gastric-type ECA with p16 (variable in HPVI), HR-HPV ISH (negative in HPVI), and p53 (almost always "wild-type" in HPVA and frequently aberrant in HPVI). HIK1083, TFF2, Claudin 18, and MUC6 may also be helpful for this differential diagnosis.[37,38] For differentiating between HPVA mucinous-type and endometrial mucinous adenocarcinoma, ER/PR staining may suffice, but note that an immunohistochemical diagnostic algorithm was recently proposed.[39] Metastases from other organs should always be excluded in tumors with abundant intracytoplasmic mucin, and clinically and radiologically relevant information together with ancillary tests, including a panel of immunohistochemical markers and HPV testing, can be used. Tumors with ISMC morphology may resemble SCC and adenosquamous carcinoma. Absence of definitive squamous differentiation on histologic (intercellular junctions, keratinization) and immunohistochemical (p63/p40, CK5/6) examination is helpful in excluding these diagnoses.

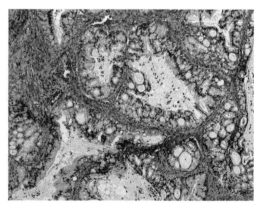

Fig. 11. ECA mucinous NOS.

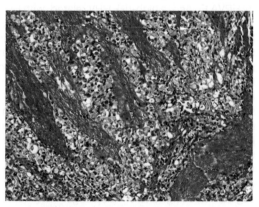

Fig. 13. ECA with signet-ring pattern.

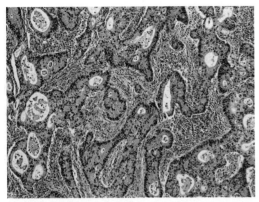

Fig. 14. Invasive stratified mucinous carcinoma pattern.

NOS type is any tumor that could not be classified by IECC or WHO criteria but in which both p16 and HPV testing are positive (**Fig. 15**).

HUMAN PAPILLOMAVIRUS-INDEPENDENT ENDOCERVICAL ADENOCARCINOMA

This category is represented by gastric-type, clear cell, endometrioid, mesonephric, and NOS adenocarcinomas. Causes are largely unknown, but different associated molecular abnormalities have been demonstrated recently, particularly for gastric, mesonephric, and clear cell adenocarcinomas. Although not unique to HPVI ECA, prevalent genetic alterations include mutations in *PIK3CA*, *KRAS*, and *PTEN*, and all members of PI3K/Akt/mTOR signaling cascade have been demonstrated in this tumor category, some of them with predictive and prognostic value.[40–43] A genetic predisposition for the development of gastric type adenocarcinoma was found in women with Peutz-Jeghers syndrome.[44–46] Most gastric-type ECAs develop within the transformation zone with a minority of cases located within the endocervical canal, or adjacent to or involving the lower uterine segment. Mesonephric ECA develops more frequently deep in the lateral part of the cervical wall, where mesonephric remnants are usually found. Similarly, the extraordinarily rare primary cervical endometrioid ECAs are thought to develop in the deep part of the cervical wall, possibly from cervical endometriosis. Macroscopically and clinically, the tumors are similar to HPVA ECAs with the exception of gastric type, where watery vaginal discharge may be a presenting symptom.

Gastric type is the second most common type of ECA and the most common HPVI, particularly in Japan. Gastric type may have a diverse cytomorphology, but most cases display abundant clear/pale eosinophilic cytoplasm, distinct cytoplasmic borders, and irregular basally located and rounded nuclei, sometimes with a distinct nucleolus (**Fig. 16**). Atypia ranges from minimal to marked. Cases previously diagnosed as minimal deviation mucinous adenocarcinomas are now termed "well-differentiated gastric-type ECA." The differential diagnosis includes usual, serous, mesonephric, or clear cell-type ECAs and metastasis. The distinction is primarily based on morphology, but immunohistochemistry can be helpful. Gastric-type carcinoma is usually negative for p16 (although one-third of cases can be positive) and positive for MUC 6, HIK1083, and more recently demonstrated, for Claudin 18 and TFF2.[37,38,47] When distinguishing between morphologically well-differentiated variants of gastric-type ECA and a variety of benign cervical glandular lesions, deep placement of glands along with mild nuclear atypia, presence of at least focal stromal desmoplasia, and ER/PR staining can be useful, as gastric-type tumors are usually negative, whereas most benign glandular lesions, with the exception of LEGH and mesonephric remnants, are positive for these markers.[48]

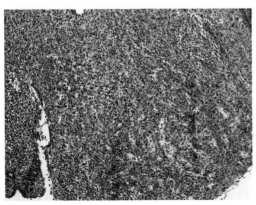

Fig. 15. ECA NOS HPVA type.

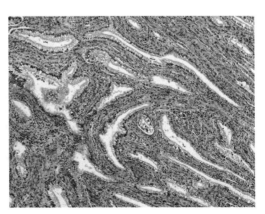

Fig. 16. ECA gastric type.

Clear cell carcinoma primary to the cervix is very rare, nowadays mostly sporadic, and seen in adult women with a mean age of 55 years at presentation. Cases related to in utero diethylstilbestrol exposure have steadily decreased over time. Like endometrial and ovarian counterparts, cervical clear cell carcinoma is characterized by solid, papillary, and tubulocystic architecture with polygonal or flattened tumor cells with clear or eosinophilic cytoplasm and highly atypical but uniform nuclei (**Fig. 17**). The main differential diagnosis is gastric-type ECA (see above) and, as mentioned above, HIK1083, TFF2, and Claudin 18 could be helpful, as these markers are negative in clear cell type. Racemase (AMACR) and Napsin A are positive in clear cell ECA, but staining may be focal and, therefore, not informative when "negative" in small biopsies. Clear cell ECA can also mimic benign glandular lesions, such as microglandular hyperplasia and Arias-Stella reaction, but the presence of a tumor mass in association with nuclear atypia and stromal desmoplasia favors clear cell adenocarcinoma.[48] As a pitfall, Arias-Stella reaction is often positive for Napsin A and HNF1-beta and shows reduction of ER expression.[49] Emerging evidence indicates that cervical clear cell carcinoma has worse disease-free and overall survival compared with HPVA ECAs, and similar survival compared with gastric-type ECAs.

Mesonephric carcinoma is usually represented by an admixture of various architectural growth patterns (**Fig. 18**). Tumor cells have scant cytoplasm and atypical hyperchromatic nuclei, with mild to moderate atypia, sometimes optically clear and grooved, resembling those of papillary thyroid carcinoma. Mesonephric remnants or hyperplasia can sometimes be identified in the tumor's periphery. Endometrioid, clear cell, usual-type ECAs, and serous carcinoma are in the differential, and ancillary tests can assist in their differentiation, including GATA 3, TFF1, and CD 10.[39]

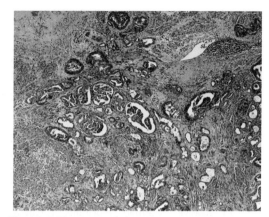

Fig. 18. ECA mesonephric type.

A diagnosis of *endometrioid carcinoma* requires confirmatory endometrioid features (low-grade endometrioid glandular component, columnar cells with mucin depletion, pseudostratified nuclei with no more than moderate atypia with or without squamous or ciliated differentiation) (**Fig. 19**).[3] When uterine corpus and primary ovary tumors are excluded, endometrioid carcinoma of the cervix is an absolutely extraordinary diagnosis. Ancillary studies do not distinguish between endometrioid carcinomas of the corpus and the cervix, but they are helpful when other entities, such as usual-type HPVA, are considered. Using modern WHO definitions, one should not make a reflexive diagnosis of endometrioid adenocarcinoma in the presence of a mucin-depleted adenocarcinoma, which is more likely to be a usual HPVA ECA.[3,50]

NOS type is represented by poorly differentiated HPVI tumors with ambiguous morphology that cannot be classified in any of the HPVI types (**Fig. 20**). P16 and/or HPV testing are required to differentiate this from HPVA NOS type.

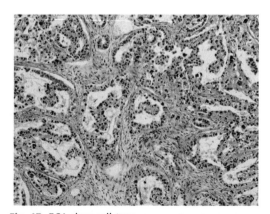

Fig. 17. ECA clear cell type.

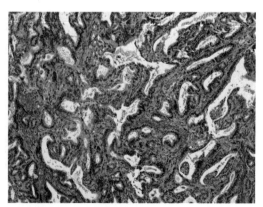

Fig. 19. ECA endometrioid type.

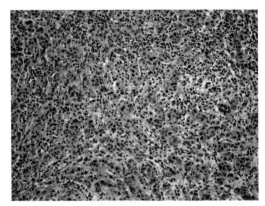

Fig. 20. ECA NOS HPVI type.

PROGNOSTIC PATHOLOGIC FACTORS IN ENDOCERVICAL ADENOCARCINOMA

Tumor grade is included in the pathologic report of ECAs even though its clinical value is controversial. Grading is not recommended by the International Society of Gynecological Pathologists (ISGyP) and ICCR for HPVI ECAs, as most of these neoplasms exhibit intrinsically aggressive behavior regardless of their morphologic appearance.[24,51] In contrast, ISGyP and ICCR recommend that HPVA adenocarcinomas should be graded using FIGO 1988 grading criteria for corpus carcinomas.[51] Tumors with a micropapillary, signet-ring, or invasive stratified mucinous carcinoma component should not be graded, as these are automatically considered high grade.[51]

FIGO stage, HPV status, Silva pattern of invasion, presence of LVI, and LNM are all prognostically significant. A pattern-based classification characterizing stromal invasion (Silva) has been introduced as an alternative or adjunct to DOI in HPVA ECAs.[52] Pattern-based classification is a powerful tool to predict LNM and, when appropriate, to spare unnecessary lymphadenectomy (Table 3).

A recent review, summarizing all studies based on Silva classification, demonstrated that no LNM, recurrences, or deaths were found in Silva pattern A cases, whereas in Silva pattern B cases, 5% had LNM, 3% had recurrences, and 1% were DOD, and in Silva pattern C cases, 22% had LNM, 19% had recurrences, and 11% of patients were death of disease (DOD).[53] Consequently, the ISGyP experts recommend the use of Silva classification in HPVA ECAs for clinical management.[53] Silva classification is not recommended for HPVI ECAs, as most are of Silva C pattern.[54] Reproducibility of pattern-based classification was addressed in 3 studies, all with similarly acceptable results.[55–57] Pattern assignment is best performed in a surgical specimen (cone/loop electrosurgical excision/hysterectomy) in which most/all the tumor is available for evaluation, rather than a biopsy.[58] Recent studies reported a higher prevalence of oncogene and tumor suppressor gene abnormalities in patterns B and C, unlike in pattern A.[59,60] This is concordance with markers of mTOR pathway activation, such as pERK, which are differentially expressed in pattern A versus pattern B/C.[61] The Silva classification is not part of the current FIGO or American Joint Committee on Cancer (AJCC) staging systems, but there are important clinical implications, as recently demonstrated in 2 studies.[62,63] The authors reported that LVI remains the most important prognosticator among FIGO stage IA and IB1 carcinomas and that a binary Silva classification can be applied by safely separating Silva low-risk cases (pattern A and B without LVI) from Silva high-risk cases (pattern B with LVI and pattern

Table 3		
Silva pattern-based classification		
Silva Pattern	**Morphologic Features**	**Proposed Binary Risk Categories**
Silva A pattern	No destructive stromal invasion, usually a lobular configuration with well-demarcated glands and rounded contours; no LVI present	Low-risk pattern: • Silva pattern A • Silva pattern B without LVI
Silva B pattern	Early (limited) destructive invasion (<4× field, no more than 5 mm in diameter) in a background Silva pattern A. LVI may be present	High-risk pattern: • Silva pattern B with LVI • Silva pattern C
Silva C pattern	Extensive and diffuse destructive stromal invasion, desmoplastic stromal response, moderately to poorly differentiated tumor; LVI may be present	

Table 4
Areas of controversies and recommendations regarding staging and reporting cervical cancer

Variable	Problem	Recommendation
Staging	Different staging systems and different societies' recommendations[67–72] Should pathologist stage cervical cancer?	Choose the staging scheme with the clinicians' and regulators' input Although it is not necessarily logical, all clinically visible lesions are at least stage IB, but this may be changed
Depth of invasion (DOI)	Difficult to measure in cases lacking AIS and in exophytic, ulcerated and glandular carcinomas Depth vs thickness Whether to provide aggregate measurements	Report thickness in such cases, but indicate that DOI cannot be measured Do not add together tumor dimensions, including DOI, from different surgical procedures[24,73] Depth of invasion reported in thirds (i.e. inner 1/3 cervical wall invasion) is used to determine need for adjuvant therapy, not for staging[74–77]
Horizontal extent (HE)	2018 FIGO removed this staging criterion for microscopic disease, but other systems have retained it How to assess HE in difficult cases	Depending on the staging system used, HE can inform the stage or merely be reported in a note (ICCR, AJCC) There is evidence that this measurement retains prognostic value in SCC and ECA[78]
Lymphovascular invasion	One of the most important prognostic factors, but NOT one that is included in any staging formulation[62,63,67,68,79–83]	Include LVI status in report Diagnose only at the periphery of the tumor Limit use of endothelial markers for cases that are favored to represent LVI on H&E sections Extracervical LVI does not upstage Not currently necessary to quantitate
Tumor size	How to measure (microscopic or macroscopic; 1, 2 or 3 dimensions)	Report the largest diameter (macroscopic if visible, microscopic if not) Consider reporting other variables in accordance with regional standards[24,73]
Multifocal invasion	Definition and significance	More than 2 mm separates foci of superficial stromal invasion[84,85] Use the largest diameter of the largest focus to stage the tumor Confirm with deeper levels[24] Discuss each difficult case in the multidisciplinary team

(*continued on next page*)

Table 4
(continued)

Variable	Problem	Recommendation
		May no longer be relevant if horizontal extent is removed from staging systems
Margins status	Shall we report? Does this affect staging?	Report margin clearance when narrow, particularly in parametrium It does affect when using FIGO 2018 system
Lymph node metastasis	Sentinel lymph node interpretation[86] Stage assignment (number of involved lymph nodes, the size of the metastasis, extracapsular spread and size of extracapsular; tumor cells involving fat tissue without presence of lymphoid tissue; pelvic, paraaortic and LNM outside regional LN)	Micro- (0.2-2.0 mm) and macrometastases are N1[87,88] Isolated tumor cells are incompletely understood and assigned N0 i+ in some but not all staging systems Consider staging regional and distant LNM in accordance with regional standards
Parametrium	Where does the parametrium begin and cervix end? What constitutes parametrial involvement? Is infiltration into anterior-posterior paracervical tissue equivalent to parametrial involvement?	Extension beyond the dense connective tissue of the deep cervical wall. Fat invasion is helpful, but not necessary Consider using prostate carcinoma criteria for determining extraprostatic (and, therefore, parametrial) extension. Stromal invasive carcinoma counts as parametrial involvement, although a positive parametrial lymph node or LVI does not count Stage infiltration into anterior-posterior paracervical tissue as for parametrial involvement[89,90]
Ovarian metastasis	M1 disease?[91] How to report different anatomic/histologic areas of adnexal involvement	No M1 disease All areas of adnexal involvement should be recorded as metastasis

C).[63] An updated FIGO staging scheme should ideally take into account not only tumor size and DOI but also LVI and Silva pattern risk stratification.[63] Treatment could be theoretically individualized using this formulation.

Despite the excellent prognosis of pattern A carcinomas without LVI and absence of LNM, both extensive adenocarcinoma situ and, theoretically, pattern A ECA can be associated with carpetlike spread through the endocervical canal and lower uterine segment with implantation in/onto one or both ovaries.[64] Consequently, it is advisable to follow such patients for ovarian recurrence. Surprisingly, some isolated ovarian metastatic HPVAs pursue a self-limited clinical course.

HPVI ECAs have a worse prognosis than HPVAs. Although this claim has mostly been based on studies whereby most HPVIs were the gastric type, it appears that clear cell and mesonephric ECA also behave differently than HPVA ECA. It was recently reported that the overall survival and relapse-free survival of both clear cell and gastric type ECAs at 5 and 10 years were similar.[65] Mesonephric adenocarcinomas also frequently present at advanced stage, develop distant recurrences, and have a predilection for pulmonary recurrences, similar to gastric and clear cell carcinoma, concluding that mesonephric, along with clear cell and gastric-type ECAs, is an aggressive type.[66] Data regarding the prognosis of endometroid ECA are lacking, mostly because of the rarity of true primary cervical endometrioid adenocarcinomas.

STAGING AND PROGNOSTIC FACTORS ISSUES AND CONTROVERSIES IN CERVICAL CARCINOMA

Both FIGO and TNM (Union for International Cancer Control and AJCC) staging systems are used. An update to the FIGO system was released in 2018, with a revision published in 2019, and this is reflected in the AJCC latest edition and the subsequently released College of American Pathologists (CAP) cancer reporting template update.[67–70] Therefore, FIGO 2018 and 2019, AJCC, and CAP systems are now in perfect concordance. The major changes, incorporated into 2018 FIGO system and areas of controversies when dealing with cervical cancer staging and diagnosis, are included in **Table 4**.

SUMMARY

SCC is the most frequent epithelial malignant tumor of the cervix and among the most frequent neoplasms affecting women worldwide. ECAs are the second most frequent epithelial malignancy of the cervix. Both tumors and their precursors are currently classified based on HPV status with prognostic and predictive value. Various prognostic biomarkers and alternative morphologic parameters have been recently described and could be used in the management of these patients. Multiple areas regarding classification, diagnosis, and staging are still controversial, and there is a need to clarify these issues in the future.

CLINICS CARE POINTS

- In situ adenocarcinoma human papillomavirus-associated is well known; in contrast, in situ adenocarcinoma human papillomavirus-independent has been only recently described and is not well characterized. Larger studies, including follow-up, will bring more data regarding its diagnosis and treatment.

- International Endocervical Adenocarcinoma Criteria and Classification 2018 and Silva classification are already incorporated into World Health Organization 2020 classifications for endocervical adenocarcinomas; both can be assessed in many cases on hematoxylin-eosin–stained slides, and both can help manage decisions.

- Immunohistochemistry and human papillomavirus testing should be used only in difficult cases for the diagnosis of endocervical adenocarcinomas.

- The FIGO staging system could potentially be improved by including lymphovascular invasion and Silva pattern when staging endocervical adenocarcinomas.

- Squamous cell carcinoma is currently classified based on human papillomavirus status, which may have prognostic and predictive value similar to what is seen in endocervical adenocarcinoma. Histologic types are now considered growth patterns, and their prognostic value is debatable; grading is no longer recommended.

- Alternative prognostic parameters will add more information about prognosis and survival regarding squamous cell carcinoma, whereas staging issues are still to be evaluated by ongoing studies.

REFERENCES

1. Bray F, Ferlay J, Soejomataram I, et al. Global cancer statistics 2018: GLOBOCAN estimates of incidence and mortality worldwide for 36 cancers in 185 countries. Cancer J Clin 2018;68(6):394–424.
2. Arbyn M, Weiderpass E, Bruni L, et al. Estimates of incidence and mortality of cervical cancer in 2018: a worldwide analysis. Lancet Glob Health 2020; 8(2):e191–203.
3. Stolnicu S, Barsan I, Hoang L, et al. International ECA criteria and classification (IECC): a new pathogenetic classification for invasive adenocarcinomas

of the endocervix. Am J Surg Pathol 2018;42: 214–26.

4. Casey S, Harley I, Jamison J, et al. A rare case of HPV-negative cervical squamous carcinoma. Int J Gynecol Pathol 2015;34(2):208–12.

5. Rodriguez-Carunchio L, Soveral I, Steenbergen RDM, et al. HPV-negative carcinoma of the uterine cervix: a distinct type of cervical cancer with poor prognosis. BJOG 2015;122(1):119–27.

6. Nicolas I, Marimon L, Barnadas E, et al. HPV-negative tumors of the uterine cervix. Mod Pathol 2019; 32(8):1189–96.

7. Herrington CS, Kim KR, Kong C, et al. Tumours of the uterine cervix. W. C. o. T. E. B. F. g. tumours. Lyon (France): International Agency for Research on Cancer; 2020.

8. Kurman RJ, Carcangiu ML, Herrington CS, et al. WHO classification of tumors of female reproductive organs. 4th edition. Lyon: IARC, WHO Press; 2014.

9. Authors listed No. NCCN Guidelines for Treatment of Cervical Cancer: National Comprehensive Cancer Network. 2014. Available at: www.nccn.org/professionals/physician_gls/pdf/cervical.pdf. Accessed April 25, 2019.

10. McBride A. Oncogenic human papillomaviruses. Philos Trans R Soc Lond B Biol Sci 2017;372(1732).

11. Halec G, Alemany L, Lloveras B, et al. Pathogenic role of the eight probably/possibly carcinogenic HPV types 26, 53, 66, 67, 68, 70, 73 and 82 in cervical cancer. J Pathol 2014;234(4):441–51.

12. Guimera N, Lloveras B, Lindeman J, et al. The occasional role of low-risk human papillomaviruses 6, 11, 42, 44 and 70 in anogenital carcinoma defined by laser capture microdissection/PCR methodology: results from a global study. Am J Surg Pathol 2013; 37(9):1299–310.

13. Tornesello ML, Annunziata C, Buonaguro L, et al. TP53 and PIK3CA gene mutations in adenocarcinoma, SCC and high-grade intraepithelial neoplasia of the cervix. J Transl Med 2014;12:255.

14. Burk RD, Chen Z, Saller C, et al. Integrated genomic and molecular characterization of cervical cancer. Nature 2017;543(7645):378–84.

15. Bais AG, Kooi S, Teune TM, et al. Lymphoepithelioma-like carcinoma of the uterine cervix: Absence of Epstein-Barr virus, but presence of multiple human papillomavirus infection. Gynecol Oncol 2005;197:716–8.

16. Chao A, Tsai CN, Hsueh LY, et al. Does Epstein-Barr virus play a role in lymphoepithelioma-like carcinoma of the uterine cervix? Int J Gynecol Pathol 2009;28:279–85.

17. Robert ME, Fu YS. SCC of the uterine cervix- a review with emphasis on prognostic factors and unusual variants. Sem Diagn Pathol 1990;7:73–189.

18. Yorganci A, Serinsoz E, Ensari A, et al. A case report of multicentric verrucous carcinoma of the female genital tract. Gynecol Oncol 2003;90(2):478–81.

19. Chung HC, Ros W, Delord JP, et al. Efficacy and safety of pembrolizumab in previous treated advanced cervical cancer: results from the phase II KEYNOTE-158 study. J Clin Oncol 2019;1470–8.

20. Frenel JS, Le Tourneau C, O'Neil B, et al. Safety and efficacy of pembrolizumab in advanced, programmed death ligand 1-positive cervical cancer: results from the phase ib KEYNOTE-028 Trial. J Clin Oncol 2017;35:4035–41.

21. Borcoman E, Le Tourneau C. Pembrolizumab in cervical cancer: latest evidence and clinical usefulness. Ther Adv Med Oncol 2017;9:431–9.

22. Cole L, Stoler MH. Issues and inconsistencies in the revised gynecologic staging systems. Semin Diagn Pathol 2012;29(3):167–73.

23. McCluggage WG. Towards developing a meaningful grading system for cervical SCC. J Pathol Clin Res 2018;4(2):81–5.

24. McCluggage WG, Judge MJ, Alvarado-Cabrero I, et al. Data set for the reporting of carcinomas of the cervix: Recommendations for the International Collaboration on Cancer Reporting (ICCR). Int J Gynecol Pathol 2018;37:205–2017.

25. Jesinghaus M, Strehl J, Boxberg M, et al. Introducing a novel highly prognostic grading scgeme based on tumor budding and cell nest size for SCC of the utetine cervix. J Pathol Clin Res 2018; 4(2):93–102.

26. Zare SY, Aisagbonhi O, Hasteh F, et al. Independent validation of tumor budding activity and cell nest size as determinants of patient outcome in squamous cell carcinoma of the uterine cervix. Am J Surg Pathol 2020;44(9):1151–60.

27. Horn LC, Fisher U, Raptis G, et al. Pattern of invasion is of prognostic value in surgically treated cervical cancer patients. Gynecol Oncol 2006;103: 906–11.

28. de Sanjose S, Quint WG, Alemany L, et al. Human Papillomavirus genotype attribution in invasive cervical cancer: a retrospective cross-sectional worldwide study. Lancet Oncol 2010;11(11):1048–56.

29. Morrison C, Catania F, Wakely P Jr, et al. High differentiated keratinizing squamous cell carcinoma of the cervix. A rare locally aggressive tumor not associated with human papillomavirus or squamous intraepithelial lesion. Am J Surg Pathol 2001; 25:1310–5.

30. Pilch H, Gunzel S, Schaffer U, et al. The presence of HPV DNA in cervical cancer: correlation with clinicopathologic parameters and prognostic significance: 10 years experience at the Department of Obstetrics and Gynecology of the Mainz University. Int J Gynecol Cancer 2001;11(1):39–48.

31. Hodgson A, Park KJ, Djordjevic B, et al. International endocervical adenocarcinoma criteria and classification: validation and interobserver reproducibility. Am J Surg Pathol 2019;43:75–83.

32. Stolnicu S, McCluggage WG. The evolving spectrum of ECA in situ (AIS). Virchows Arch 2020; 476(4):485–6.

33. Alvarado-Cabrero I, McCluggage WG, Estevez-Castro R, et al. Micropapillary cervical adenocarcinoma: a clinicopathologic study of 44 cases. Am J Surg Pathol 2019;43(6):802–9.

34. Alvarado-Cabrero I, Roma AA, Park K, et al. Factors predicting pelvic lymph node metastasis, relapse and disease outcome in pattern C endocervical adenocarcinomas. Int J Gynecol Pathol 2017;36(5): 476–85.

35. Lastra RR, Park KJ, Schoolmeester JK. Invasive stratified mucin producing carcinoma and stratified mucin-producing intraepithelial lesion (SMILE): 15 cases presenting a spectrum of cervical neoplasia with description of a distinctive variant of invasive adenocarcinoma. Am J Surg Pathol 2016;40:262–9.

36. Stolnicu S, Boros M, Segura S, et al. Invasive stratified mucinous carcinoma (iSMC) of the cervix often presents with high-risk features that are determinants of poor outcome: an international multicentric study. Am J Surg Pathol 2020. https://doi.org/10.1097/PAS.0000000000001485. Online ahead of print.

37. Kiyokawa T, Hoang L, Terinte C, et al. Trefoil Factor 2 (TFF2) as a Surrogate Marker for Endocervical Gastric-type Carcinoma. Int J Gynecol Pathol 2021;40(1):65–72.

38. Asaka S, Nakajima T, Kugo K, et al. Immunophenotype analysis using CLDN18, CDH17, and PAX8 for the subcategorization of endocervical adenocarcinomas in situ: gastric-type, intestinal-type, gastrointestinal-type, and Müllerian-type. Virchows Arch 2020;476(4):499–510.

39. Stolnicu S, Barsan I, Hoang L, et al. Diagnostic algorithmic proposal based on comprehensive immunohistochemical evaluation of 297 invasive endocervical adenocarcinomas. Am J Surg Pathol 2018;42:989–1000.

40. Ojesina AI, Lichtenstein L, Freeman SS, et al. Landscape of genomic alterations in cervical carcinomas. Nature 2014;506:371–5. https://doi.org/10.1038/nature12881.

41. Wright AA, Howitt BE, Myers AP, et al. Oncogenic mutations in cervical cancer: genomic differences between adenocarcinomas and squamous cell carcinomas of the cervix. Cancer 2013;119:3776–83. https://doi.org/10.1002/cncr.28288.

42. Lou H, Villagran G, Boland JF, et al. Genome analysis of latin American cervical cancer: frequent activation of the PIK3CA pathway. Clin Cancer Res 2015;21:5360–70. https://doi.org/10.1158/1078-0432.CCR-14-1837.

43. Tornesello ML, Annunziata C, Buonaguro L, et al. TP53 and PIK3CA gene mutations in adenocarcinoma, squamous cell carcinoma and high-grade intraepithelial neoplasia of the cervix. J Transl Med 2014;12:255. https://doi.org/10.1186/s12967-014-0255-5.

44. Castellsague X, Diaz M, de Sanjose S, et al. Worldwide human papillomavirus etiology of cervical adenocarcinoma and its cofactors: implications for screening and prevention. J Natl Cancer Inst 2006; 98:303–15. https://doi.org/10.1093/jnci/djj067.

45. Lacey JV Jr, Brinton LA, Barnes WA, et al. Use of hormone replacement therapy and adenocarcinomas and squamous cell carcinomas of the uterine cervix. Gynecol Oncol 2000;77:149–54. https://doi.org/10.1006/gyno.2000.5731.

46. Lacey JV Jr, Swanson CA, Brinton LA, et al. Obesity as a potential risk factor for adenocarcinomas and squamous cell carcinomas of the uterine cervix. Cancer 2003;98:814–21. https://doi.org/10.1002/cncr.11567.

47. Pirog EC, Park KJ, Kiyokawa T, et al. Gastric-type adenocarcinoma of the cervix: tumor with wide range of histologic appearance. Adv Anat Pathol 2018;26(1):1–12.

48. Stolnicu S. Cervical cancer. What's new in classification, morphology, molecular findings and prognosis of glandular precursor and invasive lesions. Diagnostic Histopathology 2021, in press.

49. Ip PPC, Wang SY, Wong OGW, et al. Hepatocytic Nuclear Factor-1-Beta (HNF-1beta), Estrogen and Progesterone receptors Expression in Arias-Stella Reaction. Am J Surg Pathol 2019;43(3):325–33.

50. Stolnicu S, Park KJ, Kyiokawa T, et al. Tumor typing on endocervical adenocarcinoma: contemporary review and recommendations from the International Society of Gynecological Pathologists. Int J Gynecol Pathol 2021;40(suppl 1):S75–91.

51. Talia KL, Oliva S, Rabban JT, et al. Grading on endocervical adenocarcinomas: review of the literature and recommendation from the International Society of Gynecological Pathologists. Int J Gynecol Pathol 2021;40(suppl 1):S66–74.

52. Diaz De Vivar A, Roma AA, Park KJ, et al. Invasive ECA: proposal for a new pattern-based classification system with significant clinical implications: a multi-institutional study. Int J Gynecol Pathol 2013; 32(6):592–601.

53. Alvarado-Cabrero I, Parra-Herran C, Stolnicu S, et al. The Silva pattern-based classification for HPV-associated invasive endocervical adenocarcinoma and the ditinction between in situ and invasive adenocarcinoma: relevant issues and recommendations from the International Society of Gynecological Pathologists. Int J Gynecol Pathol 2021;40(suppl 1): S48–65.

54. Stolnicu S, Barsan I, Hoang L, et al. Stromal invasion pattern identifies patients at lowest risk of lymph node metastasis in HPV-associated endocervical adenocarcinomas but is irrelevant in

adenocarcinomas unassociated with HPV. Gynecol Oncol 2018;150:56–60.

55. Paquette C, Jeffus SK, Quick CM, et al. Interobserver variability in the application of a proposed histologic subclassification of endocervical adenocarcinoma. Am J Surg Pathol 2015;39:93–100.

56. Parra-Herran C, Taljaard M, Djordjevic B, et al. Pattern-based classification of invasive endocervical adenocarcinoma, depth of invasion measurement and distinction from adenocarcinoma in situ: interobserver variation among gynecologic pathologists. Mod Pathol 2016;29:879–92.

57. Rutgers JKL, Roma AA, Park KJ, et al. Pattern classification of endocervical adenocarcinoma: reproducibility and review of criteria. Mod Pathol 2016; 29:1083–94.

58. Djordjevic B, Parra-Herran C. Application of a Pattern-based Classification System for Invasive Endocervical Adenocarcinoma in Cervical Biopsy, Cone and Loop Electrosurgical Excision (LEEP) Material: Pattern on Cone and LEEP is Predictive of Pattern in the Overall Tumor. Int J Gynecol Pathol 2016;35:456–66.

59. Hodgson A, Amemiya Y, Seth A, et al. Genomic abnormalities in invasive adenocarcinoma correlate with pattern of invasion: biologic and clinical implications. Mod Pathol 2017;30:1633–41.

60. Spaans VM, Scheunhage DA, Barzaghi B, et al. Independent validation of the prognostic significance of invasion patterns in endocercvical adenocarcinoma: pattern A predicts excellent survival. Gynecol Oncol 2018;151(2):196–201.

61. Segura S, Stolnicu S, Boros M, et al. mTOR activation assessed by immunohistochemostry in cervical biopsies of HPV-associated endocervical adenocarcinomas (HPVA): correlation with Silva invasion patterns. Appl Immunohistochem Mol Morphol 2021. https://doi.org/10.1097/PAI.0000000000000915.

62. Stolnicu S, Boros M, Hoang L, et al. FIGO 2018 stage IB ECAs: a detailed international study of clinical outcomes informed by prognostic biomarkers, including human papillomavirus (HPV) status. Int J Gynecol Cancer 2020;31(2):177–84.

63. Stolnicu S, Boros M, Hoang L, et al. Clinical Correlation of Silva Patterns of Invasion and 2019 FIGO Low-Stage (IA and IB1) in ECA (ECA). USCAP meeting abstract book 2021.

64. Ronnett BM, Yemelyanova AV, Vang R, et al. Endocervical adenocarcinomas with ovarian metastases: analysis of 29 cases with emphasis on minimally invasive cervical tumors and the ability of the metastases to simulate primary ovarian neoplasms. Am J Surg Pathol 2008;32:1835–53.

65. Stolnicu S, Boros M, Karpathiou G, et al. Clear cell carcinoma (CCC) of the cervix is a Human Pappilomavirus (HPV)-independent tumor associated with poor prognosis. Gotheburg Sweden: Abstract

accepted for European Congress of Pathology; 2021.

66. Pors J, Segura S, Chiu DS, Almadani N, Ren H, Fix DJ, et al. Clinicopathologic characteristics of mesonephric adenocarcinomas and mesonephric-like adenocarcinomas in the gynecologic tract: a multiinstitutional study. Am J Surg Pathol 2021; 45(5):498–506.

67. Bhatla N, Aoki D, Sharma DN, et al. Cancer of the cervix uteri. Int J Gynecol Obstet 2018;143:22–36.

68. Bhatla N, Berek JS, Cuello Fredes M, et al. Revised FIGO staging for carcinoma of the cervix uteri. Int J Gynecol Obstet 2019;145:129–35.

69. College of American Pathologists Protocol for the examination of resection specimens from patients with primary carcinoma of the uterine cervix. Version: uterine cervix resection 4.3.0.0. 2020. Available at: http://www.cap.org. Accessed September 4, 2020.

70. Olawaiye AB, Baker TP, Washington K, et al. The new (version 9) American Joint Committee on Cancer tumor, node, metastasis staging for cervical cancer. CA Cancer J Clin 2021;71:287–98.

71. Cibula D, Potter R, Planchamp F, et al. The European Society of Gynaecological Oncology/European Society for Radiotherapy and Oncology/European Society of Pathology Guidelines for the Management of Patients with Cervical Cancer. Virchows Arch 2018;472:919–36.

72. Amin MB, Edge S, Greene F, et al. AJCC cancer staging manual. 8th edition. Switzerland: Springer International Publishing: American Joint Commission on Cancer; 2017.

73. Parra-Herran C, Malpica A, Oliva E, et al. Endocervical adenocarcinoma, gross examination and processing including intraoperative evaluation: recommendations from the International Society of Gynecological Pathologists. Int J Gynecol Pathol 2021;40(suppl 1):S24–47.

74. Van de Putte G, Lie AK, Vach W, et al. Risk grouping in stage IB squamous cell cervical carcinoma. Gynecol Oncol 2005;99:106–12.

75. Delgado G, Bundy BN, Fowler WC, et al. A prospective surgical pathological study of stage I squamous carcinoma of the cervix: a Gynecologic Oncology Group study. Gynecol Oncol 1989;35:314–20.

76. Ryu SY, Kim MH, Nam BH, et al. Intermediate-risk grouping of cervical cancer patients treated with radical hysterectomy: a Korean Gynecologic Oncology Group study. Br J Cancer 2014;110:278–85.

77. Samlal RA, van der Velden J, Ten Kate FJ, et al. Surgical pathologic factors that predict recurrence in stage IB and IIA cervical carcinoma patients with negative pelvic lymph nodes. Cancer 1997;80: 1234–40.

78. Zyla RE, Gien LT, Vicus D, et al. The prognostic role of horizontal and circumferential tumor extend in

cervical cancer: implications for the 2019 FIGO staging system. GynecolOncol 2020;158:266–72.

79. Sevin BU, Nadji M, Averette HE, et al. Microinvasive carcinoma of the cervix. Cancer 1992;70:2121–8.

80. Elliott P, Coppleson M, Russell P, et al. Early invasive (FIGO stage IA) carcinoma of the cervix: a clinico-pathologic study of 476 cases. Int J Gynecol Cancer 2000;10:42–52.

81. Zaino R, Ward S, Delgado G, et al. Histopathologic Predictors of the Behavior of Surgically Treated Stage IB SCC of the Cervix. A Gynecologic Oncology Group Study. Cancer 1992;69(7):1750–8.

82. Obermair A, Wanner C, Bilgi S, et al. The influence of vascular space involvement on the prognosis of patients with stage IB cervical carcinoma: correlation of results from hematoxylin and eosin staining with results from immunostaining for factor VIII-related antigen. Cancer 1998;82(4):689–96.

83. Morice P, Piovesan P, Rey A, et al. Prognostic value of lymphovascular space invasion determined with hematoxylin-eosin staining in early stage cervical carcinoma: results of a multivariate analysis. Ann Oncol 2003;14(10):1511–7.

84. Day E, Duffy S, Bryson G, et al. Multifocal FIGO stage IA1 squamous carcinoma of the cervix: Criteria for identification, staging and its good clinical outcome. Int J Gynecol Pathol 2016;35:467–74.

85. McIlwaine P, Nagar H, McCluggage WG. Multifocal FIGO stage IA1 cervical squamous carcimomas have an extremely good prognosis equivalent to uni-focal lesions. Int J Gynecol Pathol 2014;33:213–7.

86. Cibula D, McCluggage WG. Sentinel lymph node (SLN) concept in cervical cancer: current limitations and unanswered questions. Gynecol Oncol 2019; 152:202–7.

87. Guani B, Dorez M, Magaud L, et al. Impact of micrometastasis or isolated tumor cells on recurrence and survival in patients with early cervical cancer: SENTICOL Trial. Int J Gynecol Cancer 2019;29: 447–52.

88. Holman LL, Levenback CF, Frumovitz M, et al. Sentinel lymph evaluation in women with cervical cancer. J Minim Invasive Gynecol 2014;21:540–5.

89. Park KJ, Roma A, Singh N, et al. Tumor staging of endocervical adenocarcinoma: recommendations from the International Society of Gynecological Pathologists. Int J Gynecol Pathol 2021;40:S92–101.

90. Stendahl U, Willen H, Willen R. Invasive SCC of the uterine cervix. I. Definition of parameters in a histo-pathologic malignancy grading system. Acta Radiol Oncol 1980;19:467–80.

91. Shimada M, Kigawa J, Nishimura R, et al. Ovarian metastasis in carcinoma of the uterine cervix. Gynecol Oncol 2006;101:234–7.

Squamous and Glandular Lesions of the Vulva and Vagina
What's New and What Remains Unanswered?

Kelly X. Wei, BSc[a], Lynn N. Hoang, MD[b],*

KEYWORDS

- Vulva • Vagina • Squamous cell carcinoma • Differentiated vulvar intraepithelial neoplasia
- Differentiated exophytic vulvar intraepithelial lesion • Vulvar aberrant maturation • Adenocarcinoma

Key points

- In-situ and invasive squamous neoplasia of the vulva and vagina are now divided into HPV-associated and HPV-independent types, harmonizing the categorization adopted across all lower genital sites prone to HPV infection.

- Morphology-based assessment alone will be unreliable in the distinction between HPV-associated and HPV-independent invasive and in-situ squamous neoplasia in the vulva, in a subset of cases.

- All invasive squamous cell carcinomas of the vulva and vagina should be stratified by p16 immunohistochemistry, as a surrogate marker for high-risk HPV.

- The most recent FIGO uses the alternate method of measuring depth of invasion in invasive squamous cell carcinoma, which differs from the traditional method used by other cancer reporting organizations.

- Glandular lesions of the vagina now encompass HPV-independent gastric type adenocarcinoma, gastric type adenosis, and HPV-associated adenocarcinoma.

ABSTRACT

A number of changes have been introduced into the 5th Edition of the World Health Organization (WHO) Classification of squamous and glandular neoplasms of the vulva and vagina. This review highlights the major shifts in tumor classification, new entities that have been introduced, recommendations for p16 immunohistochemical testing, biomarker use, molecular findings and practical points for pathologists which will affect clinical care. It also touches upon several issues that still remain answered in these rare but undeniably important women's cancers.

OVERVIEW

Cancers of the vulva and vagina reside within the exceptional minority when considered in the broad scope of gynecologic malignancies. Cancers of the vulva (mons pubis, labia majora, labia minora, clitoris, vestibular bulbs, vestibule, Bartholin's glands, and Skene's glands) represent 3% to 5% of gynecologic malignancies in developed countries.[1,2] Vulvar cancers have an annual incidence of 1.9 per 100,000 and accounted for 7046 cases and 1745 deaths in North America in 2020.[3] Vaginal cancers are even rarer, representing 1% to 2% of gynecologic malignancies, an annual incidence of 0.44

[a] MD Undergraduate Program, Faculty of Medicine, University of British Columbia, Vancouver, British Columbia, Canada; [b] Vancouver General Hospital and University of British Columbia, Vancouver, British Columbia, Canada
* Corresponding author. Department of Anatomical Pathology, Vancouver General Hospital, 910 West 10 Avenue, Vancouver, British Columbia V5Z 1M9, Canada.
E-mail address: Lien.Hoang@vch.ca

Surgical Pathology 15 (2022) 389–405
https://doi.org/10.1016/j.path.2022.02.011
1875-9181/22/© 2022 Elsevier Inc. All rights reserved.

per 100,000, and 1627 cases and 471 deaths in North America in 2020.[4] At both sites, the most common type of malignancy is squamous cell carcinoma (>90%), followed by adenocarcinoma and rare tumor types. Despite their relative rarity, epithelial malignancies in these locations comprise a heterogenous group from a biological and clinical perspective, requiring an accurate categorization by the pathologist. This review highlights the major changes and challenges in tumor classification of squamous and glandular lesions of the vulva and vagina introduced into the 5th Edition of the World Health Organization Blue Book (2020, WHO Classification of Tumors: Female Genital Tumors[5]).

INVASIVE SQUAMOUS CELL CARCINOMA

Unlike the major strides in tumor sub-classification achieved in ovarian and endometrial carcinomas, prompted by a wealth of advanced molecular studies, molecular sub-classification of vulvar carcinomas has only recently gained momentum. The first major sub-classification in vulvar squamous cell carcinoma (SCC) is based on human papillomavirus (HPV)-status, spurred by the paradigm shift realized in SCC of the head and neck region, where HPV-associated oropharyngeal SCC has been shown to be highly chemo- and radiosensitive and prognostically favorable.[6] The National Cancer Comprehensive Network (NCCN) treatment guidelines require p16 testing on all oropharyngeal SCC, as a surrogate marker for high-risk HPV infection, and consider treatment de-escalation for p16 (HPV) positive tumors.[6,7] HPV/p16 testing for all oropharyngeal SCC has also been endorsed by the American Society for Clinical Oncology (ASCO) and the College of American Pathologists (CAP).[8] In the vulva, similar attributes (increased sensitivity to chemo- and radiation therapy and improved prognosis) have been observed in HPV-associated vulvar SCC compared to HPV-independent vulvar SCC; the 5-year overall survival for HPV-associated vulvar SCCs ranges from 59% to 89% versus 38% to 63% for HPV-independent vulvar SCCs, while the 5-year recurrence free survival ranges from 54% to 90% and 45% to 64% for HPV-associated and HPV-independent vulvar SCCs, respectively.[9–16] In response to this growing body of literature, the most recent edition of the WHO Blue Book now endorses that SCC be divided into HPV-associated (HPVA) and HPV-independent (HPVI) groups.[5]

CLINICAL FEATURES

HPVA vulvar SCCs are usually found in younger women (19–97 years, median: 58–62 years),

approximately a decade younger than their HPVI SCC counterparts (18–104 years, median of 64–75 years).[9–11,13,17–20] In two studies that subdivided HPVI based on p53 status, those with p53 wild-type (p53wt) tumors occurred at an intermediate age (35–93 years, median: 68–73 years) compared to HPVA (19–92 years, median: 59–62 years) and HPVI p53 mutant (p53abn) SCCs (23–98 years, median: 74–75) **(Table 1)**.[10,11] Approximately 44% of patients with HPVA SCC or HPV-associated vulvar intraepithelial neoplasia (VIN) will also have synchronous or metachronous cervical neoplasia.[21]

Vulvar SCCs form exophytic masses that can be ulcerated. HPVA SCC is more often multifocal, while HPVI SCC is more often unifocal and associated with longstanding inflammation and lichen sclerosus.[22–25]

MICROSCOPIC EVALUATION & IMPLICATIONS FOR PATIENT CARE

HISTOLOGIC SUBTYPE

The latest edition of the WHO moves away from the traditional morphologic descriptors for vulvar SCC (basaloid, warty, verrucous, keratinizing, non-keratinizing), and toward an etiologic-based classification system: HPVA and HPVI **(Fig. 1)**.[5] This shift reflects an increased appreciation for the biology and prognosis of these tumors, and harmonizes the categorization taken across all lower genital sites prone to HPV infection.

Historically, HPVA tumors are generally more basaloid or warty ("blue" on histologic examination due to the loss of maturation and increased nucleus-to-cytoplasm ratio), while HPVI tumors are well-differentiated and keratinizing ("pink" imparted by the retained squamous maturation).[26,27] HPVA tumors are also more likely to exhibit necrosis, moderate/marked pleomorphism, koilocytic changes, and invasive fronts in a nested pattern compared to their HPVI counterparts.[17] The significance of tumor budding has not yet been formally examined in vulvar SCCs. However, we now recognize that the distinction between an HPVA and HPVI SCC is difficult because overlap exists between the two, complicating histological-based distinction **(Figs. 2 and 3)**.[17,28] In the largest study to date (n = 1594), Rakislova *and colleagues* (2017) found that 36.5% of HPVA tumors had keratinizing features (typically associated with HPVI tumors) and 5.2% of HPVI vulvar SCCs displayed basaloid or warty characteristics (usually associated with HPVA tumors).[17] These findings align with the conundrum of morphologic overlap described previously.[9,28]

Table 1
Summary of HPV-associated and HPV-independent vulvar SCC attributes

	HPV-Associated	HPV-Independent TP53 Wild-Type	HPV-Independent TP53 Mutant
Proportion of all SCC	16%–60%	10%–32%	30%–67%
Age (years)	58–62	68–73	74–75
Precursor Lesions	HPVA VIN (HSIL)	HPVI VIN (VAAD/DEVIL)	HPVI VIN (DVIN)
Histologic Appearance	Basaloid or warty	Well-differentiated (verrucous)	Typically keratinizing
Biomarkers (p16 IHC, p53 IHC)	p16 positive (strong block-like) p53 reduced (basal sparing/ mid-epithelial or reduced staining)	p16 negative p53 scattered pattern	p16 negative p53 mutant pattern (basal overexpression, parabasal/diffuse overexpression, absent, or cytoplasmic)
Mutations[a]			
TP53	0%–46%	0%	100%
HRAS	7%–14%	6%–57%	0%–21%
NOTCH1	0%	33%–50%	37%
PIK3CA	7%–34%	0%–29%	5%–25%
CDKN2A	17%	11%–12%	11%–33%
FBXW7	0%–17%	12%–33%	8%–11%
FGFR3	0%–1%	33%	0%
PTEN	1%–8%	0%	0%
FAT1	0%	22%	11%
APC	0%	11%	22%
Prognosis	Good	Intermediate	Poor
Treatment Implications	Antiviral treatments (e.g., Imiquimod) HPV vaccination More sensitive to adjuvant therapy		Potential for immune checkpoint inhibitors More likely to have positive margins
Relative Survival (hazards ratio)[11]	1	2.16	3.43

[a] Based on studies which separated HPVI into *TP53* mutated and *TP53* wild-type. [10,43,59,60,65]

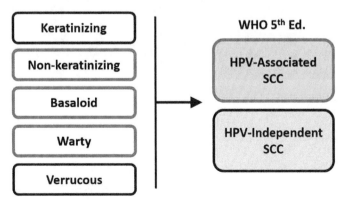

Fig. 1. Change in the WHO classification for squamous cell carcinoma (SCC) of the vulva and vagina. The traditional morphology-based classification is now replaced by dichotomization, as per human papillomavirus (HPV) status, into HPV-associated (HPVA) and HPV-independent (HPVI) types.

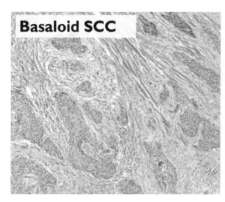 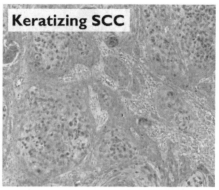

Fig. 2. Vulvar squamous cell carcinoma. Both of these examples of squamous cell carcinoma (*Left*: Basaloid, *Right*: Keratinizing) are associated with HPV, negating the concept that morphology alone can always accurately predict HPV status.

Although the presence of a precursor lesion can help inform HPV status, even these lesions can be morphologically misleading as detailed below. As a result, p16 has been recommended for the routine stratification of SCC of the vulva and vagina and is incorporated in the 2021 International Collaboration on Cancer Reporting (ICCR) guidelines and 2021 International Federation of Gynecology and Obstetrics (FIGO).[29,30]

The proportion of vulvar SCCs, that are associated with HPV infections, varies widely between 16%–60%.[11,17,22,31] Similarly, the proportion of HPVI SCCs of the vagina ranges widely between 0%–79%.[32] It is anticipated that the proportion of HPVA SCC will decrease over time due to uptake of the national HPV vaccination programs.[33,34] Collaterally, the relative proportion and corresponding treatment and diagnostic related difficulties stemming from HPVI SCC will be of increasing importance.

As with many movements in histologic classification, shifts in treatment approach have yet to follow. The latest NCCN guidelines for the treatment of vulvar cancer consider stage, tumor size, depth of invasion, lymph node status, margin status, lymphovascular space invasion, and even spray/diffuse infiltrative pattern, but do not yet separate treatment based on HPV status. However, it is foreseeable that this will change in the future, given the findings noted above and below.

DEPTH OF INVASION

Depth of invasion is an important histologic parameter, as it will dictate lymph node sampling or dissection at most institutions. A tumor measuring less than 2 cm in size and with a depth of invasion ≤1 mm (FIGO stage 1A) can be managed with wide local excision, without the need for groin lymph node dissection. A depth of invasion greater than 1 mm, however, will warrant sentinel lymph node biopsy or inguinofemoral lymphadenoectomy.[35–37]

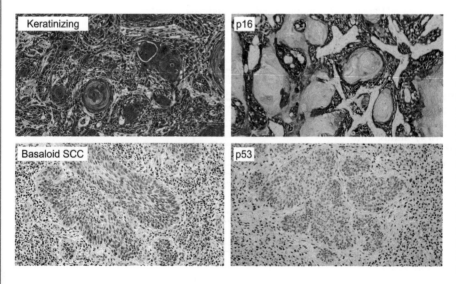

Fig. 3. Vulvar squamous cell carcinoma. Additional examples of cases in which the morphology is discrepant with the classically expected immunophenotype, including a keratinizing squamous cell carcinoma with p16 overexpression indicating association with HPV (*top*) and a basaloid squamous cell carcinoma with abnormal (null) p53 staining (*bottom*).

The depth of invasion has been traditionally defined as the distance from the most superficial dermal papilla adjacent to the tumor to the deepest point of invasion. There is an alternate method of measurement, which starts from the basement membrane of the deepest adjacent tumor-free rete ridge or dysplastic rete ridge to the deepest point of invasion. This alternate method downstages approximately 20% of stage IB tumors to stage 1A; importantly, these down-staged tumors experienced less local recurrences compared to tumors that remained stage IB.[38] This alternate system has recently been adopted by FIGO in 2021, while the traditional method is currently used by the American Joint Committee on Cancer (AJCC) and ICCR. It remains uncertain whether there will be enough compelling evidence to harmonize this change across all cancer reporting agencies.

MARGIN ASSESSMENT

The majority of guidelines recommend a clinical gross margin of 1 to 2 cm, which corresponds to at least 8 mm after tissue shrinkage due to formalin fixation.[35,36,39] More conservative margins can be taken to preserve anatomic function of midline structures. Margins less than 8 mm or positive margins may warrant re-excision or adjuvant radiotherapy.[36] Margin distances should be performed in a straight line (not along tissue curves) from the peripheral edge of the invasive nests to the nearest inked peripheral margin. This peripheral margin may be the epithelial surface or the stromal edge, whichever is closest.[40]

While the 8 mm rule is endorsed by the majority of guidelines, the literature has yielded mixed results in what determines adequate minimal margin distance.[41,42] The issue of adequate margin clearance to reduce local recurrence risk remains one of the vitally important unanswered questions in the treatment of vulvar SCC. It is very likely that a 'field cancerization' effect plays a major role in local recurrence, particularly in HPVI tumors.[43,44] With the added use of p53 immunohistochemistry (IHC) for mapping, p53-abnormal epithelial cells adjacent to the tumor frequently extend beyond the morphologic bounds detected by the unaided pathologist eye. When p53 IHC is used, it can highlight p53 abnormal cells in initially unrecognized DVIN or cells which look almost morphologically normal, akin to a p53 signature lesion in the fallopian tube.[44] These p53-abnormal cells can extend to the margins, changing margin status from "negative" to "positive" in approximately one-third of cases.[44,45] The risk of local recurrence when cells bearing abnormal p53 are present at a surgical margin is astonishingly 73%, the same rate as when *bone fide* differentiated vulvar intraepithelial neoplasia (DVIN) is present at a surgical margin and a risk two-times higher compared to when no lesion is identified at a margin.[44] McAlpine *et al.* reported extremely persuasive data, where outcomes for HPVA and HPVI SCC were similar before 1995 (when all patients had radical surgeries with wide margins) compared to after 1995, where outcomes for HPVI SCC were significantly worse than HPVA SCC (when there was a move toward more conservative surgery).[9] All of these facets raise an important question: Should margin clearance be defined differently for HPVA and HPVI tumors?

ANCILLARY STUDIES

P16 AND HUMAN PAPILLOMAVIRUS DETECTION STUDIES

At lower anogenital sites, p16 IHC is a reliable surrogate marker for high-risk HPV infection (**Table 2**). p16 (also known as p16^{INK4A}) is a protein encoded by the *CDKN2A* gene locus and functions by inhibiting cyclin-dependent kinase 4 (CDK4) and 6 (CDK6). CDK4/6 normally phosphorylates retinoblastoma protein (pRb), inactivating it and permitting the cell to enter the cell cycle.[46] The inhibition of pRb phosphorylation by p16 thus results in cell cycle arrest. E6 and E7 are HPV oncoproteins that inactivate p53 and pRb, respectively, allowing for cell cycle progression. As a result, p16 levels rise to compensate under these conditions, leading to p16 overexpression in lesions and tumors associated with high-risk HPV infections.[46] The Lower Anogenital Squamous Terminology (LAST) Standardization Project proposes that p16 is considered positive when there is continuous block-like staining in at least the lower third of the squamous epithelium.[47] In some cases of HPVA tumors, p16 can be negative (false negative staining) due to methylation and loss of heterozygosity.[48] In these situations, HPV testing by PCR or in-situ hybridization (ISH) is informative. RNA-based ISH is preferred to DNA-based ISH as the former has been shown to have more accurate detection in

Table 2		
Concordance of p16 IHC and HPV DNA PCR in vulvar SCC[15,17,112–115]		
	p16 +	**p16 -**
HPV DNA+	83%–100%	0%–17%
HPV DNA-	1%–16%	84%–99%

tumors with low to intermediate (50–100 copies/cell) viral copy numbers. ISH has also been found to be more accurate than PCR detection, which can be confounded by environmental contamination and the need for specialized equipment and technical skills.[49,50]

P53

p53, famously nicknamed 'the guardian of the genome', detects DNA damage and either orchestrates DNA repair or initiates apoptosis. p53 IHC can serve as a surrogate marker for *TP53* mutation status. Ovarian and endometrial adenocarcinomas use a proportion and intensity cut-off (i.e., strong staining in >80% of tumor cells).[51,52] This is not applicable to squamous neoplasia because it exhibits architectural maturation in both in-situ and invasive lesions. Instead, p53 IHC needs to be interpreted as a "pattern" rather than a simplistic "positive". The lack of uniformity in p53 interpretation in the literature has unfortunately led to mixed results in the ability of p53 IHC to predict *TP53* mutation status, leaving many observers with protracted skepticism.[53–55] Only recently has a reliable framework been developed to interpret p53 IHC in squamous neoplasia of the vulva.[56,57] In HPVI squamous neoplasia, p53 wild-type staining was seen as patchy heterogeneous staining in the basal layer of the epithelium or invasive squamous nest. For *TP53* mutant cases, there are four patterns: 1) basal overexpression (strong, uniform nuclear staining in ≥ 80% of the basal cells without significant parabasal staining), 2) parabasal/diffuse overexpression (strong, uniform nuclear staining in ≥ 80% of the basal cells in addition to strong extension to parabasal or more superficial layers), 3) absent (completely absent [null] staining in the presence of a positive internal control), and 4) cytoplasmic expression. This framework was reliably applicable to both in-situ and invasive lesions, yielding 93% to 95% IHC to mutation-status concordance[56] and strong agreement amongst expert observers.[57] As with any IHC, titration is important, particularly in distinguishing between basal-overexpression patterns and strong wild-type patterns (one of the most challenging scenarios). It is helpful to compare the p53 staining in the lesion of question to the adjacent normal skin or hair follicles, which usually demonstrate wild-type staining.

One should be aware that the interpretation of p53 IHC in HPVA lesions is quite different.[56–58] p53 IHC expression is reduced (p53 is degraded due to HPV oncoprotein E6). This is seen as mid-epithelial (basal-sparing) and reduced (diminished intensity) IHC staining patterns.[22,56] In contrast to normal skin, HPVA in-situ and invasive SCC show an absence of staining in the basal layer (normal skin will show patchy positive staining in the basal layer). This absence of staining in the basal layer can be juxtaposed to variable (often very strong) staining in the parabasal layers, and thus is named 'basal sparing' and should not be misinterpreted to reflect a missense mutation. This basal-sparing pattern can also have a variety of forms. There can be an absence of staining in the basal layer only, in the basal-layer and portion of parabasal layers and even the full-thickness of the epithelium (a pattern we have called the markedly reduced – "null-like" pattern). The "null-like" pattern is especially confusing, as an unexpecting pathologist may confuse this with a true null-mutation pattern. In this situation, a positive p16 stain or HPV ISH can be a clue that the reduced staining is due to HPVA infection and p53 protein degradation, not a true null-mutation. In the context of HPVA squamous neoplasia, there are two clues that are generally helpful: (1) Lesions which show top-heavy p53 (stronger at the top of the epithelium compared to the bottom of the epithelium in VIN, or stronger in the central portion of the squamous nests compared to the periphery of the nests in invasive carcinoma) are usually indicative of a high-risk HPV infection. Normal squamous epithelium, reactive lesions, and HPVI VIN will all show stronger p53 at the base of the epithelium, which tapers/diminishes in intensity toward the surface. (2) Lesions which demonstrate very strong p53 IHC throughout are unlikely to be HPV-associated (because HPV should degrade the p53 protein).

MOLECULAR FINDINGS & PROGNOSTICATION

Unlike some other gynecologic malignancies, vulvar SCC does not have a defining molecular mutation. Vaginal squamous neoplasia, due to its even greater rarity, has only been explored to a limited extent.

HPVI vulvar SCCs have higher mutational loads compared to HPVA SCCs, but copy number alterations and mutation signatures do not differ between the groups.[59] HPVI SCCs have higher rates of *TP53* mutations, but the difference in mutation frequencies affecting other genes is variable (see **Table 1**).[10,18,60–63] In the largest study to date (n = 280 vulvar squamous cell carcinomas, 406 cancer-related genes), Williams *and colleagues* found that 61% of HPVA tumors had alterations in the PI3K/AKT/mTOR pathway, compared to 27% of HPVI tumors (*P* < .0001). Several studies have found higher frequencies of *NOTCH1*,[10,18,63,64] *FAT1*,[18,59,64] *TERT*,[64] and *FBXW7*[60,65] in HPVI compared to HPVA SCCs. In the HPVI group, those that are p53 wild-type tend to have higher mutational frequencies in *HRAS, BRAF,* and *CDK2NA*.[2,10,43,59,66] In the HPVI group, Williams *and colleagues* also found higher rates of PD-L1 high-positive IHC staining and *PDL1/PDL2* amplifications, which may suggest potential for immune checkpoint inhibitor therapies.[18]

In the past few years, there has been interest in further sub-stratifying HPVI SCCs into *TP53* mutated and *TP53* wild-type tumors, as *TP53* mutations tend to portend a worse prognosis.[9–12] In 2017, Nooij *and colleagues* studied 36 SCC and 82 precursors using a targeted gene panel encompassing 17 genes. They subsequently examined the prognostic significance of three identified subtypes (HPV+, HPV-/p53wt, and HPV-/p53abn) in a follow up cohort of 236 vulvar cancer patients. They found that there was a statistically significant lower local recurrence rate for HPV+ tumors (5.3%) compared to HPV$^-$/p53wt tumors (16.3%) and HPV$^-$/p53abn tumors (22.6%) ($P = .044$).[10] However, there was no statistically significant difference between the HPV-/p53wt and HPV-/p53abn patient groups, although a trend did exist. Five-year overall survivals for HPV+, HPV-/p53wt, and HPV-/p53abn patient groups were 75%, 67.2%, and 56.3%, respectively, with the difference between HPV+ and both HPV- groups reaching statistical significance.[10] Subsequent to this, Korkekaas *and colleagues* studied 413 primary SCC cases obtained from two Dutch university hospitals (Leiden University Medical Center and ErasmusMC Rotterdam) that were treated between 2000 to 2015.[11] In their univariate analysis, the HPV-/p53abn group had statistically significant worse overall survival (hazards ratio [HR]: 3.43), relative survival (relative excess risk [RER]: 4.02), and recurrence-free period (HR: 3.76) compared to the HPV+ group ($P < .05$ for all comparisons). For the HPV-/p53wt group, the only statistically significant difference was in overall survival (HR: 3.16, $P < .049$). In a smaller study by Kashofer *and colleagues*, 14 of 45 (31%) patients with *TP53* mutated HPVI SCC died of disease within the 5 year study period (mean 12 months, range 2–24 months after diagnosis), compared to 0/13 patients with HPVA SCC and 0/14 patients with HPVI *TP53* wild-type SCC.[67] Regauer *and colleagues* also found that disease-free intervals differed greatly depending on *TP53* gene status (33 months for *TP53* mutated SCC vs 65 months for *TP53* wild type primary SCC).[68] These findings are compelling and are worth validating as they would suggest that all SCCs should also have p53 IHC performed.

We are only at the early stages in understanding the role of *TP53* in vulvar SCC. Approximately 7% to 27% of vulvar SCCs have more than one *TP53* mutation.[2,63,67,68] In tumors that recur, *TP53* mutations can be identical to the primary or recur with additional or more complex *TP53* gene mutations.[68,69] Some patients with primary *TP53* wild-type SCC can recur with an acquired *TP53* mutation and, peculiarly, primary *TP53* mutant SCC can recur or metastasize with *TP53* wild-type SCC.[63,68,70] Whether this represents a true event, tumor heterogeneity/sampling or a new primary tumor warrants validation in larger studies.

IN-SITU SQUAMOUS NEOPLASIA

According to the 2020 WHO classification, and similarly to the invasive SCC counterparts, vulvar in-situ squamous precursors are divided into HPV-associated and HPV-independent types (**Table 3**). The preferred terminology is "squamous intraepithelial lesion (SIL)" for HPVA lesions and "vulvar intraepithelial neoplasia (VIN)" for HPVI lesions. Of note, the term *usual type* VIN (uVIN) is also acceptable for HPVA lesions as per the WHO. For simplicity, we will refer to both HPVA and HPVI lesions using VIN nomenclature. In the vagina, only HPVA lesions are currently recognized and also follow the SIL nomenclature (with equivalent vaginal intraepithelial neoplasia - VaIN terminology).

HUMAN PAPILLOMAVIRUS-ASSOCIATED VULVAR INTRAEPITHELIAL NEOPLASIA

HPVA VIN (uVIN) now follows the Bethesda structure which divides lesions into low grade squamous intraepithelial lesion (LSIL) and high-grade squamous intraepithelial lesion (HSIL). LSIL is equivalent to VIN1, and HSIL equivalent to VIN2 and VIN3. This new terminology antiquates the flurry of terms used to describe HPVA lesions in the vulva (i.e., Bowen's dysplasia/disease, Mobus Bowen, erythroplasiform dyskeratosis, erythroplasia de Queyrat, dedifferentiated VIN, classic VIN, carcinoma in-situ).[71] The same binary categorization applies to vaginal lesions, which were formerly classified as vaginal intraepithelial neoplasia (VaIN): LSIL corresponds to VaIN1 and HSIL to VaIN2/3.

LSIL is associated with low-risk HPV types and is found more frequently in women in their 40s and 50s.[72,73] The majority in the vulva are exophytic, in the form of condyloma acuminatum. LSILs in the vulva are rarely flat. They are classically knuckle-shaped and have koilocytosis, binucleation, irregular nuclear contours, and are negative for p16 (no staining or patchy

Table 3
Summary of HPV-associated and HPV-independent in-situ neoplasia attributes

	HPV-Associated VIN -LSIL	HPV-Associated VIN -HSIL	HPV-Independent VIN VAAD/DEVIL [*TP53* Wild-Type]	HPV-Independent VIN DVIN [*TP53* Mutant]
Age	42–51	40–44	41–96	60–80
Histologic Appearance	Koilocytosis, binucleation, basal atypia	Warty, basaloid, hyperchromatic, high NC ratios, suprabasilar mitoses, apoptotic bodies	Absence of basal atypia, marked acanthosis with flat (VAAD) or exophytic (DE-VIL) surface, verruciform architecture, superficial epithelial cell pallor, loss of the granular cell layer, multilayered parakeratosis	Marked nuclear atypia, abnormal keratinocyte maturation in the form, dyskeratosis, hyperkeratosis, parakeratosis, prominent intercellular bridges, anastomotic rete ridges
Biomarkers (p16 IHC, p53 IHC)	p16 negative	p16 positive (confluent and strong staining in at least the lower one-third of the epithelium) p53 wild-type (basal sparing, mid-epithelial pattern)	p16 negative p53 mostly wild-type (scattered staining)	p16 negative p53 mostly abnormal (basal/diffuse overexpression, absent, cytoplasmic)
Mutations				
TP53		10.5%	14.3%	47.5%–90%
NOTCH		10.5%	28.6%	20%
HRAS		5.3%	71.4%	10%
PIK3CA		-	33%–100%	31%
BRAF		-	9%	
Prognosis	Negligible chance of progression	9%–16% progression to SCC for untreated cases (3% for treated cases)	44% progression to SCC	30%–90% progression to SCC
Precursor lesion to invasive carcinoma (time for transformation)	6–7 y	41 mo	22–65 mo	23–44 mo

staining).[73–75] LSILs have a low/negligible risk of progression to HPV-associated vulvar SCC, and thus are recommended to be treated only if symptomatic.[76–78]

HSIL is associated with high-risk HPV types.[77,79,80] It is more commonly found in women aged 40 to 44.[81] Historically, HSILs can be subdivided into warty (condylomatous), basaloid, or mixed types based on appearance.[77,81] They exhibit suprabasilar mitoses, hyperchromasia, pleomorphism, high nuclear-to-cytoplasmic ratios, apoptotic bodies, and multinucleated cells.[77,81] p16 IHC staining is usually positive (strong and block-like), while p53 stains in a wild-type (basal sparing) pattern.[77,81,82] If untreated, approximately 9% to 16% of HSILs will progress into vulvar SCCs; the rate drops to 3% for treated cases.[81] Treatment is usually via imiquimod, excision, or laser.[83]

Fig. 4. Change in the WHO classification for vulvar intraepithelial neoplasia (VIN), which is now divided into HPV-associated (HPVA) and HPVI-independent (HPVI) types.

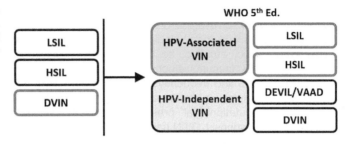

HUMAN PAPILLOMAVIRUS-INDEPENDENT VULVAR INTRAEPITHELIAL NEOPLASIA

Unlike the classification of HPVA VIN, which has gained clarity over the recent years, the nomenclature for HPVI VIN is less clear. In the WHO, HPVI VIN encompasses three broad entities: differentiated vulvar intraepithelial neoplasia (DVIN), vulvar acanthosis with altered differentiation (VAAD), and differentiated exophytic vulvar intraepithelial lesion (DEVIL) (**Figs. 4** and **5**).

DVIN is found more commonly in the 6th to 8th decades of life.[81] It is more often associated with pruritis and multifocality, compared to DE-VIL/VAAD.[84] The common denominator feature for DVIN is the presence of basal cytologic atypia, in the form of hyperchromatic or vesicular chromatin, pleomorphism, nuclear enlargement, and prominent nucleoli.[2,84,85] A variety of other features have been described, such as spongiosis (prominent intercellular bridges), parakeratosis, hyperkeratosis, acanthosis, dyskeratosis, atypical mitoses, abnormal stroma, and rete ridge elongation with anastomoses.[77,81,86] Not all of these features are necessary for the diagnosis of DVIN, and often the nuclear atypia is more subtle than described in textbooks.[2] The atypia can better be appreciated if compared to the background normal epithelium. DVIN is often overlooked if there is superimposed inflammation or non-

Fig. 5. Classic morphologic features for DVIN with corresponding abnormal p53 IHC pattern, DE-VIL, VAAD, and corresponding wild-type p53 IHC pattern in DE-VIL.

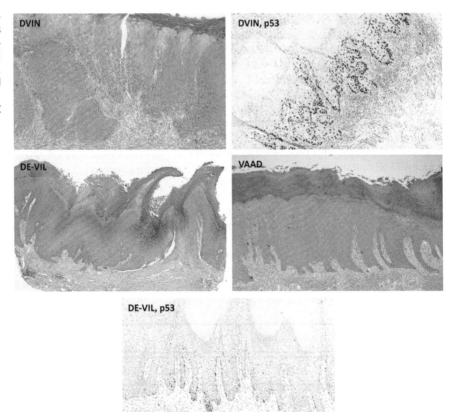

acanthotic skin (atrophic).[2] The International Society for the Study of Vulvovaginal Diseases (ISSVD) has described several morphologic variants for DVIN: hypertrophic, atrophic, acantholytic, and subtle forms.[87] By immunohistochemistry, DVIN is negative for p16 and frequently harbors *TP53* mutations.[2,10,85] However, abnormal p53 expression or *TP53* mutations, at present, are not required for the diagnosis. DVIN has a higher rate of progression to vulvar SCC compared to HPVA precursor lesions, with rates between 30% to 90% and a shorter time to progression.[88] The wide percentages likely reflect the difficulties in the morphologic diagnosis of DVIN.[89–91] The majority of DVIN are treated with surgical excision but variation in management modalities exists.[83]

The terms VAAD and DE-VIL were described in 2004 and 2017, respectively, as postulated precursor lesions to verrucous carcinoma and other forms of HPVI SCC.[66,92] VAAD is characterized by marked acanthosis, absence of cytologic atypia, variable verruciform architecture, superficial epithelial cell pallor, loss of the granular cell layer, and multilayered parakeratosis.[92] DE-VIL has been reported to have exophytic growth, absence of HPV histology, prominent verruciform/acanthotic architecture, and absence of significant basal atypia.[86] Although VAAD and DE-VIL are described separately in some studies, the seminal characterization of DE-VIL included cases within the morphologic spectrum of VAAD, and both terms are understood as part of the same disease spectrum.[43,66,86] Both VAAD and/or DE-VIL harbor mutations in *PIK3CA*, *HRAS*, and *NOTCH1*.[2,10,43,66] In general, VAAD/DE-VILs exhibit wild-type *TP53*, but rare cases with abnormal *TP53* have been described.[10,93] In addition, some VAAD/DE-VILs progress into SCCs that acquire *TP53* mutations.[66] The prognosis and natural history for VAAD/DEVIL are not well-known. In a small series by Akbari *and colleagues*, the times to progression from DE-VIL to verrucous carcinoma in 3 patients were 22, 33, and 65 months.[43] A recent series by Roy *and colleagues* showed lesion recurrence in 44% (12/27) of patients with initial diagnosis of VAAD/DE-VIL or verruciform lichen simplex chronicus.[94] Moreover, progression to a squamous cell carcinoma diagnosis was documented in 37% (10/27) of patients, being more frequent in VAAD/DE-VIL (10/16) than in verruciform lichen simplex chronicus (2/11).[94] Most recently, a publication by the ISSVD coined the term vulvar aberrant maturation (VAM) to replace VAAD/DE-VIL and to encompass the umbrella of lesions exhibiting aberrant maturation but lacking the atypia seen in DVIN.

The entire scope of HPVI preneoplasia poses an incredible challenge to pathologists due to significant overlaps in morphologic characteristics between entities and benign lesions. Rare conditions such as hypertrophic lichen sclerosus[95] and verruciform lichen simplex chronicus[94] have been reported to give rise to HPVI SCC, suggesting that some of these lesions may represent underdiagnosed squamous precursors. To this end, DE-VIL cases described by Watkins *and colleagues* were initially diagnosed as "verruciform lichen simplex chronicus". Moreover, a recent study by Roy *and colleagues* documented morphologic changes, recurrence, and progression to SCC in verruciform lichen simplex chronicus similar to VAAD/DE-VIL, in support of considering these lesions as pre-cancerous.[94] Despite the variations in nomenclature, it is likely all these lesions exist on the same spectrum of HPVI intraepithelial neoplasia. It would be reasonable to consider a simplified framework where DVIN is synonymous to HPVI p53-mutant VIN, and DE-VIL or VAM synonymous to HPVI p53-wt VIN. This would avoid much of the interobserver-related variations in diagnosis and would likely have more direct clinical relevance (**Fig. 6**).

MICROSCOPIC CHALLENGES IN THE INTERPRETATION OF VULVAR INTRAEPITHELIAL NEOPLASIA AND RELATED LESIONS

It is also important to re-emphasize that the histologic features of HPVA and HPVI VIN can overlap. There is a morphologic variant of DVIN (basaloid VIN) which appears quite "blue", highly resembling HSIL. Likewise, a morphologic variant of HSIL (HSIL with superimposed lichen simplex

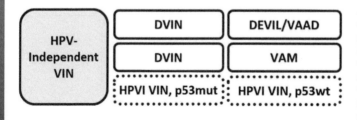

Fig. 6. Different systems for the classification of HPV-independent vulvar intraepithelial neoplasia (VIN). DVIN and DEVIL/VAAD are terms used in the WHO Classification, while DVIN and VAM are recommended by the ISSVD. We propose that stratification via p53 status would be more consistent and clinically meaningful.

Fig. 7. Variant morphologic features in vulvar intraepithelial neoplasia (VIN). HSIL with superimposed lichen simplex chronicus changes can have a very low-power pink appearance, but the positive block-like p16 and basal-sparing p53 patterns help determine that this is an HPV-associated VIN lesion. DVIN can have a basaloid or atrophic appearance, usually with an abnormal p53 pattern (basal/diffuse overexpression).

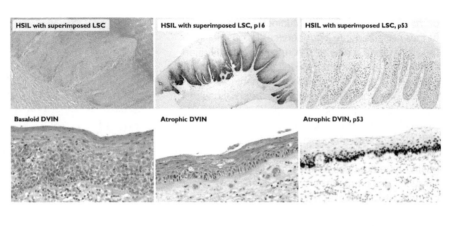

chronicus) that appears quite "pink" has also been described (**Fig. 7**).[96,97] Approximately 5% of HSIL has been shown to mimick DVIN[98] and with 18% of DVIN mimicking HSIL.[99] As alluded to above, p16 IHC is useful for accurately subdividing precursor lesions into HPVA and HPVI.[98,99] p53 IHC is also helpful, as HSIL will demonstrate a basal-sparing pattern.[58,100] HPV-associated VIN may show features mimicking the appearance of HPV-independent VIN, and adjacent lichen sclerosus is seen in up to 50% of HPV-associated VINs.[100]

In a sizable study of 779 HPVI SCCs by the HPV VAAP (international survey on HPV prevalence and type distribution in vulvar, vaginal, anal and penile neoplasms) study group (38 countries), 68% of vulvar SCCs had abnormal p53 IHC patterns in both the SCC and adjacent skin lesion, and 21% had abnormal p53 IHC in the SCC and wild type staining in the adjacent skin lesion. These adjacent skin lesions were mostly inflammatory, but they may have also represented p53-wild type neoplasia.[93] Moreover, approximately 15% of the lesions designated as inflammatory exhibited an abnormal p53 IHC pattern.[93] This highlights the continued challenges in p53 IHC and preneoplasia interpretation. We have found that inflammatory lesions such as lichen sclerosus, lichen simplex chronicus, lichen planus, and spongiotic dermatitis can show increased p53 staining, sometimes resulting in basal-only overexpression.[101] In this setting, DVIN can be considered only in the right morphologic context. Other p53 patterns attributed to *TP53* mutations (strong parabasal/diffuse,

absent, cytoplasmic) are not found, and their presence is therefore compatible with DVIN.[101]

p53 status is notoriously difficult to interpret in lichen sclerosus. Lichen sclerosus has been shown to harbor *TP53* mutations that match the *TP53* mutation in the invasive SCC.[53,54] This again raises several important unanswered questions: What is the clinical significance (natural history) of *TP53*-mutant lichen sclerosus? Should they be diagnosed and treated like *TP53*-mutant DVIN?

GLANDULAR LESIONS OF THE VULVA

Glandular lesions of the vulva have not changed substantially since the previous edition of the WHO. They are divided into (1) mammary-type glandular lesions, (2) Bartholin gland related lesions and adenocarcinomas associated with (3) Paget disease, (4) sweat gland origin, and (5) intestinal-type origin. The only significant update is the expansion of molecular subtypes within adenocarcinomas of mammary-gland type. These adenocarcinomas are considered analogous to those that arise with the breast, and similarly exhibit four molecular subtypes (luminal A, luminal B, HER2 enriched, basal-like).[102] For this reason, ancillary biomarker testing (ER, PR, and HER2/neu) is recommended.

GLANDULAR LESIONS OF THE VAGINA

The 2020 edition of the WHO Classification of Tumors now separates the histopathological gland types of vaginal adenosis into tuboendometrioid or mucinous patterns.[103] Mucinous patterns are further classified into endocervical or gastric, with the latter being a new addition to the classification scheme.[103,104] The morphologic characteristics of gastric-type adenosis include prominent cell membranes, pale eosinophilic cytoplasm, and occasionally intestinal differentiation with Goblet cells.[104] Atypical gastric adenosis has also been reported, with suggestions that gastric adenosis can progress through atypical gastric adenosis into gastric-type adenocarcinoma.[103–105]

Mucinous carcinoma of the vagina is now divided into gastric and intestinal types. Gastric type mucinous carcinoma is a primary mucinous adenocarcinoma of the vagina with gastric differentiation, similar to its cervical counterpart. These are also rare neoplasms that are found in patients aged 41 to 69 years (mean of 56 years).[104,106,107] The etiology remains largely unknown, though associations with congenital genitourinary malformations have been suggested. Gastric type mucinous carcinoma may arise from gastric type adenosis through atypical adenosis.[104–106] Histologically, the tumor cells exhibit eosinophilic/foamy, voluminous pale/clear cytoplasm, variable nuclear atypia, and prominent cell membranes. Intestinal/neuroendocrine differentiation may be seen as well.[104,106,107] Positive IHC staining is usually seen for MUC6, HIK1083, CDX2, CK7, CEA, CA125, and CA19-9, with more variable staining for CK20 and PAX8. p16 is negative (or focally positive), hormone receptors are negative, and approximately half of cases show abnormal p53.[106] Data on prognosis are again limited, though the tumors appear to be aggressive.[104] Intestinal type mucinous carcinoma is a primary adenocarcinoma of the vagina with similar characteristics to colorectal carcinomas. They usually occur in older women (36 to 86 years; median of 56 years) and are usually found in the lower, posterior vagina.[108,109] Although the etiology is unknown, some cases occur in association with intestinal-type adenomas and/or adenosis, potentially suggesting they follow an adenoma-carcinoma sequence.[108,109] Histologically, they exhibit intestinal adenocarcinoma features, including Goblet cells and intracytoplasmic mucin. Neuroendocrine cells have also been reported.[108,109] They typically express CK20 and CDX2, have variable staining for CK7, and are negative for ER. Limited data exists on long term follow-up, though recurrences and deaths have been reported in one study.[108,109]

HPVA adenocarcinoma of the vagina is another new addition to the 2020 WHO Classification of Tumors. It is defined as an HPVA glandular tumor with exophytic expansile-type invasion and/or

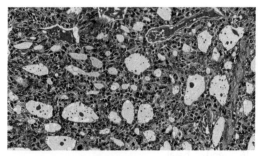

Fig. 8. HPV-associated adenocarcinoma of the vagina. These rare lesions have the same morphology seen in usual HPV-associated adenocarcinomas of the cervix. Typically, the tumor is comprised of mucin-depleted cells with hyperchromatic irregular nuclei and brisk mitoses.

invasion of the stroma after exclusion of cervical adenocarcinoma.[110] These neoplasms have been found in patients aged 38 to 51 years and are quite rare.[110] These carcinomas exhibit histologic characteristics similar to those seen in HPVA adenocarcinomas of the cervix: Papillary, glandular, and/or villoglandular architecture, columnar cells that show mucinous or mucin-poor characteristics, nuclei that are hyperchromatic, irregular, and cigar to ovoid shaped, conspicuous apical mitoses and apoptotic debris, and diffuse p16 positivity.[110,111] (**Fig. 8**).

SUMMARY

As our access to large clinical databases and biomarker/omics strategies to refine diagnosis continues to grow, we will continue to see shifts in tumor classifications that will improve treatment decisions. Although the magnitude of movements in vulvar and vaginal lesions is slow compared to other gynecologic giants, significant shifts to include HPV status and HPVI squamous and glandular lesions have been made.

CLINICS CARE POINTS

- Stratification of vulvar squamous cell carcinoma by HPV (p16) and p53 has implications for prognosis, surgical margins and adjuvant treatment
- Depth of invasion is important in determining the need for lymph node sampling

DISCLOSURE

The authors have nothing to disclose.

REFERENCES

1. Halec G, Alemany L, Quiros B, et al. Biological relevance of human papillomaviruses in vulvar cancer. Mod Pathol 2017;30(4):549–62.

2. Tessier-Cloutier B, Pors J, Thompson E, et al. Molecular characterization of invasive and in situ squamous neoplasia of the vulva and implications for morphologic diagnosis and outcome. Mod Pathol Off J U S Can Acad Pathol Inc 2021;34(2): 508–18.

3. 21-Vulva-fact-sheet.pdf. Available at: https://gco. iarc.fr/today/data/factsheets/cancers/21-Vulva--fact-sheet.pdf. Accessed May 11, 2021.

4. 22-Vagina-fact-sheet.pdf. Available at: https://gco. iarc.fr/today/data/factsheets/cancers/22-Vagina--fact-sheet.pdf. Accessed June 16, 2021.

5. BlueBooksOnline. Available at: https://tumourclassification.iarc.who.int/paragraphcontent/34/525. Accessed May 11, 2021.

6. Perri F, Longo F, Caponigro F, et al. Management of HPV-Related Squamous Cell Carcinoma of the Head and Neck: Pitfalls and Caveat. Cancers 2020;12(4):E975.

7. Guidelines Detail. NCCN. Available at: https://www. nccn.org/guidelines/guidelines-detail. Accessed October 11, 2021.

8. Fakhry C, Lacchetti C, Rooper LM, et al. Human Papillomavirus Testing in Head and Neck Carcinomas: ASCO Clinical Practice Guideline Endorsement of the College of American Pathologists Guideline. J Clin Oncol Off J Am Soc Clin Oncol 2018;36(31):3152–61.

9. McAlpine JN, Leung SCY, Cheng A, et al. Human papillomavirus (HPV)-independent vulvar squamous cell carcinoma has a worse prognosis than HPV-associated disease: a retrospective cohort study. Histopathology 2017;71(2):238–46. https://doi.org/10.1111/his.13205.

10. Nooij LS, ter Haar NT, Ruano D, et al. Genomic Characterization of Vulvar (Pre)cancers Identifies Distinct Molecular Subtypes with Prognostic Significance. Clin Cancer Res 2017;23(22):6781–9.

11. Kortekaas KE, Bastiaannet E, van Doorn HC, et al. Vulvar cancer subclassification by HPV and p53 status results in three clinically distinct subtypes. Gynecol Oncol 2020;159(3):649–56.

12. HPV-independent Vulvar Squamous Cell Carcinoma is Associated With Significantly Worse Prognosis Compared With HPV-associated Tumors | Ovid. Available at: https://oce-ovid-com.ezproxy.library.ubc.ca/article/00004347-202007000-00013/HTML. Accessed May 11, 2021.

13. Hinten F, Molijn A, Eckhardt L, et al. Vulvar cancer: Two pathways with different localization and prognosis. Gynecol Oncol 2018;149(2):310–7.

14. Wang T, Bhargava R, Zhiqiang C, et al. A five-year retrospective clinicopathological analsysis of vulvar squamous cell carcinoma in a large tertiary care women's hospital. Abstracts from USCAP 2020: Gynecologic and Obstetric Pathology (1047-1234). Mod Pathol 2020;33(2):1164–337.

15. Barlow EL, Lambie N, Donoghoe MW, et al. The Clinical Relevance of p16 and p53 Status in Patients with Squamous Cell Carcinoma of the Vulva. J Oncol 2020;2020:e3739075.

16. Woelber L, Prieske K, Eulenburg C, et al. p53 and p16 expression profiles in vulvar cancer: a translational analysis by the Arbeitsgemeinschaft Gynäkologische Onkologie Chemo and Radiotherapy in Epithelial Vulvar Cancer study group. Am J Obstet Gynecol 2021;224(6):595.e1–11.

17. Rakislova N, Clavero O, Alemany L, et al. Histological characteristics of HPV-associated and -independent squamous cell carcinomas of the vulva: A study of 1,594 cases. Int J Cancer 2017; 141(12):2517–27.

18. Williams EA, Werth AJ, Sharaf R, et al. Vulvar Squamous Cell Carcinoma: Comprehensive Genomic Profiling of HPV+ Versus HPV– Forms Reveals Distinct Sets of Potentially Actionable Molecular Targets. JCO Precis Oncol 2020;(4):647–61.

19. Dohopolski MJ, Horne ZD, Pradhan D, et al. The Prognostic Significance of p16 Status in Patients With Vulvar Cancer Treated With Vulvectomy and Adjuvant Radiation. Int J Radiat Oncol 2019;103(1):152–60.

20. Horne ZD, Dohopolski MJ, Pradhan D, et al. Human papillomavirus infection mediates response and outcome of vulvar squamous cell carcinomas treated with radiation therapy. Gynecol Oncol 2018;151(1):96–101.

21. Hording U, Daugaard S, Junge J, et al. Human papillomaviruses and multifocal genital neoplasia. Int J Gynecol Pathol Off J Int Soc Gynecol Pathol 1996;15(3):230–4.

22. Almadani N, Thompson EF, Tessier-Cloutier B, et al. An update of molecular pathology and shifting systems of classification in tumours of the female genital tract. Diagn Histopathol 2020;26(6):278–88.

23. Léonard B, Kridelka F, Delbecque K, et al. A Clinical and Pathological Overview of Vulvar Condyloma Acuminatum, Intraepithelial Neoplasia, and Squamous Cell Carcinoma. Biomed Res Int 2014; 2014. https://doi.org/10.1155/2014/480573.

24. BlueBooksOnline. Available at: https://tumourclassification.iarc.who.int/chaptercontent/34/373. Accessed May 13, 2021.

25. BlueBooksOnline. Available at: https://tumourclassification.iarc.who.int/chaptercontent/34/500. Accessed May 30, 2021.

26. Kurman RJ, Toki T, Schiffman MH. Basaloid and warty carcinomas of the vulva. Distinctive types of squamous cell carcinoma frequently associated

with human papillomaviruses. Am J Surg Pathol 1993;17(2):133–45.

27. Toki T, Kurman RJ, Park JS, et al. Probable nonpapillomavirus etiology of squamous cell carcinoma of the vulva in older women: a clinicopathologic study using in situ hybridization and polymerase chain reaction. Int J Gynecol Pathol Off J Int Soc Gynecol Pathol 1991;10(2):107–25.

28. Dong F, Kojiro S, Borger DR, et al. Squamous Cell Carcinoma of the Vulva: A Subclassification of 97 Cases by Clinicopathologic, Immunohistochemical, and Molecular Features (p16, p53, and EGFR). Am J Surg Pathol 2015;39(8):1045–53.

29. Carcinomas of the Vulva - International Collaboration on Cancer Reporting. Available at: http://www.iccr-cancer.org/datasets/published-datasets/female-reproductive/carcinoma-of-the-vulva. Accessed October 11, 2021.

30. Olawaiye AB, Cotler J, Cuello MA, et al. FIGO staging for carcinoma of the vulva: 2021 revision. Int J Gynaecol Obstet Off Organ Int Fed Gynaecol Obstet 2021;155(1):43–7.

31. Age, treatment and prognosis of patients with squamous cell vulvar cancer (VSCC) - analysis of the AGO-CaRE-1 study- ClinicalKey. Available at: https://www-clinicalkey-com.ezproxy.library.ubc.ca/#!/content/playContent/1-s2.0-S0090825821001700?returnurl=null&referrer=null. Accessed May 13, 2021.

32. BlueBooksOnline. Available at: https://tumourclassification.iarc.who.int/chaptercontent/34/489. Accessed June 17, 2021.

33. Drolet M, É Bénard, Pérez N, et al. Population-level impact and herd effects following the introduction of human papillomavirus vaccination programmes: updated systematic review and meta-analysis. Lancet 2019;394(10197):497–509.

34. van de Nieuwenhof HP, van Kempen LCLT, de Hullu JA, et al. The Etiologic Role of HPV in Vulvar Squamous Cell Carcinoma Fine Tuned. Cancer Epidemiol Prev Biomark 2009;18(7):2061–7.

35. Dellinger TH, Hakim AA, Lee SJ, et al. Surgical Management of Vulvar Cancer. J Natl Compr Cancer Netw JNCCN 2017;15(1):121–8.

36. Rogers LJ, Cuello MA. Cancer of the vulva. Int J Gynaecol Obstet Off Organ Int Fed Gynaecol Obstet 2018;143(Suppl 2):4–13.

37. Van der Zee AGJ, Oonk MH, De Hullu JA, et al. Sentinel node dissection is safe in the treatment of early-stage vulvar cancer. J Clin Oncol Off J Am Soc Clin Oncol 2008;26(6):884–9.

38. van den Einden LCG, Massuger LFAG, Jonkman JK, et al. An alternative way to measure the depth of invasion of vulvar squamous cell carcinoma in relation to prognosis. Mod Pathol Off J U S Can Acad Pathol Inc 2015;28(2):295–302.

39. Francis JA, Eiriksson L, Dean E, et al. 370-Management of Squamous Cell Cancer of the Vulva. J Obstet Gynaecol Can JOGC J Obstet Gynecol Can JOGC 2019;41(1):89–101.

40. Kortekaas KE, Van de Vijver KK, van Poelgeest MIE, et al. Practical Guidance for Measuring and Reporting Surgical Margins in Vulvar Cancer. Int J Gynecol Pathol Off J Int Soc Gynecol Pathol 2020;39(5):420–7.

41. Nooij LS, van der Slot MA, Dekkers OM, et al. Tumour-free margins in vulvar squamous cell carcinoma: Does distance really matter? Eur J Cancer Oxf Engl 1990 2016;65:139–49.

42. Julia CJ, Hoang LN. A review of prognostic factors in squamous cell carcinoma of the vulva: Evidence from the last decade. Semin Diagn Pathol 2021;38(1):37–49.

43. Akbari A, Pinto A, Amemiya Y, et al. Differentiated exophytic vulvar intraepithelial lesion: Clinicopathologic and molecular analysis documenting its relationship with verrucous carcinoma of the vulva. Mod Pathol 2020;33(10):2011–8.

44. Thompson E, Jamieson A, Huvila J, Wong RWC, Trevisan G, Almadani N, Senz J, Ho J, C., Gilks B, Mcalpine JN, Hoang L, Thompson E P. PROGNOSTIC SIGNIFICANCE OF 'P53 SIGNATURE' (FIELDS OF DYSPLASIA) AND IN SITU MARGIN STATUS IN ORGAN-CONFINED HPV-INDEPENDENT P53 ABNORMAL VULVAR SQUAMOUS CELL CARCINOMAIGCS 2021 Abstracts: Oral Plenary Sessions. Presented at: 2021; IGSC.

45. Singh N, Leen SL, Han G, et al. Expanding the morphologic spectrum of differentiated VIN (dVIN) through detailed mapping of cases with p53 loss. Am J Surg Pathol 2015;39(1):52–60.

46. Wing-Cheuk Wong R, Palicelli A, Hoang L, et al. Interpretation of p16, p53 and mismatch repair protein immunohistochemistry in gynaecological neoplasia. Diagn Histopathol 2020;26(6):257–77.

47. Darragh TM, Colgan TJ, Cox JT, et al. The Lower Anogenital Squamous Terminology Standardization Project for HPV-Associated Lesions: Background and Consensus Recommendations From the College of American Pathologists and the American Society for Colposcopy and Cervical Pathology. J Low Genit Tract Dis 2012;16(3):205–42.

48. Nicolás I, Saco A, Barnadas E, et al. Prognostic implications of genotyping and p16 immunostaining in HPV-positive tumors of the uterine cervix. Mod Pathol 2020;33(1):128–37.

49. Keung ES, Souers RJ, Bridge JA, et al. Comparative Performance of High-Risk Human Papillomavirus RNA and DNA In Situ Hybridization on College of American Pathologists Proficiency Tests. Arch Pathol Lab Med 2020;144(3):344–9.

50. Craig SG, Anderson LA, Moran M, et al. Comparison of Molecular Assays for HPV Testing in

Oropharyngeal Squamous Cell Carcinomas: A Population-Based Study in Northern Ireland. Cancer Epidemiol Biomarkers Prev 2020;29(1):31–8.

51. Singh N, Piskorz AM, Bosse T, et al. p53 immuno-histochemistry is an accurate surrogate for TP53 mutational analysis in endometrial carcinoma biopsies. J Pathol 2020;250(3):336–45.

52. Köbel M, Kang EY. The Many Uses of p53 Immunohistochemistry in Gynecological Pathology: Proceedings of the ISGyP Companion Society Session at the 2020 USCAP Annual9 Meeting. Int J Gynecol Pathol Off J Int Soc Gynecol Pathol 2021;40(1):32–40.

53. Vanin K, Scurry J, Thorne H, et al. Overexpression of wild-type p53 in lichen sclerosus adjacent to human papillomavirus-negative vulvar cancer. J Invest Dermatol 2002;119(5):1027–33.

54. Rolfe KJ, MacLean AB, Crow JC, et al. TP53 mutations in vulval lichen sclerosus adjacent to squamous cell carcinoma of the vulva. Br J Cancer 2003;89(12):2249–53.

55. Choschzick M, Hantaredja W, Tennstedt P, et al. Role of TP53 mutations in vulvar carcinomas. Int J Gynecol Pathol Off J Int Soc Gynecol Pathol 2011;30(5):497–504.

56. Tessier-Cloutier B, Kortekaas KE, Thompson E, et al. Major p53 immunohistochemical patterns in in situ and invasive squamous cell carcinomas of the vulva and correlation with TP53 mutation status. Mod Pathol 2020;33(8):1595–605.

57. Kortekaas KE, Solleveld-Westerink N, Tessier-Cloutier B, et al. Performance of the pattern-based interpretation of p53 immunohistochemistry as a surrogate for TP53 mutations in vulvar squamous cell carcinoma. Histopathology 2020;77(1):92–9.

58. Thompson EF, Chen J, Huvila J, et al. p53 Immunohistochemical patterns in HPV-related neoplasms of the female lower genital tract can be mistaken for TP53 null or missense mutational patterns. Mod Pathol Off J U S Can Acad Pathol Inc 2020;33(9):1649–59.

59. Han MR, Shin S, Park HC, et al. Mutational signatures and chromosome alteration profiles of squamous cell carcinomas of the vulva. Exp Mol Med 2018;50(2):e442.

60. Prieske K, Alawi M, Oliveira-Ferrer L, et al. Genomic characterization of vulvar squamous cell carcinoma. Gynecol Oncol 2020;158(3):547–54.

61. Trietsch MD, Spaans VM, ter Haar NT, et al. CDKN2A(p16) and HRAS are frequently mutated in vulvar squamous cell carcinoma. Gynecol Oncol 2014;135(1):149–55.

62. Weberpals JI, Lo B, Duciaume MM, et al. Vulvar Squamous Cell Carcinoma (VSCC) as Two Diseases: HPV Status Identifies Distinct Mutational Profiles Including Oncogenic Fibroblast Growth Factor Receptor 3. Clin Cancer Res Off J Am Assoc Cancer Res 2017;23(15):4501–10.

63. Xing D, Liu Y, Park HJ, et al. Recurrent genetic alterations and biomarker expression in primary and metastatic squamous cell carcinomas of the vulva. Hum Pathol 2019;92:67–80. https://doi.org/10.1016/j.humpath.2019.08.003.

64. Salama A, Momeni Boroujeni A, Vanderbilt C, et al. Molecular landscape of HPV negative vulvar squamous cell carcinoma including NOTCH alterations. Abstracts from USCAP 2020: Gynecologic and Obstetric Pathology (1047-1234). Mod Pathol 2020;33(2):1164–337.

65. Zięba S, Kowalik A, Zalewski K, et al. Somatic mutation profiling of vulvar cancer: Exploring therapeutic targets. Gynecol Oncol 2018;150(3):552–61.

66. Watkins JC, Howitt BE, Horowitz NS, et al. Differentiated exophytic vulvar intraepithelial lesions are genetically distinct from keratinizing squamous cell carcinomas and contain mutations in PIK3CA. Mod Pathol 2017;30(3):448–58.

67. Kashofer K, Regauer S. Analysis of full coding sequence of the TP53 gene in invasive vulvar cancers: Implications for therapy. Gynecol Oncol 2017;146(2):314–8.

68. Regauer S, Kashofer K, Reich O. Time series analysis of TP53 gene mutations in recurrent HPV-negative vulvar squamous cell carcinoma. Mod Pathol Off J U S Can Acad Pathol Inc 2019;32(3):415–22.

69. Pors J, Tessier-Cloutier B, Thompson E, et al. Targeted Molecular Sequencing of Recurrent and Multifocal Non-HPV-associated Squamous Cell Carcinoma of the Vulva. Int J Gynecol Pathol Off J Int Soc Gynecol Pathol 2020. https://doi.org/10.1097/PGP.0000000000000742.

70. Lerias S, Ferreira J, Silva F, et al. P%# Pattern-based immunohistochemistry classification in primary squamous cell vulvar carcinoma correlates with prognosis and can change during disease progression. Abstracts from USCAP 2021: Gynecologic and Obstetric Pathology (532-634). Mod Pathol 2021;34(2):767–888.

71. Wilkinson EJ, Cox JT, Selim MA, et al. Evolution of terminology for human-papillomavirus-infection-related vulvar squamous intraepithelial lesions. J Low Genit Tract Dis 2015;19(1):81–7.

72. Riethdorf S, Neffen EF, Cviko A, et al. p16INK4A expression as biomarker for HPV 16-related vulvar neoplasias. Hum Pathol 2004;35(12):1477–83.

73. Lewis N, Blanco LZ, Maniar KP. p16 Expression and Biological Behavior of Flat Vulvar Low-grade Squamous Intraepithelial Lesions (LSIL). Int J Gynecol Pathol Off J Int Soc Gynecol Pathol 2017;36(5):486–92.

74. Management of Vulvar Intraepithelial Neoplasia. (675):5.

75. Rufforny I, Wilkinson EJ, Liu C, et al. Human papillomavirus infection and p16(INK4a) protein

expression in vulvar intraepithelial neoplasia and invasive squamous cell carcinoma. J Low Genit Tract Dis 2005;9(2):108–13.

76. Bornstein J, Bogliatto F, Haefner HK, et al. The 2015 International Society for the Study of Vulvovaginal Disease (ISSVD) Terminology of Vulvar Squamous Intraepithelial Lesions. Obstet Gynecol 2016; 127(2):264–8.

77. Hoang LN, Park KJ, Soslow RA, et al. Squamous precursor lesions of the vulva: current classification and diagnostic challenges. Pathology (Phila) 2016; 48(4):291–302.

78. Nooij LS, Dreef EJ, Smit VTHBM, et al. Stathmin is a highly sensitive and specific biomarker for vulvar high-grade squamous intraepithelial lesions. J Clin Pathol 2016;69(12):1070–5.

79. Tan A, Bieber AK, Stein JA, et al. Diagnosis and management of vulvar cancer: A review. J Am Acad Dermatol 2019;81(6):1387–96.

80. Maniar KP, Ronnett BM, Vang R, et al. Coexisting high-grade vulvar intraepithelial neoplasia (VIN) and condyloma acuminatum: independent lesions due to different HPV types occurring in immunocompromised patients. Am J Surg Pathol 2013; 37(1):53–60.

81. Dasgupta S, Ewing-Graham PC, Swagemakers SMA, et al. Precursor lesions of vulvar squamous cell carcinoma – histology and biomarkers: A systematic review. Crit Rev Oncol Hematol 2020;147:102866. https://doi.org/10.1016/j.critrevonc.2020.102866.

82. Cohen PA, Anderson L, Eva L, et al. Clinical and molecular classification of vulvar squamous precancers. Int J Gynecol Cancer 2019;29(4). https://doi.org/10.1136/ijgc-2018-000135.

83. Green N, Adedipe T, Dmytryshyn J, et al. Management of Vulvar Cancer Precursors: A Survey of the International Society for the Study of Vulvovaginal Disease. J Low Genit Tract Dis 2020;24(4):387–91.

84. Day T, Marzol A, Pagano R, et al. Clinicopathologic Diagnosis of Differentiated Vulvar Intraepithelial Neoplasia and Vulvar Aberrant Maturation. J Low Genit Tract Dis 2020;24(4):392–8.

85. Pinto AP, Miron A, Yassin Y, et al. Differentiated vulvar intraepithelial neoplasia contains Tp53 mutations and is genetically linked to vulvar squamous cell carcinoma. Mod Pathol Off J U S Can Acad Pathol Inc 2010;23(3):404–12.

86. Watkins JC. Human Papillomavirus–Independent Squamous Lesions of the Vulva. Surg Pathol Clin 2019;12(2):249–61.

87. Heller DS, Day T, Allbritton JI, et al. Diagnostic Criteria for Differentiated Vulvar Intraepithelial Neoplasia and Vulvar Aberrant Maturation. J Low Genit Tract Dis 2021;25(1):57–70.

88. van de Nieuwenhof HP, Bulten J, Hollema H, et al. Differentiated vulvar intraepithelial neoplasia is often found in lesions, previously diagnosed as lichen sclerosus, which have progressed to vulvar squamous cell carcinoma. Mod Pathol Off J U S Can Acad Pathol Inc 2011;24(2):297–305.

89. Dasgupta S, de Jonge E, Van Bockstal MR, et al. Histological interpretation of differentiated vulvar intraepithelial neoplasia (dVIN) remains challenging-observations from a bi-national ring-study. Virchows Arch Int J Pathol 2021;479(2):305–15.

90. van den Einden LCG, de Hullu JA, Massuger LFAG, et al. Interobserver variability and the effect of education in the histopathological diagnosis of differentiated vulvar intraepithelial neoplasia. Mod Pathol Off J U S Can Acad Pathol Inc 2013;26(6):874–80.

91. Bigby SM, Eva LJ, Fong KL, et al. The Natural History of Vulvar Intraepithelial Neoplasia, Differentiated Type: Evidence for Progression and Diagnostic Challenges. Int J Gynecol Pathol Off J Int Soc Gynecol Pathol 2016;35(6):574–84.

92. Nascimento AF, Granter SR, Cviko A, et al. Vulvar Acanthosis With Altered Differentiation: A Precursor to Verrucous Carcinoma? Am J Surg Pathol 2004; 28(5):638–43.

93. Rakislova N, Alemany L, Clavero O, et al. p53 Immunohistochemical Patterns in HPV-Independent Squamous Cell Carcinomas of the Vulva and the Associated Skin Lesions: A Study of 779 Cases. Int J Mol Sci 2020;(21):21. https://doi.org/10.3390/ijms21218091.

94. Roy SF, Wong J, Le Page C, et al. DEVIL, VAAD and vLSC constitute a spectrum of HPV-independent, p53-independent intra-epithelial neoplasia of the vulva. Histopathology 2021. https://doi.org/10.1111/his.14451.

95. Campbell K, Shalin S, Quick C. Hypertrophic lichen sclerosus: A putative precursor to squamous cell carcinoma in the vulva. Abstracts from USCAP 2021: Gynecologic and Obstetric Pathology (532-634). Mod Pathol 2021;34(2):767–888.

96. Ordi J, Alejo M, Fusté V, et al. HPV-negative vulvar intraepithelial neoplasia (VIN) with basaloid histologic pattern: an unrecognized variant of simplex (differentiated) VIN. Am J Surg Pathol 2009; 33(11):1659–65.

97. Watkins JC, Yang E, Crum CP, et al. Classic Vulvar Intraepithelial Neoplasia With Superimposed Lichen Simplex Chronicus: A Unique Variant Mimicking Differentiated Vulvar Intraepithelial Neoplasia. Int J Gynecol Pathol Off J Int Soc Gynecol Pathol 2019;38(2):175–82.

98. Rakislova N, Alemany L, Clavero O, et al. Differentiated Vulvar Intraepithelial Neoplasia-like and Lichen Sclerosus-like Lesions in HPV-associated Squamous Cell Carcinomas of the Vulva. Am J Surg Pathol 2018;42(6):828–35.

99. Rakislova N, Alemany L, Clavero O, et al. HPV-independent Precursors Mimicking High-grade

Squamous Intraepithelial Lesions (HSIL) of the Vulva. Am J Surg Pathol 2020;44(11):1506–14.

100. Griesinger LM, Walline H, Wang GY, et al. Expanding the Morphologic, Immunohistochemical, and HPV Genotypic Features of High-grade Squamous Intraepithelial Lesions of the Vulva With Morphology Mimicking Differentiated Vulvar Intraepithelial Neoplasia and/or Lichen Sclerosus. Int J Gynecol Pathol Off J Int Soc Gynecol Pathol 2020. https://doi.org/10.1097/PGP.0000000000000708.

101. Liu YA, Ji JX, Almadani N, et al. Comparison of p53 immunohistochemical staining in differentiated vulvar intraepithelial neoplasia (dVIN) with that in inflammatory dermatoses and benign squamous lesions in the vulva. Histopathology 2021;78(3):424–33.

102. Tessier-Cloutier B, Asleh-Aburaya K, Shah V, et al. Molecular subtyping of mammary-like adenocarcinoma of the vulva shows molecular similarity to breast carcinomas. Histopathology 2017;71(3):446–52.

103. BlueBooksOnline. Available at: https://tumourclassification.iarc.who.int/chaptercontent/34/340. Accessed June 16, 2021.

104. Wong RWC, Moore M, Talia KL, et al. Primary Vaginal Gastric-type Adenocarcinoma and Vaginal Adenosis Exhibiting Gastric Differentiation: Report of a Series With Detailed Immunohistochemical Analysis. Am J Surg Pathol 2018;42(7):958–70.

105. Talia KL, Scurry J, Manolitsas T, et al. Primary vaginal mucinous adenocarcinoma of gastric type arising in adenosis: a report of 2 cases, 1 associated with uterus didelphys. Int J Gynecol Pathol Off J Int Soc Gynecol Pathol 2012;31(2):184–91.

106. BlueBooksOnline. Available at: https://tumourclassification.iarc.who.int/chaptercontent/34/347. Accessed June 17, 2021.

107. Talia KL, Wong RWC, McCluggage WG. Expression of Markers of Müllerian Clear Cell Carcinoma in Primary Cervical and Vaginal Gastric-type Adenocarcinomas. Int J Gynecol Pathol Off J Int Soc Gynecol Pathol 2019;38(3):276–82.

108. BlueBooksOnline. Available at: https://tumourclassification.iarc.who.int/chaptercontent/34/285. Accessed June 17, 2021.

109. Staats PN, McCluggage WG, Clement PB, et al. Primary intestinal-type glandular lesions of the vagina: clinical, pathologic, and immunohistochemical features of 14 cases ranging from benign polyp to adenoma to adenocarcinoma. Am J Surg Pathol 2014;38(5):593–603.

110. BlueBooksOnline. Available at: https://tumourclassification.iarc.who.int/chaptercontent/34/317. Accessed June 17, 2021.

111. Voltaggio L, McCluggage WG, Iding JS, et al. A novel group of HPV-related adenocarcinomas of the lower anogenital tract (vagina, vulva, and anorectum) in women and men resembling HPV-related endocervical adenocarcinomas. Mod Pathol Off J U S Can Acad Pathol Inc 2020;33(5):944–52.

112. Santos M, Landolfi S, Olivella A, et al. p16 overexpression identifies HPV-positive vulvar squamous cell carcinomas. Am J Surg Pathol 2006;30(11):1347–56.

113. de Sanjosé S, Alemany L, Ordi J, et al. Worldwide human papillomavirus genotype attribution in over 2000 cases of intraepithelial and invasive lesions of the vulva. Eur J Cancer Oxf Engl 1990 2013;49(16):3450–61.

114. Lee LJ, Howitt B, Catalano P, et al. Prognostic importance of human papillomavirus (HPV) and p16 positivity in squamous cell carcinoma of the vulva treated with radiotherapy. Gynecol Oncol 2016;142(2):293–8.

115. Allo G, Yap ML, Cuartero J, et al. HPV-independent Vulvar Squamous Cell Carcinoma is Associated With Significantly Worse Prognosis Compared With HPV-associated Tumors. Int J Gynecol Pathol 2020;39(4):391–9.

Neuroendocrine Neoplasia of the Female Genital Tract

Karen L. Talia, MBBS(Hons), FRCPA[a],*, Raji Ganesan, FRCPath[b]

KEYWORDS

- Neuroendocrine neoplasia • Neuroendocrine tumor • Neuroendocrine carcinoma • Carcinoid tumor
- Merkel cell carcinoma

Key points

- The fifth edition World Health Organization Classification of Tumors establishes a common nomenclature for neuroendocrine neoplasia across all organ systems. This divides tumors into low-to-intermediate grade neuroendocrine tumors (NETs) and high-grade neuroendocrine carcinomas (NECs).
- Female genital tract (FGT) neuroendocrine neoplasms are uncommon to rare and may occur at any site.
- NETs predominate in the ovary, where the term "carcinoid tumor" is retained; these are extremely rare in other FGT sites. Tumors of the cervix, endometrium, and vulva are more frequently NEC, with non-NEC admixed with NEC more prevalent than pure NEC.

ABSTRACT

Neuroendocrine neoplasia is relatively uncommon in the female genital tract (FGT) and occurs at any site, most often the ovary and cervix. A unified dichotomous nomenclature, introduced by the World Health Organization Classification of Tumors in all fifth edition volumes, divides neuroendocrine neoplasms (NENs) into well-differentiated neuroendocrine tumors (NETs) and poorly differentiated neuroendocrine carcinomas (NECs). The term carcinoid tumor is retained in the ovary and represents the commonest FGT NEN. NEC is most common in the cervix and is usually admixed with another human papillomavirus-associated epithelial neoplasm. Despite shared neuroendocrine differentiation, NET and NEC show diverse etiology, morphology, and clinical behavior.

OVERVIEW

Neuroendocrine neoplasms (NENs) may arise at any site in the female genital tract (FGT) and constitute an uncommon and diverse group of tumors, accounting for 2% of all gynecological malignancies.[1] The morphology of these tumors is largely constant across different organ systems, justifying the introduction of a unified nomenclature in fifth edition volumes of the World Health Organization (WHO) Classification of Tumors. NENs are stratified into neuroendocrine tumors (NETs) and neuroendocrine carcinoma (NECs), and although both exhibit neuroendocrine differentiation immunohistochemically, by most other measures, these tumors are distinct and should not be considered a tumor spectrum. Herein, we examine the morphology, immunohistochemistry, and molecular findings in NENs, with a focus on site-specific aspects including the varied histogenesis and clinical behavior of these lesions.

Both authors contributed equally to this article.
[a] Department of Pathology, Royal Women's Hospital and Australian Centre for the Prevention of Cervical Cancer, Melbourne, Victoria, Australia; [b] Department of Cellular Pathology, Birmingham Women's Hospital, Birmingham, United Kingdom
* Corresponding author. Department of Pathology, The Royal Women's Hospital, Level 5, 20 Flemington Road, Parkville, Victoria 3052, Australia.
E-mail address: Karen.Talia2@rch.org.au

Surgical Pathology 15 (2022) 407–420
https://doi.org/10.1016/j.path.2022.02.012

TERMINOLOGY AND CLASSIFICATION OF NEUROENDOCRINE NEOPLASIA

Historically, classification of NENs has been problematic due to varied nomenclature used across different organ systems. The 2014 WHO Classification of Tumors of Female Reproductive Organs revised the terminology for NENs at most sites to reflect that used in the fourth edition Classification of Tumors of the Digestive System,[2,3] adopting the terms NET and NEC. This system assumed that all NENs have malignant potential and graded them into NET, further subdivided into Grade 1 and 2, and NEC (Grade 3), based on the proliferative activity of the tumor, as measured by both mitotic count and Ki-67 labeling index.

In 2017, an International Agency for Research on Cancer consensus conference devised a common classification framework for NENs at all anatomic locations, and this harmonized approach is now implemented in all fifth edition volumes of the WHO Classification of Tumors.[4] A key feature is the dichotomous division of tumors into well-differentiated NET, also designated carcinoid tumors in some sites, and poorly differentiated NEC. NETs, encompassing typical and atypical carcinoid tumor, are low-to-intermediate grade with a uniform cell population arranged in organoid patterns. In some organ systems, NETs are graded based on mitotic count, Ki-67 labeling index, and the presence of necrosis. NECs are, by definition, high-grade. This subdivision is supported by genetic, clinical, epidemiologic, histologic, and prognostic differences, and the intention of this initiative is to facilitate consistent patient management, allowing for organ-specific differences in tumor biology, and enable comparison of different entities.[4]

The 2020 WHO Classification of Female Genital Tumors addresses NENs jointly in a dedicated chapter rather than in each genital site.[5] An exception is made in the ovary, where the term "carcinoid tumor" is retained, justified by its excellent prognosis, which renders grading unwarranted, and a section discussing this entity is included in the ovary chapter. In all other genital sites, the terms NET and NEC are used, with NETs graded as Grade 1 or 2, encompassing carcinoid and atypical carcinoid, also acceptable terminology. NEC is subclassified into small cell NEC (SCNEC) or large cell NEC (LCNEC). A category of carcinoma (nonneuroendocrine) admixed with NEC is also included. In the 2014 classification, what we now understand as ovarian SCNEC was then referred to as NEC "pulmonary type," to reflect the morphologic similarity with NEC of the lung and to distinguish it from ovarian small cell carcinoma of hypercalcemic type. The latter has now been recognized as an undifferentiated tumor associated with *SMARCA4* mutations and not a NET, and therefore is not categorized as NEC in the 2020 WHO classification. Consequently, NEC pulmonary type is now SCNEC under the new classification. **Table 1** compares the 2014 and 2020 WHO Classification systems for FGT NENs.

HISTOGENESIS AND CELL OF ORIGIN OF NEUROENDOCRINE NEOPLASIA

NENs are diverse in their histogenesis, with varied cells of origin postulated in different sites. NENs are commonest in the gastrointestinal and respiratory tracts, where neuroendocrine cells are normally identifiable and represent the presumed cell of origin. Similarly, pancreatic NENs originate in the alpha and beta cells of the Islets of Langerhans.[6] By comparison, FGT neuroendocrine cells are not normally visualized, although their presence has been demonstrated immunohistochemically in normal Bartholin glands and the fallopian tube.[7,8] The subset of vulval SCNECs representing Merkel cell carcinomas (MCC) are presumed to derive from sensory Merkel cells found in the skin.[9] In the cervix, it is suggested that neuroendocrine cells reside in small numbers in the squamous or glandular epithelium.[10] In the ovary, carcinoid tumors arise from neuroendocrine cells within intestinal type epithelium of mature cystic teratomas.[5] Primary ovarian paragangliomas are similarly thought to derive from teratomas or extra-adrenal paraganglia in the region of the ovary.[11] In carcinoma admixed with NEC, the neuroendocrine component likely represents divergent differentiation within the carcinoma; this is supported by a recent molecular study of mixed endometrial tumors showing both components share common mutations.[12]

The pathogenesis of NEC in cervical and non-Merkel vulvar SCNECs is attributed to high-risk human papillomavirus (HPV), most often HPV 16 and 18[7,13]; HPV is also implicated in rare cervical carcinoid tumors.[14] Most MCC is caused by the monoclonal integration of Merkel cell polyomavirus, with the remainder associated with ultraviolet light exposure.[9] Mutations in genes promoting neuroendocrine carcinogenesis occur in multiple neuroendocrine neoplasia (MEN) types 1 and 2 and von Hippel-Landau syndrome,[15] with a rare association with MEN 1 reported in ovarian carcinoid tumors.[16] The pathogenetic mechanisms underpinning NENs at other gynecological sites are unknown.[5]

Table 1
Comparison of the 2014 and 2020 WHO Classifications of neuroendocrine neoplasms of female genital organs

Site	2014 Tumor Category	2014 Tumor Type	2020[a]
Ovary	Monodermal teratoma and somatic-type tumors arising from a dermoid cyst Miscellaneous tumors	Carcinoid (subtypes strumal and mucinous carcinoid) Small cell carcinoma, pulmonary type (SCNEC) Paraganglioma	Carcinoid tumor NEC, Carcinoma admixed with NEC
Uterine corpus	Neuroendocrine tumors	Low-grade NET (carcinoid) High-grade NEC (SCNEC, LCNEC)	NET NEC (SCNEC, LCNEC), Carcinoma admixed with NEC
Uterine cervix	Neuroendocrine tumors Glandular tumors and precursors	Low-grade NET (carcinoid, atypical carcinoid) High-grade NEC (SCNEC, LCNEC) Adenocarcinoma admixed with NEC	NET NEC (SCNEC, LCNEC) Carcinoma admixed with NEC
Vagina	Other rare tumors High-grade neuroendocrine carcinoma	Carcinoid tumor, Mixed adenocarcinoma-neuroendocrine tumor SCNEC LCNEC	NET NEC (SCNEC, LCNEC)
Vulva	Neuroendocrine tumors	High-grade NEC (SCNEC, LCNEC), Merkel cell tumor	NEC (SCNEC, LCNEC)

Abbreviations: LCNEC, large cell neuroendocrine carcinoma; NEC, neuroendocrine carcinoma; NET, neuroendocrine tumor; SCNEC, small cell neuroendocrine carcinoma.

[a] The 2020 WHO classification uses the same terminology for neuroendocrine neoplasia at all body sites except the ovary.

MORPHOLOGY OF NEUROENDOCRINE NEOPLASIA

NEUROENDOCRINE TUMOR

NETs are low or intermediate-grade epithelial tumors with morphologic and immunohistochemical evidence of neuroendocrine differentiation. They have been reported in the cervix,[10] uterine corpus,[17] fallopian tube,[8] and vagina[18] but occur most often in the ovary, where the term carcinoid tumor is still used.[5] The cells constituting NETs are polygonal in shape with round or ovoid nuclei exhibiting so-called salt and pepper chromatin. Cytoplasm is abundant and eosinophilic cytoplasmic granules may be seen. The cells lack cytologic atypia and mitotic activity is low. In Grade 1 tumors, mitotic figures are rare (0–5 mitoses per 2.4 mm²; 2.4 mm² equating to 10 high power fields, each 0.55 mm in diameter), whereas in Grade 2 tumors 5 to 10 mitotic figures per 2.4 mm² are allowed. Necrosis is acceptable in Grade 2 tumours, which are regarded as atypical carcinoids. **Table 2** lists current histologic criteria for diagnosis of NET (Grades 1 and 2), SCNEC, and LCNEC.

CARCINOID TUMOR (WELL-DIFFERENTIATED NEUROENDOCRINE TUMOR, GRADE 1)

Morphologically, there are 4 patterns of primary ovarian carcinoid tumor[19]—insular (commonest), strumal, trabecular, and mucinous (goblet cell) (**Figs. 1–3**). Insular carcinoids are composed of solid nests of cells with a peripheral rim of punctated acini that may resemble glands. Carcinoid tumors arising in association with or intimately admixed with thyroid tissue are referred to as strumal carcinoids; in about 40% of these cases these are associated with mucinous glands. Trabecular and mucinous carcinoid tumors are rare. Trabecular carcinoids are composed of parallel trabeculae or wavy ribbons of cells. Mucinous carcinoids show small glands or acini lined by columnar or cuboidal epithelium with variable numbers of goblet cells. Extracellular mucin fills the gland lumina and deposits at the periphery of glands and acini, which may be displaced by the mucin. Atypical mucinous carcinoids show crowded glands, confluent growth and cribriforming. In insular and trabecular variants, the stroma may be conspicuous and hyaline, whereas in

Table 2
Diagnostic criteria for neuroendocrine tumor (grades 1 and 2, corresponding to carcinoid and atypical carcinoid tumor), small cell neuroendocrine carcinoma, and large cell neuroendocrine carcinoma

	G1 NET	G2 NET	SCNEC	LCNEC
Cell morphology	Monomorphic with variable amounts of cytoplasm	Monomorphic with variable amounts of cytoplasm	Highly atypical cells with scanty cytoplasm	Highly atypical cells with moderate to abundant cytoplasm
Nuclear morphology	Regular with uniform chromatin and small nucleoli	Variable in size and shape with irregularly distributed chromatin	Ovoid to slightly spindled nuclei with hyperchromatic and dispersed chromatin. Nuclear molding	Large nuclei with coarse chromatin and prominent nucleoli
Mitotic count	None or rare	Up to 5–10 mitotic figures/2 mm^2 (5–10 mitotic figures/10 HPF of 0.5 mm in diameter and 0.2 mm^2 in area)	Numerous	Numerous
Necrosis	No	Yes	Yes, also apoptoses	Yes, geographic
Immunohistochemistry[a]	Positive	Positive	Often positive Not required for diagnosis if characteristic morphologic features are present	Often positive Positive staining for at least one marker needed for diagnosis

[a] With neuroendocrine markers chromogranin, synaptophysin, CD56.

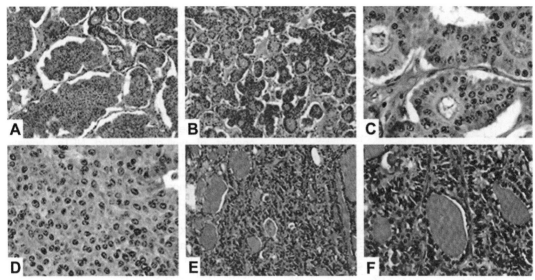

Fig. 1. Ovarian carcinoid tumor showing insular (*A*) and acinar (*B*) patterns of growth. Tumor cells show uniform round nuclei, granular "salt and pepper" chromatin and few mitoses (*C, D*). Strumal carcinoid is composed of a carcinoid tumor admixed with mature thyroid follicular tissue (*E, F*).

mucinous carcinoids, the pools of extravasated mucin are characteristic.

NEUROENDOCRINE CARCINOMA

SMALL CELL NEUROENDOCRINE CARCINOMA

SCNEC is composed of sheets of hyperchromatic, atypical cells with ovoid or somewhat spindled hyperchromatic nuclei. Cytoplasm is scant and barely appreciable. Nuclei often exhibit molding. Extensive crush artifact, brisk mitotic activity, and numerous apoptotic bodies are seen (**Fig. 4**). Necrosis is common. The growth pattern is commonly as solid sheets, but nests, trabeculae, and pseudoglandular and pseudorosette formations can also be encountered.

LARGE CELL NEUROENDOCRINE CARCINOMA

LCNEC is characterized by large polygonal cells with moderate amounts of cytoplasm, low nuclear to cytoplasmic ratio, large nuclei with coarse chromatin, and prominent nucleoli. Growth patterns include solid, pseudoglandular, nested, and trabecular. A solid pattern is common but multiple growth patterns often coexist. Brisk mitotic activity and extensive geographic necrosis are seen.

CARCINOMA ADMIXED WITH NEUROENDOCRINE CARCINOMA

This term denotes NEC admixed with a non-NEC of histotype typically seen at the body site of origin. Mixed tumors are most frequent in the cervix, endometrium, and ovary and are rare in the vulva and vagina.[5] In the cervix, the commonest non-NET component is HPV-associated adenocarcinoma followed by squamous cell carcinoma (**Fig. 5**). In the endometrium, endometrioid followed by serous carcinoma are the most common morphologies, whereas in the ovary, any ovarian epithelial tumor type may be seen. In this context, the nature of each tumor component and their relative proportion should be stated in the report as even a small (<10%) NEC component conveys an adverse outcome.[20] Vulvar NECs differ in that they usually occur in pure form. In the largest series of vulvar NECs, 1 of 16 cases was mixed with a moderately differentiated adenocarcinoma associated with the Bartholin gland.[7] Only 2 other case reports of vulvar mixed NEC are published in the literature, representing MCCs combined with squamous cell carcinomas.[21,22]

IMMUNOHISTOCHEMISTRY OF NEUROENDOCRINE NEOPLASIA

Commonly used immunohistochemical markers of neuroendocrine differentiation are chromogranin, synaptophysin, and CD56. CD56 and synaptophysin are the most sensitive, but CD56 lacks specificity. Chromogranin is the most specific neuroendocrine marker but lacks sensitivity, with only 50% of SCNECs exhibiting positive staining,[23] which may be very focal punctate cytoplasmic reactivity, visible only on high power.

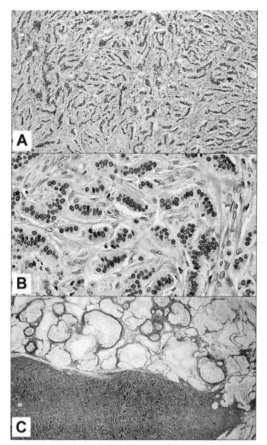

Fig. 2. Ovarian carcinoid tumor showing trabecular (*A, B*) and mucinous (*C*) growth patterns. Trabecular carcinoid is composed of "rows" or elongated nests (*A*). Cells show the typical neuroendocrine cytomorphology with "salt and pepper" nuclei and granular cytoplasm (*B*). This example has trabecular carcinoid (*bottom*), struma (*bottom*), and mucinous (*top*) morphologies (*C*).

Insulinoma-associated protein 1 (INSM1) has been increasingly shown to be a specific and sensitive marker of neuroendocrine differentiation.[24] SCNEC is variably positive with neuroendocrine markers, although this diagnosis can be made in the absence of neuroendocrine marker positivity if the morphology is typical. SCNEC may be only focally positive (often punctuate cytoplasmic staining) or even negative with broad spectrum cytokeratins (CKs). A diagnosis of LCNEC requires positive staining with at least one neuroendocrine marker in the appropriate morphologic context, and most LCNECs are diffusely positive with broad spectrum CKs. Importantly, neuroendocrine marker positivity, usually focal, can be seen in poorly differentiated carcinomas and should not be interpreted as diagnostic of NEC if the morphology is not classic or at least highly suggestive of neuroendocrine differentiation.[25]

Immunohistochemistry may help identify the primary site of origin of a NEN and guide management with targeted therapies.[26,27] Thyroid transcription factor 1 (TTF1), initially regarded as specific for pulmonary NENs, is seen in a variety of extrapulmonary sites, notably in NEC of the cervix.[23] Consequently, TTF1 is of no value in distinguishing a primary cervical NEC from a pulmonary metastasis. TTF1 can be used in the context of well-differentiated NETs, however, because positive staining is expected in pulmonary NETs and, in turn, is very rare in gastrointestinal and pancreatic primaries. Of note, case reports of primary gynecologic NETs have recorded lack of expression of TTF1 in these tumors.[28,29] PAX8 is a commonly used marker in gynecological pathology; however, polyclonal PAX8 expression is seen in gastrointestinal and lung NENs. Therefore, a monoclonal antibody should be used if specificity for gynecologic origin is needed. Diffuse block-type p16 expression is seen in cervical NEC, reflecting the etiological association with high-risk HPV. Importantly, diffuse p16 staining may also occur in NEC via HPV-independent mechanisms, and molecular methods for HPV detection may be required in this context. Loss of expression of mismatch repair (MMR) proteins, notably MLH1 and PMS2 has been seen in endometrial and cervical NEC,[30] which may enable checkpoint inhibitor therapy.[12,31]

Similar to LCNEC, NETs express at least one of chromogranin, synaptophysin, or CD56 (**Fig. 6**). Ovarian carcinoid tumors of insular type are usually diffusely positive with all 3 markers, whereas trabecular carcinoids may be chromogranin negative. Insular and mucinous carcinoids are often positive with CDX2.[32] Insular and trabecular carcinoids are typically CK 7 positive and CK20 negative, whereas mucinous carcinoids are often CK20 positive and CK7 negative. Strumal carcinoids exhibit positive staining with neuroendocrine markers in the carcinoid component and thyroglobulin and TTF1 in the thyroid component. **Table 3** summarizes markers commonly used in neuroendocrine neoplasia in the FGT.

SITE-SPECIFIC ASPECTS OF NEUROENDOCRINE NEOPLASIA

OVARY AND FALLOPIAN TUBE

Ovarian carcinoid tumor, the most frequent primary NEN in the FGT, is uncommon, representing 1% of ovarian tumors. Most arise within a mature teratoma, although foci of carcinoid tumor rarely occur in other epithelial, germ cell, or sex-cord

Fig. *3.* Ovarian mucinous (goblet cell) carcinoid. This rare variant is characterized by multiple glandular elements associated with abundant extravasated mucin (*A*). The glands are well formed and often sit at the periphery of the mucin pools, with subtle elongation or "comma" shape appearance (*B*). The glands are lined by simple columnar epithelium with intestinal goblet cell differentiation (*C*), which can be confirmed with intestinal markers such as CDX2 (*D*). Neuroendocrine markers including chromogranin (*E*) and INSM1 (*F*) are positive.

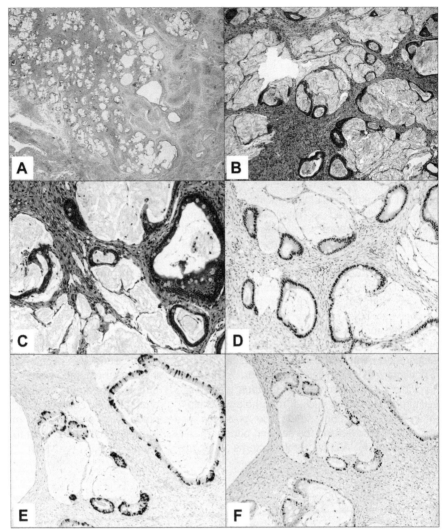

stromal tumors.[19] Tumors usually occur postmenopause and may produce mass-related symptoms,[5] with carcinoid syndrome seen in up to one-third of cases despite absence of metastases; the incidence may be higher with large tumors.[33] Most tumors are unilateral and macroscopically inapparent, representing an incidental component of a dermoid cyst; larger tumors may be recognized as having a solid yellow-tan cut surface. Most carcinoid tumors of the ovary are well-differentiated (Grade 1) and "atypical" carcinoids are in turn exceedingly rare. Nonetheless, in a

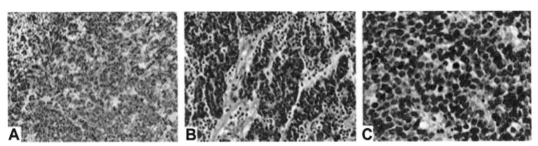

Fig. 4. Cervical SCNEC showing a solid and trabecular proliferation (*A*, *B*) of small cells with scant cytoplasm, molded nuclei, granular chromatin, and frequent apoptotic bodies (*C*).

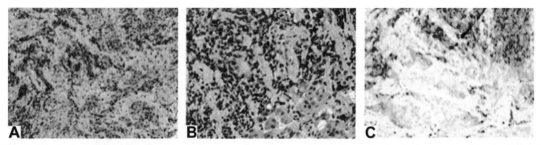

Fig. 5. Cervical SCNEC admixed with squamous cell carcinoma (*A*, *B*). Synaptophysin is expressed in the SCNEC component and absent in the nests of squamous cell carcinoma (*C*).

series of 17 carcinoids of the mucinous type, 3 tumors were classified as "atypical" (interestingly, the remaining tumors were described as "well differentiated" or "carcinoma arising in mucinous carcinoid").[34] Primary ovarian carcinoid must be distinguished from a metastasis, usually of gastrointestinal origin. An associated primary ovarian tumor or admixed thyroid elements indicating strumal carcinoid confirms an ovarian primary. Metastatic tumors are usually bilateral, with surface involvement, lymphovascular permeation, widespread peritoneal disease, and usually occur in patients with known carcinoid tumor.[19,33] Insular carcinoid tumors may mimic an adult granulosa cell tumor (GCT). The nuclear morphology is helpful in this distinction, noting the presence or absence of grooves and the salt and pepper chromatin in NET. Architectural patterns and an

immunohistochemical panel including inhibin, calretinin (positive in GCT), and neuroendocrine markers (negative in GCT) are also instrumental in resolving this dilemma. Trabecular carcinoids may be confused with Sertoli cell tumor, which can also have trabecular architecture. This is especially the case when trabecular carcinoids are chromogranin negative. Addition of inhibin and calretinin (Sertoli cell tumors are positive) and synaptophysin (Sertoli cell tumors are negative) will help differentiate these tumors. The differential diagnosis of mucinous carcinoid tumor includes metastatic adenocarcinoma (Krükenberg tumor) and primary ovarian mucinous tumors. The characteristic appearance of mucinous carcinoids, with extravasated mucin pools and well-formed glands pushed to their side, is a morphologic clue which should prompt

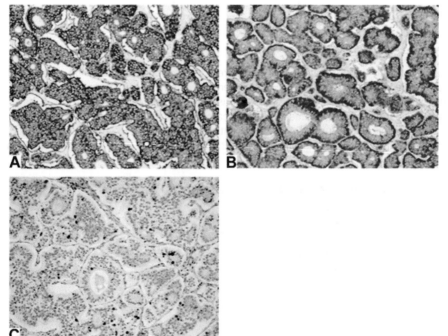

Fig. 6. Ovarian carcinoid tumor exhibiting diffuse expression of chromogranin (*A*) and synaptophysin (*B*) and an extremely low proliferation index with Ki-67 (<1%) (*C*).

Table 3
Commonly used markers in neuroendocrine neoplasia of the female genital tract

Tumor Type	Chr	Syn	CD56	CDX2	CK7	CK20	TTF1	p16	Other
NET									
Ovarian carcinoid									
Insular	+	+	+	+	+	-	NA	NA	
Trabecular	−/+	+	+	-	+	-	NA	NA	
Mucinous	+	+	+	+	−/+	+/−			
NET Cervix	+/−	+/−	+/−	*	*	*	*	*	
Endometrium									
Other FGT									
NEC									
Cervix	+/−	+/−	+/−	+/−	−/+	*	−/+	+	HPV ISH positive
Other FGT	+/−	+/−	+/−	*	*	*	−/+	−/+	Endometrium MMR loss

* Limited or no data available.

Abbreviations: Chr, chromogranin; FGT, female genital tract; HPV ISH, human papillomavirus in situ hybridization; MMR, mismatch repair; NA, not applicable; NEC, neuroendocrine carcinoma; NET, neuroendocrine tumor; Syn, synaptophysin.

immunohistochemistry for neuroendocrine markers and additional sampling (as it may reveal other carcinoid morphologies, making the diagnosis straightforward). One special consideration is metastatic mucinous carcinoid tumor to the ovary, usually of gastrointestinal/appendiceal origin. This tumour closely resembles a primary mucinous carcinoid, and the clinical context can be highly informative: features suggesting metastases include previous or concurrent appendiceal or gastrointestinal neoplasia, bilateral ovarian involvement, multinodular growth, among others.

Ovarian SCNEC (formerly known as "pulmonary type") is extremely rare and in a series of 11 patients, occurred at a mean age of 59, was bilateral in 5 patients, with spread beyond the ovary in 7 patients at presentation. Tumors were large (mean 13.5 cm), mostly solid and often admixed with a typical ovarian carcinoma.[35] Occasional case reports of SCNEC arising in teratomas have been published.[36] Small series and case reports of LCNECs, either admixed with another epithelial tumor or arising in a teratoma, also exist.[37,38] In one series of 11 patients, the mean age at presentation was 46.7 years and most tumors were unilateral with a mean size of 16.2 cm.[37] Rare reports document ovarian paragangliomas, both primary and associated with a mature cystic teratoma.[11,39] Finally, it is important to note that small cell ovarian carcinoma of hypercalcemic type is not a NEN and generally lacks neuroendocrine staining with immunohistochemistry.[19]

NENs of the fallopian tube are extremely rare. The only published series of such tumors reported 4 cases of probable primary NENs comprising 2 NETs and 2 NECs; additional isolated case reports document primary tubal NECs and a carcinoid tumor arising in a tubal teratoma.[8]

CERVIX

The cervix is the commonest site of FGT NEC, most representing SCNEC rather than LCNEC, although occasionally mixed SCNEC and LCNEC is observed. SCNECs represent approximately 2% of all cervical carcinomas[40] and most are associated with high-risk HPV.[13] NEC admixed with non-NEC is more prevalent than pure NEC. Patients often present with an abnormal cervical screening test or vaginal bleeding at a mean age of 48.1 years for SCNEC and 37 years for LCNEC. There may be metastatic disease at presentation.[5,41,42]

In the cervix, in addition to other small round blue cell tumors such as lymphoma, melanoma, and Ewing sarcoma, the differential diagnosis of SCNEC includes squamous cell carcinoma with small cell morphology. Diffuse positive nuclear staining with p63 favors a small cell variant of squamous cell carcinoma, noting that occasional NECs exhibit positive staining with p63[19]; in addition, squamous cell carcinoma lacks positive staining with neuroendocrine markers. LCNEC must be distinguished from poorly differentiated HPV-associated squamous cell carcinoma and adenocarcinoma. Again, the demonstration of significant neuroendocrine marker positivity assists in recognition of LCNEC.

Carcinoid tumors of the cervix are far less prevalent than NEC, and the subject of isolated case reports, although these neoplasms are potentially underrecognized and may be mistaken for adenocarcinoma.[10,43] Reported cases have occurred in the fifth decade, with HPV 16 and 18 identified in a cervical carcinoid and several atypical carcinoid tumors.[14]

ENDOMETRIUM

Endometrial NENs are uncommon, and most are NECs, with only extremely rare reports of endometrial NETs. Most reported endometrial NECs, which account for less than 1% of all endometrial carcinomas, comprise NEC admixed with non-NEC.[19] Clinically, uterine NECs present with abnormal bleeding and, in a series of 25 patients, the median age at diagnosis was 57 years.[30] Interestingly, in this series, in 89% of consultation cases, NEC was underrecognized and mostly LCNEC admixed with other histotypes. Tumors were mostly PAX8 negative with aberrant MMR protein expression in 8 of 18 patients.[30] Most other reports document a predominance of SCNEC.[19] The differential diagnosis includes other small round blue cell tumors and cervical NEC secondarily involving the endometrium. As mentioned, NECs arising independent of HPV exhibit diffuse p16 expression, and HPV testing may be required to resolve this differential. Distinguishing between NEC and high-grade non-NECs may be problematic, particularly as neuroendocrine marker expression occurs relatively commonly in these tumors. In a series of 71 endometrioid, serous, clear cell, undifferentiated/dedifferentiated carcinomas and carcinosarcomas, 66% of tumors expressed one or more neuroendocrine marker, usually focally.[25] In another series of 46 patients with undifferentiated endometrial carcinomas, 41% exhibited neuroendocrine expression. This was diffuse in 9% and in the remainder, limited to less than 10% of the tumor.[44] Diagnosis of NEC, therefore, requires convincing morphology in a discrete component of the tumor, and with the appropriate immunohistochemical neuroendocrine marker expression.

VULVA AND VAGINA

High-grade NECs of the vulva and vagina are extremely rare, with fewer than 80 cases reported in the literature.[7,45] Consequently, a diagnosis of vulvovaginal NEC mandates exclusion of a metastasis from another site. Most reported cases are SCNEC, often in postmenopausal women.[7,46] Vaginal tumors present with discharge or symptoms due to metastasis, usually with a clinically evident mass. Vulval tumors present as a palpable lesion most often involving the labium majus, with reported tumor size up to 9 cm.[7,46] Vulval NECs, a small subset of which derive from the Bartholin gland, have historically been considered to represent MCCs,[19] and although the 2014 WHO Classification allowed for subclassification into MCC and NEC (non-Merkel), these tumors are collectively classified as NEC in the 2020 edition.[2,5] A recently published series of 16 patients, the largest reported to date, demonstrated that most vulvar NECs are pure (94%) and exhibit SCNEC morphology (88%).[7] Based on immunohistochemistry, only 43% were classified as MCC, with the remainder representing non-Merkel NEC; the authors point out that many previously reported vulvar MCCs were not rigorously investigated with MCC-defining immunohistochemical stains. A diagnosis of MCC requires SCNEC morphology combined with expression of CK20, Cam 5.2, and neurofilament (NF) in a paranuclear dot or ring-like pattern and/or expression of Merkel cell polyoma virus large T-antigen (MCPyLTAg).[7] To reliably distinguish MCC from non-Merkel SCNEC, a panel of stains including CK20, Cam5.2, NF, TTF1, and MCPyLTAg combined with high-risk-HPV in situ hybridization is proposed.[7] NF is typically negative in non-Merkel SCNEC, whereas the opposite staining profile (MCC negative, SCNEC positive) is expected with TTF1. Importantly, p16 staining lacks discriminatory value, as previously discussed. This distinction may have clinical significance as metastatic MCC may be responsive to immune checkpoint inhibition.

Isolated reports document carcinoid tumors occurring in the vulva and vagina.[18,47] Interestingly, in a series of 3 patients with primary vulvar carcinoid tumor, 2 patients exhibited exclusively clear cell morphology with the third also including a clear cell component; the authors conclude that carcinoid tumor should be considered in the differential of vulvar tumors with clear cell change.[47]

CYTOLOGY OF NEUROENDOCRINE NEOPLASIA

Discussion is confined to cervical NEC. Cervical cytology, both conventional and liquid-based (LBC), is a relatively insensitive and nonspecific method for detection of SCNEC, although primary diagnosis on cytology may be achieved by performing immunocytochemistry on residual LBC material.[48–50] The cytologic appearance of SCNEC mirrors that in other body sites. Preparations are moderately to highly cellular, comprising clusters of small neoplastic cells forming crowded sheets or presenting singly and lacking specific architectural features although gland-like clusters and peripheral feathering, mimicking adenocarcinoma in situ, have been described.[48] Cytoplasm is scant, nuclei are round and hyperchromatic with finely stippled chromatin, and nucleoli are usually inconspicuous although may occasionally be seen. Nuclear molding, prominent nuclear pleomorphism, artifactual chromatin smearing, and tumor diathesis may occur. In LBC, the morphology differs slightly, mostly due to the absence of smearing artifact,[51] with a lack of pseudoglandular formations and more monomorphic nuclear features also described.[52] The cytologic differential diagnosis is broad and a confident diagnosis of SCNEC on cytology may be difficult, with SCNEC potentially mimicking inflammatory cells, endometrial cells, lymphoma and squamous or glandular preneoplasia/neoplasia.[48]

Cytologically, cervical LCNEC comprises rosetted or pseudoglandular clusters of large cells with ovoid nuclei, fine chromatin, and prominent nucleoli. There is moderate to abundant cytoplasm and prominent diathesis. These features overlap with adenocarcinoma and definitive diagnosis may not be possible without immunocytochemistry.[53]

In adenocarcinoma mixed with SCNEC, 2 distinct cell populations may be appreciated, with the SCNEC cells of smaller size than adenocarcinoma cells that may form gland-like structures and show prominent nucleoli.[40]

MOLECULAR PATHOLOGY OF NEUROENDOCRINE NEOPLASIA

Given the rarity of FGT NENs, studies of their molecular characteristics comprise small case series. The most widely studied are lung NENs, where the main abnormalities detected are in *MEN1*, *TP53*, *RB1*, *EGFR*, *PIK3CA*, *PTEN*, *NOTCH1*, *KMT2A*, *MYC*, and *FGFR1*.[54] In the FGT, cervical NECs are the most studied. Recurrent somatic mutations have been described in SCNEC of the cervix and include changes in *MAPK*, PIK3/AK7/mTOR, and p53/BRCA pathways.[55] Loss of heterozygosity in chromosome 3p occurs in cervical SCNEC and gains or amplifications in chromosome 3q in cervical LCNEC.[55,56] Molecular analysis of endometrial NEC by next generation sequencing classified tumors into the 4 The Cancer Genome Atlas groups.[12] Nearly 50% were microsatellite unstable/hypermutated, about a third showed no specific molecular profile and the remainder were *POLE*-mutated/ultramutated or *TP53* mutated/copy number high.

CLINICAL BEHAVIOR OF NEUROENDOCRINE NEOPLASIA

Most FGT NECs pursue an aggressive clinical course, often presenting with local nodal and widespread distant metastases, even when diagnosed at an early stage or in cases where the NEC represents a minor component of a mixed tumor.[12,41,57] A multimodality treatment strategy using radical surgery (if early-stage disease), platinum and etoposide-based chemotherapy, and radiation is often used; tumors in sites such as the adnexa, uterus, and vulva may be more amenable to surgical excision. The outcome of NECs of the cervix is significantly worse than non-NEC, with a median survival of 33.3 months compared with 315 months for cervical non-NEC in one study.[58] Another population-based study of SCNEC treated with radical chemoradiation found a 5-year survival of 50%.[59] Adverse prognostic factors include age, high tumor stage, smoking, pure SCNEC histology, and insufficient use of chemotherapy.[60,61] Although chemotherapy is associated with improved survival in NEC, it is less effective against cervical carcinoid tumors, with atypical carcinoid tumor reported to have the same prognosis as NEC.[42,60] Expression of PD-L1 has been demonstrated in 7 out of 10 cervical SCNECs in one study, mostly focal.[31] However, controlled evidence for the efficacy of immunotherapy in cervical NEC is lacking.[62]

Endometrial NECs usually behave aggressively, although in the largest published series, 28% of patients survived at least 5 years.[30] A significant subset of these tumors are MMR deficient[12,30] and these stains should be performed because patients may be amenable to checkpoint inhibition therapy. Vaginal lesions are similarly aggressive with a short median survival.[46] In the largest published series of vulvar NEC, most patients (10/15) presented with International Federation of Gynecology and Obstetrics (FIGO) stage III or IV disease with a median overall survival of 24 months and 12% 5-year survival; usual metastatic sites were inguinal lymph node, liver, bone, and lung.[7] In the vulva, recognition of MCC may have therapeutic implications with reports that immune checkpoint inhibition has proven effective in treating patients with metastatic MCC, although not all had a durable response.[7]

In the largest published series of ovarian SCNEC, 7 of 11 patients presented with spread beyond the ovary and in 5 of 7 patients with follow-up the mean survival was 8 months.[35] In a series of ovarian LCNEC, the disease pursued an aggressive course with tendency to progress to advanced stage and cause death within a mean of 17 months from diagnosis.[37] The prognosis of ovarian carcinoid tumor is usually excellent, particularly when small and incidental although spread beyond the ovary may occur with insular and mucinous variants.[5,19,33,34]

Paraneoplastic carcinoid syndrome has been described in the setting of liver metastases associated with an atypical carcinoid tumor of the cervix,[43] although it may also occur in the absence of metastasis with ovarian carcinoid tumors.[33] An association with Cushing syndrome has been rarely reported in endometrial and vaginal NECs, with this being the mode of presentation in some cases.[19,63,64]

CONFLICTS OF INTEREST

The authors declare no conflicts of interest.

REFERENCES

1. Rouzbahman M, Clarke B. Neuroendocrine tumors of the gynecologic tract: select topics. Semin Diagn Pathol 2013;30(3):224–33.
2. International Agency for Research on Cancer, World Health Organization. In: Kurman RJ, editor. WHO classification of tumours of female reproductive organs. 4th edition. International Agency for Research on Cancer; 2014.
3. Bosman F, Carneiro F, Hruban RH, et al. WHO classification of tumours of the digestive system. 4th edition. IARC Press; 2010.
4. Rindi G, Klimstra DS, Abedi-Ardekani B, et al. A common classification framework for neuroendocrine neoplasms: an International Agency for Research on Cancer (IARC) and World Health Organization (WHO) expert consensus proposal. Mod Pathol 2018;31(12):1770–86.
5. International Agency for Research on Cancer. World Health organisation classification of tumours of female reproductive organs. 5th edition. IARC; 2020.
6. Di Domenico A, Pipinikas CP, Maire RS, et al. Epigenetic landscape of pancreatic neuroendocrine tumours reveals distinct cells of origin and means of tumour progression. Commun Biol 2020;3(1):740.
7. Chen PP, Ramalingam P, Alvarado-Cabrero I, et al. High-grade neuroendocrine carcinomas of the vulva: a clinicopathologic study of 16 cases. Am J Surg Pathol 2021;45(3):304–16.
8. Grondin K, Lidang M, Boenelycke M, et al. Neuroendocrine tumors of the fallopian tube: report of a case series and review of the literature. Int J Gynecol Pathol 2019;38(1):78–84.
9. Harms PW, Harms KL, Moore PS, et al. The biology and treatment of Merkel cell carcinoma: current understanding and research priorities. Nat Rev Clin Oncol 2018;15(12):763–76.
10. Papatsimpas G, Samaras I, Theodosiou P, et al. A case of cervical carcinoid and review of the literature. Case Rep Oncol 2017;10(2):737–42.
11. McCluggage WG, Young RH. Paraganglioma of the ovary: report of three cases of a rare ovarian neoplasm, including two exhibiting inhibin positivity. Am J Surg Pathol 2006;30(5):600–5.
12. Howitt BE, Dong F, Vivero M, et al. Molecular characterization of neuroendocrine carcinomas of the endometrium: representation in all 4 TCGA groups. Am J Surg Pathol 2020;44(11):1541–8.
13. Castle PE, Pierz A, Stoler MH. A systematic review and meta-analysis on the attribution of human papillomavirus (HPV) in neuroendocrine cancers of the cervix. Gynecol Oncol 2018;148(2):422–9.
14. Alejo M, Alemany L, Clavero O, et al. Contribution of Human papillomavirus in neuroendocrine tumors from a series of 10,575 invasive cervical cancer cases. Papillomavirus Res 2018;5:134–42.
15. Sharma A, Mukewar S, Vege SS. Clinical profile of pancreatic cystic lesions in von hippel-lindau disease: a series of 48 patients seen at a tertiary institution. Pancreas 2017;46(7):948–52.
16. Spaulding R, Alatassi H, Stewart Metzinger D, et al. Ependymoma and carcinoid tumor associated with ovarian mature cystic teratoma in a patient with multiple endocrine neoplasia I. Case Rep Obstet Gynecol 2014;2014:712657.
17. Chetty R, Clark SP, Bhathal PS. Carcinoid tumour of the uterine corpus. Virchows Arch A Pathol Anat Histopathol 1993;422(1):93–5.
18. Sulak P, Barnhill D, Heller P, et al. Nonsquamous cancer of the vagina. Gynecol Oncol 1988;29(3):309–20.
19. Howitt BE, Kelly P, McCluggage WG. Pathology of neuroendocrine tumours of the female genital tract. Curr Oncol Rep 2017;19(9):59.
20. Horn L-C, Hentschel B, Bilek K, et al. Mixed small cell carcinomas of the uterine cervix: prognostic impact of focal neuroendocrine differentiation but not of Ki-67 labeling index. Ann Diagn Pathol 2006; 10(3):140–3.
21. Tang CK, Toker C, Nedwich A, et al. Unusual cutaneous carcinoma with features of small cell (oat cell-like) and squamous cell carcinomas. A variant of malignant Merkel cell neoplasm. Am J Dermatopathol 1982;4(6):537–48.
22. Chen C-H, Wu Y-Y, Kuo K-T, et al. Combined squamous cell carcinoma and Merkel cell carcinoma of the vulva: role of human papillomavirus and Merkel cell polyomavirus. JAAD Case Rep 2015;1(4):196–9.
23. McCluggage WG, Kennedy K, Busam KJ. An immunohistochemical study of cervical neuroendocrine carcinomas: neoplasms that are commonly TTF1

positive and which may express CK20 and P63. Am J Surg Pathol 2010;34(4):525–32.

24. Bellizzi AM. Immunohistochemistry in the diagnosis and classification of neuroendocrine neoplasms: what can brown do for you? Hum Pathol 2020;96: 8–33.

25. Moritz AW, Schlumbrecht MP, Nadji M, et al. Expression of neuroendocrine markers in non-neuroendocrine endometrial carcinomas. Pathology 2019;51(4):369–74.

26. Pavel M, Baudin E, Couvelard A, et al. ENETS Consensus Guidelines for the management of patients with liver and other distant metastases from neuroendocrine neoplasms of foregut, midgut, hindgut, and unknown primary. Neuroendocrinology 2012;95(2):157–76.

27. Koo J, Dhall D. Problems with the diagnosis of metastatic neuroendocrine neoplasms. Which diagnostic criteria should we use to determine tumor origin and help guide therapy? Semin Diagn Pathol 2015;32(6):456–68.

28. Katafuchi T, Kawakami F, Iwagoi Y, et al. Neuroendocrine tumor grade 3 (NET G3)" of the uterine cervix: a report of 2 cases. Int J Gynecol Pathol 2021. https://doi.org/10.1097/PGP.0000000000000828.

29. Inzani F, Santoro A, Angelico G, et al. Neuroendocrine tumor (NET) of the vagina in the light of WHO 2020 2-tiered grading system: clinicopathological report of the first described case. Virchows Arch 2021. https://doi.org/10.1007/s00428-021-03078-6.

30. Pocrnich CE, Ramalingam P, Euscher ED, et al. Neuroendocrine carcinoma of the endometrium: a clinicopathologic study of 25 cases. Am J Surg Pathol 2016;40(5):577–86.

31. Morgan S, Slodkowska E, Parra-Herran C, et al. PD-L1, RB1 and mismatch repair protein immunohistochemical expression in neuroendocrine carcinoma, small cell type, of the uterine cervix. Histopathology 2019;74(7):997–1004.

32. Rabban JT, Lerwill MF, McCluggage WG, et al. Primary ovarian carcinoid tumors may express CDX-2: a potential pitfall in distinction from metastatic intestinal carcinoid tumors involving the ovary. Int J Gynecol Pathol 2009;28(1):41–8.

33. Robboy SJ, Norris HJ, Scully RE. Insular carcinoid primary in the ovary. A clinicopathologic analysis of 48 cases. Cancer 1975;36(2):404–18.

34. Baker PM, Oliva E, Young RH, et al. Ovarian mucinous carcinoids including some with a carcinomatous component: a report of 17 cases. Am J Surg Pathol 2001;25(5):557–68.

35. Eichhorn JH, Young RH, Scully RE. Primary ovarian small cell carcinoma of pulmonary type. A clinicopathologic, immunohistologic, and flow cytometric analysis of 11 cases. Am J Surg Pathol 1992; 16(10):926–38.

36. Rubio A, Schuldt M, Chamorro C, et al. Ovarian small cell carcinoma of pulmonary type arising in mature cystic teratomas with metastases to the contralateral ovary. Int J Surg Pathol 2015;23(5): 388–92.

37. Veras E, Deavers MT, Silva EG, et al. Ovarian non-small cell neuroendocrine carcinoma: a clinicopathologic and immunohistochemical study of 11 cases. Am J Surg Pathol 2007;31(5):774–82.

38. Miyamoto M, Takano M, Goto T, et al. Large cell neuroendocrine carcinoma arising in mature cystic teratoma: a case report and review of the literature. Eur J Gynaecol Oncol 2012;33(4):414–8.

39. Haag J, Hardie L, Berning A, et al. Case report of a paraganglioma arising from a mature cystic teratoma of the ovary. Gynecol Oncol Rep 2020;32: 100537.

40. Shimojo N, Hirokawa YS, Kanayama K, et al. Cytological features of adenocarcinoma admixed with small cell neuroendocrine carcinoma of the uterine cervix. Cytojournal 2017;14:12.

41. Satoh T, Takei Y, Treilleux I, et al. Gynecologic Cancer InterGroup (GCIG) consensus review for small cell carcinoma of the cervix. Int J Gynecol Cancer 2014;24(9 Suppl 3):S102–8.

42. Embry JR, Kelly MG, Post MD, et al. Large cell neuroendocrine carcinoma of the cervix: prognostic factors and survival advantage with platinum chemotherapy. Gynecol Oncol 2011;120(3):444–8.

43. Koch CA, Azumi N, Furlong MA, et al. Carcinoid syndrome caused by an atypical carcinoid of the uterine cervix. J Clin Endocrinol Metab 1999;84(11): 4209–13.

44. Taraif SH, Deavers MT, Malpica A, et al. The significance of neuroendocrine expression in undifferentiated carcinoma of the endometrium. Int J Gynecol Pathol 2009;28(2):142–7.

45. Haykal T, Pandit T, Bachuwa G, et al. Stage 1 small cell cancer of the vagina. BMJ Case Rep 2018;2018, bcr-2018-225294.

46. Kombathula SH, Rapole PS, Prem SS, et al. Primary small cell carcinoma of the vagina: a rare instance of prolonged survival. BMJ Case Rep 2019;12(3): e227100.

47. Srivastava SA, Wang Y, Vallone J, et al. Primary clear cell carcinoid tumors of the vulva. Am J Surg Pathol 2012;36(9):1371–5.

48. Zhou C, Hayes MM, Clement PB, et al. Small cell carcinoma of the uterine cervix: cytologic findings in 13 cases. Cancer 1998;84(5):281–8.

49. Kim Y, Ha H, Kim J, et al. Significance of cytologic smears in the diagnosis of small cell carcinoma of the uterine cervix. Acta Cytol 2002;46(4):637–44.

50. Giorgadze T, Kanhere R, Pang C, et al. Small cell carcinoma of the cervix in liquid-based Pap test: utilization of split-sample immunocytochemical and

molecular analysis. Diagn Cytopathol 2012;40(3): 214–9.

51. Ng W-K, Cheung LKN, Li ASM, et al. Thin-layer cytology findings of small cell carcinoma of the lower female genital tract. Review of three cases with molecular analysis. Acta Cytol 2003;47(1):56–64.

52. Ciesla MC, Guidos BJ, Selvaggi SM. Cytomorphology of small-cell (neuroendocrine) carcinoma on ThinPrep cytology as compared to conventional smears. Diagn Cytopathol 2001;24(1):46–52.

53. Nam J-H, Na J, Kim N-I, et al. A case of large cell neuroendocrine carcinoma of the uterine cervix misdiagnosed as adenocarcinoma in Thinprep cytology test. Cytojournal 2017;14:28.

54. Metovic J, Barella M, Bianchi F, et al. Morphologic and molecular classification of lung neuroendocrine neoplasms. Virchows Arch 2021;478(1):5–19.

55. Xing D, Zheng G, Schoolmeester JK, et al. Next-generation sequencing reveals recurrent somatic mutations in small cell neuroendocrine carcinoma of the uterine cervix. Am J Surg Pathol 2018;42(6): 750–60.

56. Kawauchi S, Okuda S, Morioka H, et al. Large cell neuroendocrine carcinoma of the uterine cervix with cytogenetic analysis by comparative genomic hybridization: a case study. Hum Pathol 2005; 36(10):1096–100.

57. Gardner GJ, Reidy-Lagunes D, Gehrig PA. Neuroendocrine tumors of the gynecologic tract: a Society of Gynecologic Oncology (SGO) clinical document. Gynecol Oncol 2011;122(1):190–8.

58. Ganesan R, Hirschowitz L, Dawson P, et al. Neuroendocrine carcinoma of the cervix: review of a series of cases and correlation with outcome. Int J Surg Pathol 2016;24(6):490–6.

59. Roy S, Ko JJ, Bahl G. Small cell carcinoma of cervix: a population-based study evaluating standardized provincial treatment protocols. Gynecol Oncol Rep 2019;27:54–9.

60. Ishikawa M, Kasamatsu T, Tsuda H, et al. A multi-center retrospective study of neuroendocrine tumors of the uterine cervix: Prognosis according to the new 2018 staging system, comparing outcomes for different chemotherapeutic regimens and histopathological subtypes. Gynecol Oncol 2019;155(3): 444–51.

61. Salvo G, Gonzalez Martin A, Gonzales NR, et al. Updates and management algorithm for neuroendocrine tumors of the uterine cervix. Int J Gynecol Cancer 2019;29(6):986–95.

62. Tempfer CB, Tischoff I, Dogan A, et al. Neuroendocrine carcinoma of the cervix: a systematic review of the literature. BMC Cancer 2018;18(1):530.

63. Weberpals J, Djordjevic B, Khalifa M, et al. A rare case of ectopic adrenocorticotropic hormone syndrome in small cell carcinoma of the vagina: a case report. J Low Genit Tract Dis 2008;12(2):140–5.

64. Colleran KM, Burge MR, Crooks LA, et al. Small cell carcinoma of the vagina causing Cushing's syndrome by ectopic production and secretion of ACTH: a case report. Gynecol Oncol 1997;65(3): 526–9.

Reproductive Organ Pathology of Individuals Undergoing Gender-Affirming Surgery

Justin T. Kelley, MD, MPH[a,1], Emily R. McMullen-Tabry, MD[b], Stephanie L. Skala, MD[a,*]

KEYWORDS

- Gender-affirming surgery • Transgender • Exogenous testosterone • Exogenous estrogen

Key points

- Gender-affirming surgeries are becoming increasingly common with improved access to care and growing insurance coverage.
- Pathologists reviewing specimens from gender-affirming surgeries should be familiar with the expected histologic changes resulting from gender-affirming hormone therapy.
- As patient access to electronic medical records increases, it is vital for pathologists to use appropriate terminology/language in their reports.

ABSTRACT

As gender-affirming surgeries become more routine, it is increasingly important for pathologists to recognize the expected histologic changes seen in various tissues secondary to gender-affirming hormone therapy. For example, exogenous testosterone-related squamous atrophy or transitional cell metaplasia of the cervix may be confused for high-grade squamous intraepithelial lesion. In addition to distinguishing between benign and dysplastic/malignant features, pathologists should be mindful of the phrasing of their reports and aim to use objective, nongendered language.

BACKGROUND AND CONSIDERATIONS

Gender-affirming procedures are becoming increasingly common with improved access to care, better insurance coverage, and greater recognition of gender-diverse patients.[1–5] Jacoby and colleagues reported 295 gender-affirming procedures performed in a single year at their institution alone, and 6.4% of cases showed an atypical lesion on pathologic review.[1] Procedures generating specimens for pathologist review include masculinizing surgeries, such as mastectomies, hysterectomies and salpingo-oophorectomies, or feminizing surgeries, such as orchiectomies. The procedures provide meaningful medical and mental health benefits, as demonstrated by decreased psychological distress, suicidal ideation, mental health care utilization, and substance use among patients following surgery.[6,7]

Specimens from gender-affirming procedures are routinely reviewed by pathologists to investigate incidental lesions or occult malignancies, although this practice has been debated due to the low incidence of atypical lesions in this frequently younger population.[1] According to Koltz and Girotto, screening all breast reduction

[a] Department of Pathology, University of Michigan, Ann Arbor, MI, USA; [b] Department of Pathology, Grand Traverse Pathology, PLLC, 1105 6th Street, Traverse City, MI 49684, USA
[1] Present address: 2800 Plymouth Road, Building 35, Room 35-1411, Ann Arbor, MI 48109.
* Corresponding author. 2800 Plymouth Road, Building 35, Room 36-1221-07, Ann Arbor, MI 48109.
E-mail address: sskala@med.umich.edu
Twitter: @sska_path (S.L.S.)

Surgical Pathology 15 (2022) 421–434
https://doi.org/10.1016/j.path.2022.02.013
1875-9181/22/© 2022 Elsevier Inc. All rights reserved.

specimens costs the overall health care system $236,000 per breast cancer case identified.[8] However, some authors advocate the importance of pathologic examination for gender-affirming procedures due to the potential increased risk of developing gonadal or breast cancer with exogenous hormone exposure, as observed in the cisgender (nontransgender) population,[1,9,10] although this is not established in the transgender and gender-diverse (TGD) community.[11,12] Nevertheless, pathologists should be familiar with the expected histologic changes in hormone-sensitive tissues of interest.

Patients undergoing gender-affirming procedures encompass a diverse population of genders including but not limited to transgender, nonbinary, or genderqueer individuals. The terminology accepted by the lesbian, gay, bisexual, transgender, queer, intersex, asexual, and more (LGBTQIA+) community is well discussed elsewhere.[13–16] In short, sex and gender differ in that sex is biological involving attributes like chromosomes or genitalia whereas gender is cultural encompassing qualities such as behavior and expression. Sexual orientation is different, as it encompasses a person's attraction to other people, whereas gender identity describes a person's experienced gender irrespective of their sex. Gender reassignment and sex reassignment are medical terms traditionally used in gender-affirming care, but their use now is discouraged because of their rather negative connotations.[1,16,17]

TGD individuals suffer from entrenched systemic disparities and discrimination. Disparities are present not only in the social and cultural domains but also in health status and in the health care system.[5,14,16,18–25] For example, TGD individuals were found to avoid needed health care 43.8% of the time due to factors such as lack of provider competency and fear of discrimination.[21] TGD individuals are more likely to receive poor-quality health care and to be unfairly treated when receiving health care.[19] The healthcare barriers result in gaps in routine cancer screening, adding an additional disparity to the TGD population.[23,24]

The pathologist has the vital role of evaluating for occult neoplasia and reporting their findings to the clinical teams and patients. Despite the absence of direct interaction between patients and pathologists, patients have increasing access to their electronic medical records, and laboratory results such as pathology reports are among the most frequently viewed items.[17] Objectivity in diagnostic lines, comment sections, specimen naming, and performed procedures are paramount to prevent further disenfranchisement from the healthcare system. For example, unnecessary use of gendered language should be avoided in pathology reports. Pathologists are uniquely situated to advocate for patients by thoughtfully screening all gender-affirming specimens for atypical lesions and serving as an example to other healthcare professionals through appropriate language and objective reports.[17]

UTERINE CERVIX

INTRODUCTION

- Many individuals pursuing gender-affirming therapy may choose not to undergo total hysterectomy[26]; therefore, recognition of the effects of androgens on cervical tissue is important for pathologists interpreting cervical cytology or biopsies. The American College of Obstetricians and Gynecologists (ACOG) recommends the same screening guidelines for all individuals with a cervix; however, Pap test use is lower for TGD individuals.[27] Aside from psychological issues related to discordant sex and gender, speculum insertion may be more painful because of atrophy after long-term androgen use.[28] Multiple studies have shown higher rates of unsatisfactory Pap tests in the TGD population,[29,30] and androgen-related changes may be overinterpreted as dysplasia. Compared with cisgender atrophic cohorts, transgender individuals more frequently receive abnormal Pap results including atypical squamous cells, cannot rule out high-grade squamous intraepithelial lesion (ASC-H), atypical squamous cells of undetermined significance (ASC-US), high-grade squamous intraepithelial lesion (HSIL), and low-grade squamous intraepithelial lesion (LSIL).[29,31] Accurate distinction of benign cervical changes from dysplastic features spares these patients from unnecessary procedures.

MICROSCOPIC FEATURES

- Exogenous androgen exposure commonly results in squamous atrophy, transitional cell metaplasia (**Fig. 1**A), clusters of small basophilic cells (**Fig. 1**B), and prostatic metaplasia of surface squamous epithelium (**Fig. 1**C, D).[29,31–36]
- Cervical cytology specimens from transgender individuals show dispersed and clustered parabasal cells with smooth, evenly dispersed chromatin, occasional mild nuclear

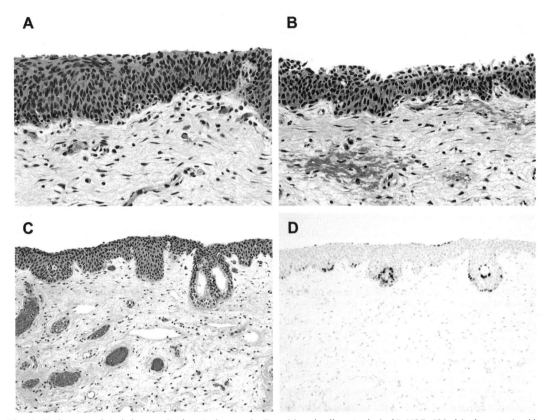

Fig. 1. Androgen-related changes in the uterine cervix. Transitional cell metaplasia (*A*, H&E, 400×) is characterized by cells with ovoid nuclei and longitudinal nuclear grooves, typically perpendicular to the basement membrane in the basal layers and parallel to the basement membrane in superficial layers. Clusters of small basophilic cells (*B*, H&E, 400×) are often seen sloughing from the surface epithelium. In this clinical context, prostatic metaplasia is usually localized to the base of the squamous epithelium (*C*, H&E, 200×) and is positive for NKX3.1 by immunohistochemistry (*D*, NKX3.1 IHC, 200×).

enlargement and irregularity, and scattered degenerated cells.[31]

- Transitional cell metaplasia and clusters of small basophilic cells are seen more often in testosterone-treated transgender cohorts.[29] Transitional cell metaplasia is characterized by ovoid nuclei with longitudinal grooves that are vertically oriented in deeper layers and streaming horizontally in superficial layers.[29,33,37–40] Nearly two-thirds of transgender men show transitional cell metaplasia in cervical epithelium although it may be unifocal.[35]
- The finding of clusters of small basophilic cells lacking normal maturation is less well characterized. On Pap, these cells have scant-to-absent cytoplasm, fine hyperchromatic chromatin, occasional indistinct nucleoli, and smooth nuclear membranes and are arranged in small, grape-like clusters.[29,33] Hysterectomy specimens may exhibit clusters of these small

basophilic cells clinging to superficial squamous epithelium.[36] There is no significant relationship between the duration of testosterone therapy and presence of transitional cell metaplasia or small basophilic cells on Pap.[29]

- Prostatic metaplasia of the surface epithelium has been documented. This change is described in the Vagina section.

DIFFERENTIAL DIAGNOSIS

- Squamous atrophy can be difficult to distinguish from dysplasia, especially in the setting of reactive atypia. In some cases, hysterectomy specimens from transgender individuals have confirmed that squamous atrophy had been mistaken for HSIL on previous biopsy.[33] Although hyperchromasia, coarse chromatin, and prominent nuclear contour irregularity are characteristic of dysplasia, reactive

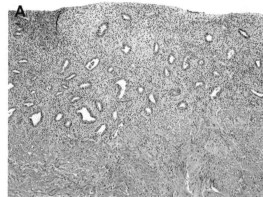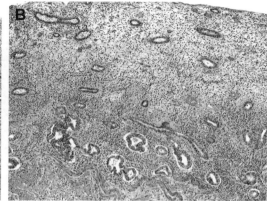

Fig. 2. Androgen-related changes in the endometrium. Exogenous testosterone therapy may result in focal areas of "decidua-like" stromal change (*A, B*, H&E, 100×), characterized by sparse glands and eosinophilic stromal cells without prominent vasculature.

parabasal cells show prominent nucleoli.[31] Similarly, transitional cell metaplasia may be misdiagnosed as HSIL.[39,40] Immunohistochemical stains for p16 and Ki-67 are useful in this distinction.

- On Pap, clusters of small basophilic squamous cells may be mistaken for endometrial cells, leading to further workup in patients >45 years old. Rather than cohesive tridimensional structures, small cells usually occur as cellular, loosely arranged aggregates.[41]

CLINICS CARE POINTS

- Squamous atrophy and transitional cell metaplasia may appear in the context of exogenous androgen therapy and may be confused for dysplasia.

- Immunohistochemical stains for p16 and Ki-67 are useful in the distinction between atrophy/metaplasia and dysplasia.

- Loose clusters of small basophilic squamous cells may be seen in the setting of exogenous androgen therapy.

UTERINE CORPUS

INTRODUCTION

- Although early reports suggested an increased risk of endometrial hyperplasia and malignancy in amenorrheic individuals on androgen therapy, this has not been a consistent finding. The World Professional Association of Transgender Health (WPATH) position is that testosterone therapy may increase the risk of endometrial cancer in transgender men, but

evidence is limited.[42] Nonetheless, there are recommendations for routine endometrial surveillance or hysterectomy in these patients.[43,44] Among individuals with abnormal uterine bleeding before the initiation of testosterone therapy, nearly one-fourth have persistent bleeding on testosterone.[45]

MICROSCOPIC FEATURES

- Endometrial samples from individuals taking exogenous testosterone typically exhibit either proliferative or atrophic/inactive endometrium.[45,46] After six months of testosterone treatment, approximately one-third of individuals have serum estrogen levels suppressed to the level seen in cisgender men.[47] Testosterone exposure increases endometrial proliferation in reproductive-age individuals[48] but has a modest antagonistic effect after menopause.[33] Atrophic endometrium may be the result of a direct androgenic effect on the endometrium[49]; however, in vitro studies have shown that androstenedione inhibits endometrial proliferation, whereas testosterone, dihydrotestosterone, and dehydroepiandrosterone do not.[50]

- Androgen is believed to enhance prolactin secretion, leading to decidualization.[51] Many cases with inactive endometrial glands show focal decidual-like endometrial stromal change (**Fig. 2**A, B) although stromal capillaries remain thin walled with no true predecidualization around them.[35]

- Endomyometrial findings are often similar to those in cisgender women and may include polyps, leiomyomata, and nonatypical hyperplasia.[45,46,52] There has been one reported case of atypical hyperplasia with focal endometrioid carcinoma.[52]

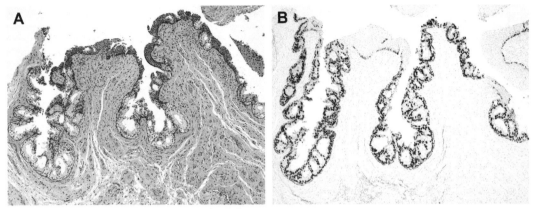

Fig. 3. Androgen-related changes in the vagina. Prostatic metaplasia is typically localized to the base of the squamous epithelium and may be extensive (*A*, H&E, 100×); the prostatic-type glands are positive for NKX3.1 (*B*, NKX 3.1 IHC, 100×).

- Although it has been reported that myometrial hypertrophy or leiomyomata are more frequent in transgender men on testosterone,[45] this has not been found in other studies.[52]

CLINICS CARE POINTS

- The endometrium of individuals taking exogenous testosterone is usually either proliferative or inactive/atrophic.

- Focal decidual-like endometrial stromal change may be seen with exogenous androgen exposure.

VAGINA

MICROSCOPIC FEATURES

- Vaginectomy specimens from individuals on long-term androgen therapy may show ectopic prostatic-type glandular differentiation throughout the basal layer of surface squamous epithelium without involvement of the lamina propria (**Fig. 3**A).[53] The prostatic-type glands may be sparse, multifocal, or confluent, and apical snouts may appear.[53] NKX3.1 and androgen receptor immunostains are positive (**Fig. 3**B) more often than prostate-specific antigen (PSA) in the context of exogenous androgen therapy; PAX8 and estrogen receptor are negative in the prostatic-type glands.[53] The squamous epithelium adjacent to these glands exhibits transitional cell metaplasia.[53] The vagina and the prostate are both derived from the urogenital sinus,[54] and mouse models have shown that androgens can induce prostatic metaplasia in the vaginal tissue.[55] The distribution of prostatic-type glands in the vaginal

tissue from transgender men is similar to that of "embryonic-type" adenosis,[56] supporting the theory that this is a metaplastic change. No masses or neoplasia have been reported in follow-up.[53]

- As in the cervix, atrophy and decreased glycogenation can be seen in the vagina.

- Vestibulovaginal sclerosis (VVS) presents as a white plaque in the vestibule or vagina and has been reported in one transgender man (without injury or traumatic sexual practices)[57] in addition to peri- and postmenopausal cisgender women.[58–60] The histologic findings are like those of lichen simplex chronicus, with focal sclerosis of subepithelial lamina propria and thickened basement membrane highlighted by PAS. Vestibulovaginal sclerosis may represent an unusual reparative stromal change, possibly related to atrophy-related vaginal irritation.[58] It has been suggested that VVS may be a variant of lichen sclerosus.

CLINICS CARE POINTS

- Vaginectomy specimens from individuals taking exogenous androgens often show ectopic prostatic-type glandular differentiation throughout the basal layer of surface squamous epithelium.

- This "surface prostatic metaplasia" can be confirmed with NKX3.1 immunohistochemistry.

VULVA

Like cisgender women, transgender men and gender diverse individuals assigned female at birth (AFAB) may develop vulvar squamous

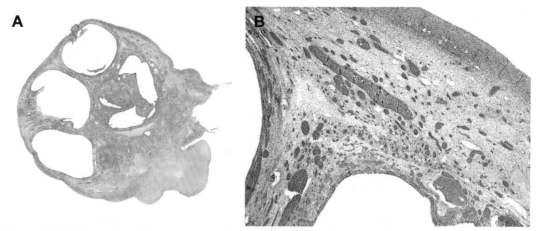

Fig. 4. Androgen-related changes in the ovary. The ovaries often develop subcortical cystic follicles (*A*, H&E, 1×) and increased stromal collagen in the cortex (*B*, H&E, 40×).

intraepithelial lesions. There is one case report of HSIL identified in the vulva of a 41-year-old transgender man during a first-stage phalloplasty.[1] It is also possible that they can develop chronic inflammatory dermatoses and eventually HPV-independent lesions, such as differentiated vulvar intraepithelial neoplasia, although such phenomena have not been yet documented in this population.

CLINICS CARE POINTS

- HPV-related lesions can be seen in the vulva of individuals taking exogenous androgens.

NEOVAGINA

INTRODUCTION

- Penile inversion vaginoplasty is the most common technique used to create a functional vagina. The neovaginal lining is composed of penile skin, and external genitalia are formed from preputial and scrotal skin. Other surgical approaches may use nongenital skin, intestine, or peritoneum for the neovaginal lining.[61]
- A study of neovaginal swabs from 54 transgender women who had undergone vaginoplasty demonstrated positivity for high-risk human papillomavirus (hrHPV) in 20% of sexually active women although no lesions or symptoms were clinically identified.[62] Of note, one woman with neovaginal hrHPV infection had a sigmoid vaginoplasty (rather than vaginoplasty with genital skin).
- Neovaginal pain in the first postoperative year is considered normal; neovaginal pain beyond that timeframe may be a sign of an HPV-associated lesion.

MICROSCOPIC FEATURES

- Symptomatic hrHPV-related neovaginal lesions are exceedingly rare (4 of 1082 patients in one study) but include condylomata and HSIL.[63]

CLINICS CARE POINTS

- High-risk HPV can affect neovaginal tissue, even when derived from intestine.

OVARY

INTRODUCTION

- When gender-affirming hysterectomies are performed, oophorectomy is often included.

MICROSCOPIC FEATURES

- Bilateral cystic follicles (**Fig. 4**A) are commonly seen in the ovaries of transgender men with preoperative androgen exposure.[35,45] These cysts are typically lined by nonluteinized granulosa cells, like those seen in the setting of polycystic ovarian syndrome (PCOS). Endometriotic cysts and simple cysts have also been reported in transgender individuals.[64] Body mass index and duration of testosterone therapy do not seem to be associated with the presence of ovarian cysts.[64]
- Androgens may stimulate the proliferation of ovarian stromal cells, resulting in enlargement and increased collagen content.[52] Indeed, patients taking exogenous testosterone have been reported to have thickened ovarian cortex, increased collagen (**Fig. 4**B), ovarian stromal hyperplasia, and ovarian stromal

luteinization.[65] Animal studies have shown that exogenous androgen supplementation leads to polycystic ovaries and reduced menstrual cycles.[66]

- Ovarian follicle density may be higher than expected for age.[35] Some investigators report a maturation shift in which most follicles are primordial[67] whereas others note an increase only in the number of atretic follicles compared to controls.[65]
- Two transgender men with prior diagnoses of PCOS on ultrasound showed resolution of some cystic follicles after testosterone therapy.[65]
- There is no convincing evidence that elevated androgen levels related to gender-affirming therapy increase the risk of ovarian cancer compared with that in cisgender women[68]; however, overweight women with PCOS and high circulating androgens have been shown to have a modest increased risk of serous borderline ovarian tumors.[69] Transmasculine individuals have been reported to develop some of the same ovarian tumors as cisgender women, including serous borderline tumor,[70,71] serous cystadenoma, mature cystic teratoma,[35] and (one) endometrioid carcinoma.[72]

CLINICS CARE POINTS

- Ovaries with exogenous androgen exposure commonly show bilateral cystic follicles and a thickened ovarian cortex.
- Ovarian neoplasms have been documented in transgender AFAB individuals.

FALLOPIAN TUBE

MICROSCOPIC FEATURES

- One instance of fallopian tube with exogenous androgen exposure has been reported to show hyperplastic paratubal mesonephric remnants with pseudostratified ciliated columnar epithelium, reminiscent of epididymis.[34]

BREAST/CHEST TISSUE (ASSIGNED FEMALE AT BIRTH [AFAB])

INTRODUCTION

- Gender-affirming therapy for AFAB individuals often includes testosterone therapy and surgical intervention to assist in the masculinization process. Chest wall contouring, typically done

by mastectomy, is the most common surgical intervention AFAB individuals seeking a flat chest choose to undergo after prolonged androgen therapy.[73,74] Temporal trends have seen an increase in chest wall contouring because of expanded access to care, reduced social stigma, and enhanced insurance coverage.[2,73] Therefore, the pathologist should be aware of the histopathologic findings that are seen in mastectomy specimens from this population.

GROSS FEATURES

- Gross abnormalities are rarely encountered.[75]
- Median recommended sampling of breast tissue ranges from two to four blocks.[75–78]
  - The most frequent suggestion is four tissue blocks per gender-affirming mastectomy, if no gross pathologic finding.[77,78] Submission of additional blocks is not associated with an increased rate of atypical findings.[78]

MICROSCOPIC FEATURES

- Androgen therapy is associated with a marked reduction of glandular tissue and increased fibrous tissue (Fig. 5A).[52]
- Commonly encountered histopathologic features in transmasculine mastectomy specimens include duct ectasia, lobular atrophy, fibrous stroma, and fibrocystic changes[75,76]
  - A longer duration of androgen therapy is associated with a higher degree of lobular atrophy.[77]
- Gynecomastoid change (Fig. 5B) can also be encountered and is thought to be a secondary effect of androgen therapy.[75,76]
- Other changes such as pseudoangiomatous stromal hyperplasia, fibroadenoma, benign vascular lesions, and papillomas have been described in individuals on exogenous androgens as well as cisgender women[76] although these findings are less often seen in individuals on long-term androgen therapy.[77]
- Although rarely encountered, atypical lesions can also be identified (1.5%–4.7% of mastectomy specimens[78]).
  - Atypical ductal hyperplasia, atypical lobular hyperplasia, lobular carcinoma in situ, flat epithelial atypia, and ductal carcinoma in situ have been reported.[75,76,78]
  - E.R.M. has also encountered an incidental high-grade ductal carcinoma in situ (Fig. 5C, D) in a gender-affirming mastectomy specimen from a transgender man,

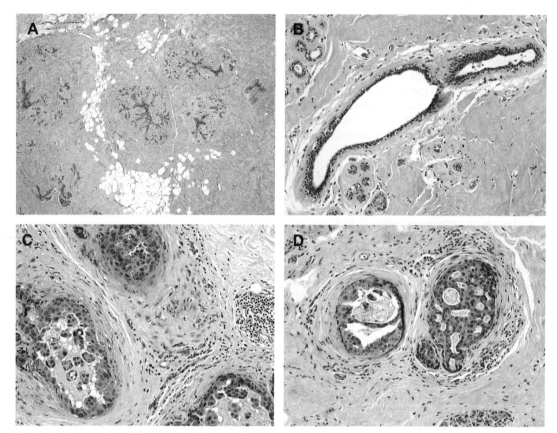

Fig. 5. Androgen-related changes in the breast/chest tissue. Testosterone therapy causes a decrease in glandular tissue and increase in fibrous tissue (*A*, H&E, 40×), as well as occasional gynecomastoid change (*B*, H&E, 200×). Rarely, ductal carcinoma in situ may be seen (*C, D*, H&E, 200×).

and the patient was subsequently referred to surgical oncology for further management.

○ Rare cases of breast carcinoma have been reported.[78–81]

CLINICS CARE POINTS

- Common histopathologic findings of mastectomy specimens from AFAB individuals include duct ectasia, lobular atrophy, fibrous stroma, and fibrocystic changes.

- Adequate sampling (approximately four tissue blocks) of mastectomy specimens should be performed to rule out an atypical lesion or invasive carcinoma.

BREAST/CHEST TISSUE (ASSIGNED MALE AT BIRTH [AMAB])

INTRODUCTION

- Gender-affirming therapy for AMAB individuals includes estradiol with or without an

antiandrogen, and feminization surgeries including breast augmentation.[82] There is minimal literature on the benign histopathologic findings in breast tissue for transfeminine individuals.

MICROSCOPIC FEATURES

- Well-developed lobules are associated with estrogen therapy.[82–85]
- Several case reports of neoplasia of the breast in AMAB individuals have been published.[82]
  ○ Thirty-eight adenocarcinomas have been reported in the literature (23 invasive ductal, 4 in situ, 1 secretory carcinoma, 1 poorly differentiated carcinoma, and 8 undescribed).[82]
  ○ There is mixed literature on the risk of development of breast cancer compared with cisgender men, with some groups reporting comparable risk[80] and others reporting increased risk.[86]
- Other findings have been reported including fibroepithelial lesions and angiolipomas.[82]

CLINICS CARE POINTS

- Well-developed breast lobules are associated with estrogen therapy.
- Neoplastic breast findings have been reported in transfeminine individuals.

TESTIS

INTRODUCTION

- Transgender women receiving hormone therapy with documented low testosterone have decreased spermatogenesis.[9,82,87–90] The recommended level of androgen suppression by the Endocrine Society is a testosterone level of less than 50 ng/dL.[91] Recovery of spermatogenesis can take months following cessation of hormone therapy.
- Grossly, reduced testicular size, weight, and volume are associated with intensity, rather than the duration, of hormone suppression.[82,88] Reduced testicular weight and volume and younger age are also correlated with both reduced and incomplete spermatogenesis.[88]

MICROSCOPIC FEATURES

- Atrophy is the most common hormone therapy-related finding in the testes. Seminiferous tubules typically show maturation arrest, reduced diameter, and thickened basement membrane (**Fig. 6**A). Compensatory Sertoli cell hyperplasia with vacuolization is commonly seen (**Fig. 6**B). The stroma typically shows increased fibrosis and Leydig cell hypoplasia with vacuolization; rare cases of Leydig cell hyperplasia have been reported (**Fig. 6**C).[9,82,90] A subset of cases showed rare, large cells with nuclei three times the size of Sertoli cell nuclei and smudged chromatin.[90] The proximal epididymis additionally showed epithelial hyperplasia, including stratification and micropapillae, in 20% of cases. Andrews and colleagues described two case reports of ectopic adrenal tissue in their review of the literature (**Fig. 6**D).[82] They found no hormone receptor expression differences between transgender women on hormone therapy and cisgender men. Barreno and colleagues reported atherosclerosis in 50% of cases, of which the patients had a mean age of 35 years without a vasculopathic clinical diagnosis.[9] They also discussed venous dilation in the mediastinum testis in 21% of cases.

- Testicular cancer is a rare finding in gender-affirming orchiectomies. Most series report no cases of premalignant or malignant lesions in the testes from transgender women on hormone therapy.[9,89,90] Only four cases have been reported, all of which were germ cell tumors (GCTs).

CLINICS CARE POINTS

- Atrophy is the most common finding in the testes of TGD individuals receiving exogenous estrogen and is associated with the concentration of exogenous hormones.
- Spermatogenesis is variable and is most often reduced with infrequent complete maturation.
- Seminiferous tubule hypoplasia with thickened basement membrane and interstitium expansion with increased fibrosis are common microscopic findings.
- Testicular cancer is exceedingly rare and all four reported cases were GCTs.

PROSTATE

INTRODUCTION

- Prostatectomies are not performed in gender-affirming surgical transitions due to risk of complications, such as incontinence and urethral stricture.[92–94] The retention of the prostate in this population prompts the need for continued awareness of the retained prostate and need for ongoing prostate cancer screening.[95–97]
- Only two cases of benign prostatic hypertrophy requiring transurethral resection have been described in transgender women following orchiectomy and on hormone therapy for more than 20 years.
- Likewise, only 11 cases of prostate cancer in transgender women on hormone therapy for at least six years (median 20 years) have been described.[94,95] However, most individuals who developed prostate cancer were over 50 years old when beginning hormone therapy, and it is unclear whether the prostate cancer was present before hormone intake.[94] Originally cited incidence of prostate cancer in transgender women on hormone therapy following orchiectomy is exceedingly rare with an incidence rate of 0.04% in all patients and 0.13% in patients initiating hormone therapy at or after 40 years of age.[98] A more

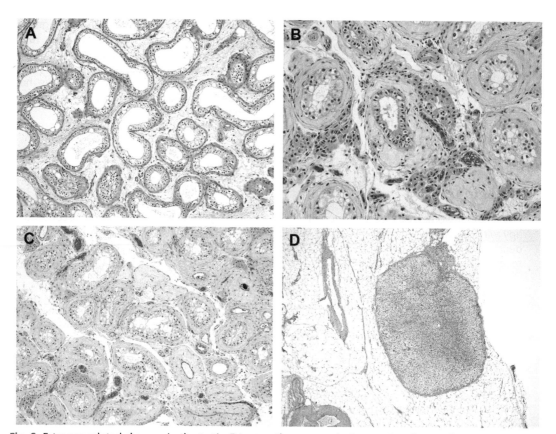

Fig. 6. Estrogen-related changes in the testis. Estrogen therapy results in atrophy of seminiferous tubules, with thickening of the basement membrane (*A*, H&E, 100×) and Sertoli cell hyperplasia with vacuolization (*B*, H&E, 200×). The quantity of Leydig cells is variable (*C*, H&E, 100×). Ectopic adrenal tissue may be seen adjacent to the testis (*D*, H&E, 40×).

recent publication shows a standardized incidence ratio of 0.20.[96,97]

- Prostate cancer screening remains controversial in cisgender men, and the literature is too sparse in transgender women to formulate appropriate screening recommendations.[95–97] The WPATH and Endocrine Society both recommend individualized screening based on personalized assessment of risk of developing prostate cancer.[42,91] The upper threshold of normal for PSA level is recommended to be set to 1 ng/mL, similar to that in androgen-deprived cisgender men, based on the largest prostate cancer incidence study in transgender women on hormone therapy following orchiectomy.[94,95,98] Furthermore, similar to cisgender men, the velocity of PSA level shift remains a significator prognosticator of malignancy.[94]

MICROSCOPIC FEATURES

- Prostate histology remains largely unaffected following hormone therapy in transgender women and gender-diverse AMAB individuals for both benign and malignant conditions. In benign prostatic tissue, the gland-to-stroma ratio remains intact without changes in the stroma. The glands, however, are more likely to demonstrate basal cell hyperplasia and squamous metaplasia, similar to atrophic findings seen in cisgender men. PSA, prostatic acid phosphatase, and androgen receptor are likely to show weak, variable staining, and estrogen receptor and progesterone receptor are more likely to demonstrate positive staining (as seen in four out of five cases examined), compared with cisgender men.[98]

- According to the largest reported case series (*n* = 11) of prostate cancers in transgender women, four were Gleason score (GS) 7, one was GS 8 and three were GS 9 (four were unknown but reported as poorly differentiated prostatic adenocarcinoma).[82,95] Metastatic disease was found at presentation in six of nine patients (two were unknown).[95] No other carcinoma types, differentiation, or special features have been reported.

CLINICS CARE POINTS

- Transgender women and gender diverse AMAB individuals retain their prostate, necessitating awareness for prostate cancer screening.

- The incidence of prostate cancer in transgender women is exceedingly rare with only 11 cases reported to date.

- Screening for prostate cancer in transgender women remains similar to that in cisgender men with an emphasis on individualized risk of developing prostate cancer.

- Prostate histology in transgender women undergoing hormone therapy and/or orchiectomy remains similar to cisgender men.

USING GENDER-INCLUSIVE TERMINOLOGY IN PATHOLOGY REPORTS

With increased and easier access to electronic health records by patients, healthcare providers must adopt the use of neutral and inclusive language in their notes and reports. Using a gender different from the patient's experienced gender can bring acute distress, particularly to transgender individuals.[98,99] To this end, using gendered language in pathology reports should be avoided (e.g., using ''female breast tissue'' in the gross description, "woman undergoing transition to man" in the clinical diagnosis, or "female genital organs with no significant pathologic change" in the final diagnosis). Gender-neutral language in pathology reports can be achieved by limiting the terminology to that related to the organs evaluated, without making any implications of patient gender or clinical diagnosis. A comprehensive discussion of this topic was recently written by Ahmad and colleagues.[17]

ACKNOWLEDGMENTS

The authors would like to thank Shanna K. Kattari, PhD, MEd, CSE, ACS, Sara Weiner, LMSW, and Hadrian Kinnear, MD, PhD candidate from the University of Michigan for their review of language/terminology used in this publication.

DISCLOSURE

The authors have nothing to disclose.

REFERENCES

1. Jacoby A, Rifkin W, Zhao LC, et al. Incidence of cancer and premalignant lesions in surgical specimens of transgender patients. Plast Reconstr Surg 2021; 147(1):194–8.

2. Canner JK, Harfouch O, Kodadek LM, et al. Temporal trends in gender-affirming surgery among transgender patients in the united states. JAMA Surg 2018;153(7):609–16.

3. Zurada A, Salandy S, Roberts W, et al. The evolution of transgender surgery. Clin Anat 2018;31:878–86.

4. Wiepjes CM, Nota NM, de Blok CJM, et al. The amsterdam cohort of gender dysphoria study (1972-2015): trends in prevalence, treatment, and regrets. J Sex Med 2018;15:582–90.

5. LGBT Policy Coordinating Committee. Advancing LGBT health and well-being: 2016 report. 2016. Available at. https://www.hhs.gov/programs/topic--sites/lgbtq/reports/health-objectives-2016.html. Accessed September 13, 2021.

6. Branstrom R, Pachankis JE. Reduction in mental health treatment utilization among transgender individuals after gender-affirming surgeries: a total population study. Am J Psychiatry 2020;177(8): 727–34.

7. Almazan AN, Keuroghlian AS. Association between gender-affirming surgeries and mental health outcomes. JAMA Surg 2021;156(7):611–8.

8. Koltz PF, Girotto JA. The price of pathology: is screening all breast reduction specimens cost effective? Plast Reconstr Surg 2010;125(5):1575–6.

9. Pena Barreno C, Gonzalez-Peramato P, Nistal M. Vascular and inflammatory effects of estrogen and anti-androgen therapy in the testis and epididymis of male to female transgender adults. Reprod Toxicol 2020;95:37–44.

10. Chandhoke G, Shayegan B, Hotte SJ. Exogenous estrogen therapy, testicular cancer, and the male to female transgender population: a case report. J Med Case Rep 2018;12:373–8.

11. Joint R, Chen ZE, Cameron S. Breast and reproductive cancers in the transgender population: a systematic review. BJOG 2018;125:1505–12.

12. McFarlane T, Zajac JD, Cheung AS. Gender-affirming hormone therapy and the risk of sex hormone-dependent tumours in transgender individuals—a systematic review. Clin Endocrinol 2018;89:700–11.

13. The Fenway guide to lesbian, gay, bisexual, and transgender health/[edited by] Harvey J. Makadon, Kenneth H. Mayer, Jennifer Potter, Hilary Goldhammer. –2nd edition. American College of Physicians: Philadelphia, PA.

14. National LGBT Health Education Center. A program of the fenway institute. understanding the health needs of LGBT people. 2016. Available at. https://www.lgbtqiahealtheducation.org/wp-content/uploads/LGBTHealthDisparitiesMar2016.pdf. Accessed September 13, 2021.

15. National LGBT Health Education Center: A Program of the Fenway Institute. LGBTQIA+ glossary of

terms for health care teams. Available at: https://www.lgbtqiahealtheducation.org/wp-content/uploads/2020/10/Glossary-2020.08.30.pdf. Accessed September 13, 2021.

16. American Psychological Association. Guidelines for psychological practice with transgender and gender nonconforming people. Am Psychol 2015;70(9): 832–64.

17. Ahmad T, Lafreniere A, Grynspan D. Incorporating transition-affirming language into anatomical pathology reporting for gender affirmation surgery. Transgend Health 2019;4(1):335–8.

18. Fish JN, Krueger EA. Reconsidering approaches to estimating health disparities across multiple measures of sexual orientation. LGBT Health 2020;7(4): 198–207.

19. Jennings L, Barcelos C, McWilliams C, et al. Inequalities in lesbian, gay, bisexual, and transgender (LGBT) health and health care access and utilization in Wisconsin. Prev Med Rep 2019;14(10084):1–7.

20. Hutchcraft ML, Teferra AA, Montemorano L, et al. Differences in health-related quality of life and health behaviors among lesbian, bisexual, and heterosexual women surviving cancer from the 2013 to 2018 national health interview study. LGBT Health 2021; 8(1):68–78.

21. Moll J, Krieger P, Heron SL, et al. Attitudes, behavior, and comfort of emergency medicine residents in caring for lgbt patients: what do we know? AEM Educ Train 2019;3(2):129–35.

22. Macapagal K, Bhatia R, Greene GJ. Differences in healthcare access, use, and experiences within a community sample of racially diverse lesbian, gay, bisexual, transgender, and questioning emerging adults. LGBT Health 2016;3(6):434–42.

23. Langston ME, Fuzzell L, Lewis-Thames MW, et al. Disparities in health information-seeking behaviors and fatalistic views of cancer by sexual orientation identity: a nationally representative study of adults in the united states. LGBT Health 2019;6(4):192–201.

24. Banerjee SC, Walters CB, Staley JM, et al. Knowledge, beliefs, and communication behavior of oncology health-care providers (HCPs) regarding lesbian, gay, bisexual, and transgender (LGBT) patient health care. J Health Commun 2018;23(4): 329–39.

25. Wilson CK, West L, Stepleman L, et al. Attitudes toward LGBT patients among students in the health professions: influence of demographics and discipline. LGBT Health 2014;1(3):204–11.

26. Bauer GR, Travers R, Scanlon K, et al. High heterogeneity of HIV-related sexual risk among transgender people in Ontario, Canada: a province-wide respondent-driven sampling survey. BMC Public Health 2012;12:292.

27. Committee on health care for underserved women. committee opinion no. 512: health care for transgender individuals. Obstet Gynecol 2011;118: 1454–8.

28. van Trotsenburg MA. Gynecological aspects of transgender healthcare. Int J Transgend 2009;11: 238–46.

29. Williams MPA, Kukkar V, Stemmer MN, et al. Cytomorphologic findings of cervical pap smears from female-to-male transgender patients on testosterone therapy. Cancer Cytopathol 2020;128:491–8.

30. Peitzmeier SM, Reisner SL, Harigopal P, et al. Female-to-male patients have high prevalence of unsatisfactory Paps compared to non-transgender females: implications for cervical cancer screening. J Gen Intern Med 2014;29:778–84.

31. Adkins BD, Barlow AB, Jack A, et al. Characteristic findings of cervical Papanicolaou tests from transgender patients on androgen therapy: Challenges in detecting dysplasia. Cytopathology 2018;29:281–7.

32. Papanicolaou GN, Ripley HS, Shorr E, et al. Suppressive action of testosterone propionate on menstruation and its effect on vaginal smears. Endocrinology 1939;24:339.

33. Miller N, Bedard YC, Cooter NB, et al. Histological changes in the genital tract in transsexual women following androgen therapy. Histopathology 1986; 10:661–9.

34. Singh K, Sung CJ, Lawrence WD, et al. Testosterone-induced "virilization" of mesonephric duct remnants and cervical squamous epithelium in female-to-male transgenders: a report of 3 cases. Int J Gynecol Pathol 2016;36:328–33.

35. Khalifa MA, Toyama A, Klein ME, et al. Histologic features of hysterectomy specimens from female-male transgender individuals. Int J Gynecol Pathol 2018;38:520–7.

36. McMullen-Tabry ER, Sciallis AP, Skala SL. Surface prostatic metaplasia, transitional cell metaplasia, and superficial clusters of small basophilic cells in the uterine cervix: prevalence in gender-affirming hysterectomies and comparison to benign hysterectomies from cisgender women. Histopathology 2021, [in production].

37. Folkes LV, Agrawal V, Parkinson MC, et al. The effects of androgen therapy on female genital tract. Mod Pathol 2005;18(suppl 1s):183A.

38. Weir MM, Bell DA. Transitional cell metaplasia of the cervix: a newly described entity in cervicovaginal smears. Diagn Cytopathol 1998;18:222–6.

39. Egan AJ, Russell P. Transitional (urothelial) cell metaplasia of the uterine cervix: morphological assessment of 31 cases. Int J Gynecol Pathol 1997;16:89–98.

40. Weir MM, Bell DA, Young RH. Transitional cell metaplasia of the uterine cervix and vagina: an underrecognized lesion that may be confused with high-grade dysplasia. a report of 59 cases. Am J Surg Pathol 1997;21:510–7.

41. DeMay RM. The pap smear (cytology of glandular epithelium). In: DeMay RM, editor. Art Sci

Cytopathology: Exfoliative Cytolvol. 1. Chicago, IL: ASCP Press; 1996. p. 122–5.

42. Coleman E, Bockting W, Botzer M, et al. Standards of care for the health of transsexual, transgender, and gender-nonconforming people, version 7. Int J Transgend 2012;13:165–232.

43. Unger CA. Care of the transgender patient: the role of the gynecologist. Am J Obstet Gynecol 2014;210:16–26.

44. Gorton R, Buth J, Spade D. Medical therapy and health maintenance for transgender men: a guide for health care providers. San Francisco: Lyon-Martin Women's Health Services; 2005. Available at: https://www.nickgorton.org/Medical%20Therapy%20and%20HM%20for%20Transgender%20Men_2005.pdf.

45. Loverro G, Resta L, Dellino M, et al. Uterine and ovarian changes during testosterone administration in young female-to-male transsexuals. Taiwan J Obstet Gynecol 2016;55:686–91.

46. Dreisler E, Stampe Sorensen S, Ibsen PH, et al. Prevalence of endometrial polyps and abnormal uterine bleeding in a Danish population aged 20–74 years. Ultrasound Obstet Gynecol 2009;33:102–8.

47. Deutsch MB, Bhakri V, Kubicek K. Effects of cross-sex hormone treatment on transgender women and men. Obstet Gynecol 2015;125:605–10.

48. Perrone AM, Cerpolini S, Maria Salfi NC, et al. Effect of long-term testosterone administration on the endometrium of female-to-male (FtM) transsexuals. J Sex Med 2009;6:3193–200.

49. Gooren LJG, Giltay EJ. Review of studies of androgen treatment of female-to-male transsexuals: effects and risks of administration of androgens to females. J Sex Med 2008;5:765–76.

50. Tuckerman EM, Okon MA, Li T-C, et al. Do androgens have a direct effect on endometrial function? an in vitro study. Fertil Steril 2000;74:771–9.

51. Futterweit W. Endocrine therapy of transsexualism and potential complications of long-term treatment. Arch Sex Behav 1998;27:209–26.

52. Grynberg M, Fanchin R, Dubost G, et al. Histology of genital tract and breast tissue after long-term testosterone administration in a female-to-male transsexual population. Reprod Biomed Online 2010;20:553–8.

53. Anderson WJ, Kolin DL, Neville G, et al. Prostatic metaplasia of the vagina and uterine cervix: an androgen-associated glandular lesion of surface squamous epithelium. Am J Surg Pathol 2020;44:1040–9.

54. Robboy SJ, Kurita T, Baskin L, et al. New insights into human female reproductive tract development. Differentiation 2017;97:9–22.

55. Boutin EL, Battle E, Cunha GR. The response of female urogenital tract epithelia to mesenchymal inductors is restricted by the germ layer origin of the epithelium: prostatic inductions. Differentiation 1991;48:99–105.

56. Robboy SJ, Hill EC, Sandberg E, et al. Vaginal adenosis in women born prior to the diethylstilbestrol era. Hum Pathol 1986;17:488–92.

57. O'Sullivan C, Day T, Scurry J. Vestibulovaginal sclerosis in a transgender man on testosterone. J Low Genit Tract Dis 2020;24:229–31.

58. Fadare O. Vaginal stromal sclerosis: a distinctive stromal change associated with vaginal atrophy. Int J Gynaecol Pathol 2011;30:295–300.

59. Day T, Burston K, Dennerstein G, et al. Vestibulovaginal sclerosis versus lichen sclerosus. Int J Gynaecol Pathol 2018;37:356–63.

60. Croker BA, Scurry JP, Petry FM, et al. Vestibular sclerosis: is this a new, distinct clinicopathological entity? J Low Genit Tract Dis 2018;22:260–3.

61. Horbach SE, Bouman MB, Smit JM, et al. Outcome of vaginoplasty in male-to-female transgenders: a systematic review of surgical techniques. J Sex Med 2015;12:1499–512.

62. van der Sluis WB, Buncamper ME, Bouman M, et al. Prevalence of neovaginal high-risk human papillomavirus among transgender women in the netherlands. Sex Transm Dis 2016;43(8):503–5.

63. van der Sluis WB, Buncamper ME, Bouman M, et al. Symptomatic HPV-related neovaginal lesions in transgender women: case series and review of literature. Sex Transm Infect 2016;92:499–501.

64. Grimstad FW, Fowler KG, New EP, et al. Ovarian histopathology in transmasculine persons on testosterone: a multicenter case series. J Sex Med 2020; 17:1807–18.

65. Ikeda K, Baba T, Noguchi H, et al. Excessive androgen exposure in female-to-male transsexual persons of reproductive age induces hyperplasia of the ovarian cortex and stroma but not polycystic ovary morphology. Hum Reprod 2013;28(2):453–61.

66. Chen MJ, Chou CH, Chen SU, et al. The effect of androgens on ovarian follicle maturation: Dihydrotestosterone suppress FSH stimulated granulosa cell proliferation by upregulating PPARg-dependent PTEN expression. Sci Rep 2015;5:18319.

67. De Roo C, Lierman S, Tilleman K, et al. Ovarian tissue cryopreservation in female-to-male transgender people: insights into ovarian histology and physiology after prolonged androgen treatment. Reprod Biomed Online 2017;34:557–66.

68. Ose J, Fortner RT, Rinaldi S, et al. Endogenous androgens and risk of epithelial invasive ovarian cancer by tumor characteristics in the european prospective investigation into cancer and nutrition. Int J Cancer 2015;136:399–410.

69. Olsen CM, Green AC, Nagle CM, et al. Epithelial ovarian cancer: testing the "androgens hypothesis". Endocr Relat Cancer 2008;15:1061–8.

70. Millington K, Hayes K, Pilcher S, et al. A serous borderline ovarian tumour in a transgender male adolescent. Br J Cancer 2021;124:567–9.

71. Hage JJ, Dekker JJML, Karim RB, et al. Ovarian cancer in female-to-male transsexuals: report of two cases. Gynecol Oncol 2000;76:413–5.

72. Dizon DS, Tejada-Berges T, Koelliker S, et al. Ovarian cancer associated with testosterone supplementation in a female-to-male transsexual patient. Gynecol Obstet Invest 2006;62:226–8.

73. Cuccolo NG, Kang CO, Boskey ER, et al. Mastectomy in Transgender and Cisgender Patients: A Comparative Analysis of Epidemiology and Postoperative Outcomes. Plast Reconstr Surg Glob Open 2019;7(6):e2316.

74. McEvenue G, Xu FZ, Cai R, et al. Female-to-male gender affirming top surgery: a single surgeon's 15-year retrospective review and treatment algorithm. Aesthet Surg J 2017;38(1):49–57.

75. East EG, Gast KM, Kuzon WM, et al. Clinicopathological findings in female-to-male gender-affirming breast surgery. Histopathology 2017;71:859–65.

76. Torous VF, Schnitt SJ. Histopathologic findings in breast surgical specimens from patients undergoing female to male gender reassignment surgery. Mod Pathol 2019;32:346–53.

77. Baker GM, Guzman-Arocho YD, Bret-Mounet VC, et al. Testosterone therapy and breast histopathological features in transgender individuals. Mod Pathol 2021;34:85–94.

78. Hernandez A, Schwarts CJ, Warfield D, et al. Pathologic Evaluation of Breast Tissue from Transmasculine individuals undergoing gender-affirming chest masculinization. Arch Pathol Lab Med 2020;144:888–93.

79. Katayama Y, Motoki T, Watanabe S, et al. A very rare case of breast cancer in a female-to-male transsexual. Breast cancer 2016;23:937–44.

80. Gooren L, Bowers M, Lips P, et al. Five New cases of breast cancer in transsexual persons. Andrologia 2015;47(10):1202–5.

81. Shao T, Grossbard ML, Lkein P. Breast cancer in female-to male transsexuals: two cases with a review of physiology and management. Clin Breast Cancer 2011;11(6):417–9.

82. Andrews AR, Kakadekar A, Schmidt RL, et al. Histologic findings in surgical pathology specimens from individuals taking feminizing hormone therapy for the purpose of gender transition. a systematic scoping review. Arch Pathol Lab Med 2021;146(2):252–61.

83. Kanhai RC, Hage JJ, van Diest PJ, et al. Short-term and long-term histologic effects of castration and estrogen treatment on breast tissue of 14 male-to-female transsexuals in comparison with two chemically castrated men. Am J Surg Pathol 2000;24(1):18–23.

84. Pritchard TJ, Pankowsky DA, Crowe JP, et al. Breast cancer in a male-to-female transsexual: a case report. JAMA 1988;259(15):2278–80.

85. Richards SM, Pine-Twaddell ED, Loffe OB, et al. A case of benign phyllodes tumor in a transgender woman receiving cross-sex hormones. Int J Surg Pathol 2018;26(4):356–9.

86. de Blok CJM, Wiepjes CM, Nota NM, et al. Breast cancer risk in transgender people receiving hormone treatment: nationwide cohort study in the Netherlands. BMJ 2019;365:l1652.

87. Vereecke G, Defreyne J, Van Saen D, et al. Characterisation of testicular function and spermatogenesis in transgender women. Hum Reprod 2021;36(1):5–15.

88. Jiang DD, Swenson E, Mason M, et al. Effects of Estrogen on Spermatogenesis in Transgender Women. J Urol 2019;132:117–22.

89. Kent MA, Winoker JS, Grotas AB. Effects of feminizing hormones on sperm production and malignant changes: microscopic examination of post orchiectomy specimens in transwomen. J Urol 2018;121:93–6.

90. Matoso A, Khandakar B, Yuan S, et al. Spectrum of findings in orchiectomy specimens of persons undergoing gender confirmation surgery. Hum Pathol 2018;76:91–9.

91. Hembree WC, Cohen-Kettenis PT, Gooren L, et al. Endocrine treatment of gender-dysphoric/gender-incongruent persons: an endocrine society clinical practice guideline. J Clin Endocrinol Metab 2017;102(11):3869–903.

92. Mahfouda S, Moore JK, Siafarikas A, et al. Gender-affirming hormones and surgery in transgender children and adolescents. Lancet Diabetes Endocrinol 2019;7:484–98.

93. Safa B, Lin WC, Salim AM, et al. Current concepts in feminizing gender surgery. Plast Reconstr Surg 2019;143(5):1081e–91e.

94. Trum HW, Hoebeke P, Gooren LJ. Sex reassignment of transsexual people from a gynecologist's and urologist's perspective. Acta Obstet Gynecol Scand 2015;94:563–7.

95. Ingham MD, Lee RJ, MacDermed D, et al. Prostate cancer in transgender women. Urol Oncol 2018;36(12):518–25.

96. de Nie I, de Blok CJM, van der Sluis TM, et al. Prostate cancer incidence under androgen deprivation: nationwide cohort study in trans women receiving hormone treatment. J Clin Endocrinol Metab 2020;105(9):e3293–9.

97. Gooren L, Morgentaler A. Prostate cancer incidence in orchidectomised male-to-female transsexual persons treated with oestrogens. Andrologia 2014;46:1156–60.

98. Deutsch MB, Buchholz D. Electronic health records and transgender patients—practical recommendations for the collection of gender identity data. J Gen Intern Med 2015;30(6):843–7.

99. Donald C, Ehrenfeld JM. The opportunity for medical systems to reduce health disparities among lesbian, gay, bisexual, transgender and intersex patients. J Med Syst 2015;39(11):178.

Printed and bound by CPI Group (UK) Ltd, Croydon, CR0 4YY

03/10/2024

01040372-0005